Introduction to Computer Systems for Health Information Technology

Nanette B. Sayles, EdD, RHIA, CCS, CHPS, FAHIMA
and
Kathy C. Trawick, EdD, RHIA

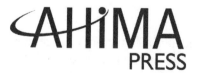

AHIMA PRESS

Copyright ©2011 by the American Health Information Management Association. All rights reserved. No part of this publication may be reproduced, stored in a retrieval system, or transmitted, in any form or by any means, electronic, photocopying, recording, or otherwise, without the prior written permission of the publisher.

ISBN: 978-1-58426-220-6
AHIMA Product No. AB103409

AHIMA Staff:
Claire Blondeau, MBA, Acquisitions Editor
Angela K. Dihn, MHA, RHIA, Reviewer
Cynthia Douglas, Developmental Editor
Katie Greenock, Editorial and Production Coordinator
Ashley Sullivan, Assistant Editor
Ken Zielske, Director of Publications

All information contained within this book, including Web sites and regulatory information, was current and valid as of the date of publication. However, Web page addresses and the information on them may change or disappear at any time and for any number of reasons. The user is encouraged to perform his or her own general Web searches to locate any site addresses listed here that are no longer valid.

American Health Information Management Association
233 North Michigan Avenue, 21st Floor
Chicago, IL 60601-5800

ahima.org

Contents

Detailed Contents

About the Editors and Authors

Nanette B. Sayles, EdD, RHIA, CCS, CHPS, FAHIMA

Dr. Sayles has a BS in Medical Record Administration, a MS in Health Information Management, a Masters in Public Administration, and a doctorate in Adult Education. Dr. Sayles has more than 10 years experience as a Health Information Management practitioner with experience in hospitals, a consulting firm, and a computer vendor. She was the 2005 American Health Information Management Association Triumph Educator award winner. She has held numerous offices and other volunteer roles for the American Health Information Management Association (AHIMA), the Georgia Health Information Management Association (GHIMA), the Alabama Association of Health Information Management (AAHIM), the Middle Georgia Health Information Management Association (MGHIMA), and the Birmingham Regional Health Information Management Association (BRHIMA). These positions include: AHIMA Educational Strategies Committee, AHIMA Co-Chair RHIA Workgroup, GHIMA Director, and President of MGHIMA. Dr. Sayles has published two books: Professional Review Guide for the CHP, CHS, and CHPS Examinations and Case Studies in Health Information Management. She is an editor for the PRG Professional Review Guide for the RHIA and RHIT Examinations. Dr. Sayles is currently the Program Director of the Health Information Management and Technology Programs and Associate Professor at Macon State College in Macon, Georgia where she has been employed for 11 years.

Kathy C. Trawick, EdD, RHIA

Dr. Kathy Trawick, RHIA, is the chairman and associate professor of the Health Information Management Department at the University of Arkansas for Medical Sciences in Little Rock, Arkansas. She is a 1985 graduate of the University of Alabama at Birmingham, Health Information Management (formerly Medical Record Administration) program. Dr. Trawick has expertise in Higher Education and in the Allied Health Sciences. Her basic research interests with keywords under the ERIC database include higher educational administration effectiveness, institutional effectiveness, and student satisfaction. Dr. Trawick has been a practitioner for 10 years in acute care facilities and an HIM educator and program chairman since 1999. Topics of instruction include healthcare statistics, legal issues, HIM systems, and the CPR, health administration, quality improvement, and cancer registry principles. She has been a contributing author of texts in medical terminology and medical law and ethics. She has authored the Statistics/Research chapter of Cengage Learning's *Professional Review Guide for the RHIA and RHIT Examinations* from the years of 2006 until the present. She has published articles in the *Journal of AHIMA* and *Advance for HIM* as well as the Educational Perspectives in Health Information Management and the Mid-South Educational Research Association Proceedings. She is a consultant to various types of healthcare facilities in Arkansas. In addition to holding offices at the state level in HIM and Cancer Registry associations, she is currently serving on the CAHIIM Panel of Reviewers for HIT/HIA program accreditation.

Acknowledgments

From Nanette Sayles:

This book is dedicated to my husband, Mark; my daughter, Rachel; my parents George and Jeanette Burchfield, my sister, Crystal Steen; and my brother, Ron Burchfield. Their support and love is a blessing from God. To my co-author Kathy Trawick, who I have known since our Medical Record Administration college days: I appreciate the hard work that you put into this book and the laughs you have given me throughout the process. Finally to my students, past and present, who were my motivation for writing this book: may you find it a useful tool in your studies.

From Kathy Trawick:

This book is dedicated to the honor and memory of my parents, Mr. and Mrs. Robert W. Cooper. May their legacy live through my work in the classroom as I prepare future students in health information management. I further dedicate this book to my sister and brother, Ara Jo and Rob for their lifelong support and to my faculty and staff, Karen Smith and Betty Montgomery who are wonderful teammates and a joy to work with daily. My final thank you goes to my husband, Wayne, who has always been my greatest supporter and who is truly my source of love and life. My deepest appreciation goes to Nanette Sayles, who asked me to co-write this text with her, she has the greatest patience and provided an unending assistance to me throughout this process. And to my students, past and future, may this book be valuable to you as a source of knowledge to open new doors in our profession.

Chapter 1
Introduction to Computers

Objectives

- Describe the functions of the basic components of the personal computer to include hardware, software, networks, and Internet technologies.

- Identify and discuss the impact of computers in healthcare in all areas within a facility.

- Discuss the history of computers in healthcare.

- Compare and contrast the similarities and differences between the Internet, Intranet, and the Extranet as used in healthcare.

- Introduce the electronic health record and the benefits of its use over the paper record in acute care facilities.

Key Terms

Accelerated Graphics Port
Address bus
Arrow keys
Backspace key
BASIC
Bit
Bluetooth port
Blu-Ray disc
Broadband bandwidth
Bus network
Byte
Cable television modem
Cache memory
Compact disc (CD)
Central processing unit (CPU)
Client/server network
COBOL
Cursor

Daisy chain network
Data bus
Data projector
Delete key
Device driver
Dial-up modem
Digital camera
Digital subscriber line (DSL) modem
Docking station
Dot-matrix printer
Dots per inch (DPI)
DRG (diagnosis-related group) groupers
Dummy terminal
Digital video disc (DVD)
Encoders
Enter key

Enterprise software
ESC key
External bus
Extensible Markup Language (XML)
Extranet
Financial applications
Firewall
Firewire port
Flash drive
Footer
Formula translation (FORTRAN)
Free and open source software (FOSS)
Function keys
Gigabyte (Gb)
Graphical user interface (GUI)
Hard drive

Header
Headphones
Home and End keys
Hypertext Markup Language
    (HTML)
Hub computer
Hybrid network
Hypertransport
Infrared Data Association (IrDA)
    port
Ink jet printer
Insert key
Interface
Internal bus
Internet
Internet service provider (ISP)
Intranet
Java
Keyboard
Keystoning
Kilobyte (Kb)
LCD screen
Laptop computer
Laser printer
Light pen
Local area network (LAN)
Mainframe computers

Markup
Megabyte (Mb)
Megahertz (MHz)
Megapixel
Memory chip
Microphone
Modem
Monitor
Motherboard
Mouse
Multitasking
Notebook computer
Operating system
Optical character recognition
Page up and Page down keys
Parallel port
PCI-Express
PDA
Peer-to-peer network
Personal computer
Pixel
Plasma screen
Plug and Play (Pnp)
Print Screen key
Printer
Programming languages
Random access memory (RAM)

Read-only memory (ROM)
Resolution
Router
Scanner
Serial port
Sound card
Standard Generalized Markup
    Language (SGML)
Star network
Stylus
System files
Tab keys
Tag
Terabyte (Tb)
Thermal printer
Token ring network
Touch screen
Tree network
Universal serial bus (USB) port
Video card
Wide area network (WAN)
Wi-Fi
Wireless card
Wireless Markup Language
    (WML)
World Wide Web (WWW)
Write once read many (WORM)

Although the history of computers is not generally thought to be closely tied to health-care, the impact of computers in patient care, public health, and research has significantly influenced the systems used since the 1960s. The health information management (HIM) profession has been reliant on data since the time of the first paper medical record. Through the decades, many changes have occurred in the way health information and related data are shared and communicated. From data interaction among individuals and departments to systemwide networks and hospital systems that span several states, computers now directly impact the healthcare industry as a whole—including patient care delivery. It is the role of the HIM professional to enter, analyze, use, and maintain data at all levels of computer systems and networks in hospitals and other healthcare facilities.

History of Computers in Healthcare

Technology changes extremely quickly, as evidenced by the development of the computer systems that have evolved over the past 60 years. The first computers in healthcare were punch-card systems used prior to the 1960s. At that time, computers were large machines that filled entire rooms and needed extreme cooling controls; these machines used vacuum tubes rather than microchips for memory. Much of the healthcare-related computer use in the 1960s involved data entry.

Data entry systems in the 1960s were mostly **financial applications**, as these were among the few software systems available and were some of the simplest software packages.

Financial applications were also packaged for other industries, so the ease of using computers in finance for healthcare at this time was well supported. In addition, most computer departments fell under the domain of a Chief Financial Officer (CFO), who likely would have welcomed a financial software package because the CFO was responsible for both the facility's monetary and technological advances. With the use of mainframes throughout hospitals, the healthcare industry was beginning to see the benefit computers could provide.

In the 1970s, as computers developed, integrated circuits replaced the vacuum tubes. Within these machines, microchips replaced the vacuum tubes and cooling systems. The memory capability of computers had improved over the decade. It was in the late 1970s when the healthcare industry began to use departmental computer systems.

Within HIM departments, computers were being brought in to help the personnel with master patient index (MPI) functions and abstracting. These were some of the earliest functions performed in the medical record departments during the late 1970s. Most of the computers were **dummy terminals**, meaning they were limited to a monitor and keyboard, and the bare minimum of hardware needed to connect it to the network using the server's PC to perform all functions (White 2008, 318). The **hard drive** is the brain of the standard PC and performs all functions of the computer, as this is where the system files are located (White 2008, 12). Thus, most of the HIM technicians in a typical department would be seen using these dummy (or dumb) terminals to look up medical record numbers or patient names.

Some advanced HIM departments in the 1970s began having abstractors input patient data into the terminals, capturing various patient or clinical data for reporting purposes. Previously, all abstracting was done by the HIM technicians on paper abstracts, which were then mailed to the various reporting agencies. The ability to abstract patient data once into a computer system, which then could be used to send the abstracts to several agencies or used to generate several reports, was seen by the HIM technicians as a new luxury. Using the old paper abstracts for reporting purposes was a time-consuming process for the personnel, and having the computer system available to print out much of the data regarding patient demographics that was already contained within the computer system saved abstractors a great deal of time. The new computer systems also decreased the possibility of errors made when transcribing by hand any notes from the primary record to a secondary source. The computerized abstract printed the reports directly from the system in available ad-hoc formats as directed so that reports could be individualized for each agency as needed.

The 1980s and 1990s saw even more advancement in computers' memory capacity and speed. Computer memory was increased at tremendous rates, as was the random access memory and read-only memory (RAM and ROM; discussed in detail later) in computers. Use of computers in business continued to increase, and purchases of home computers multiplied in this period as well. The prices of personal computers (PCs) for the consumer became more affordable, making computers something home users could enjoy and not just a tool for business and industry. The personal computer by definition is a microcomputer or a "small one-user computer system with its own central processing unit (CPU), memory, and storage devices" (Joos et al. 2006, 16). With the increased presence of computers in the home, technology literally became a household word.

Within the HIM industry, computers helped increase employee productivity. By the end of the 1990s, most HIM technicians—such as coders, abstractors, transcriptionists, release of information technicians, chart analysts, and quality analysts—used PCs at their workstations to better perform their HIM roles within the facility.

Specialized Software

Also during the 1980s and 1990s, software vendors developed specialized software to help health information specialists with their tasks, and this soon became a growing business. With the implementation of the prospective payment system (PPS) in 1985, diagnosis-related groups (DRGs) and coding for reimbursement brought the coding function to the forefront. Vendors of coding software developed numerous types of encoders and

DRG groupers to assist coding personnel in their daily tasks. **Encoders** by definition are "specialty software used to facilitate the assignment of diagnostic and procedural codes according to the rules of the coding system (Johns 2007, 964). The **DRG grouper** is a "computer software program that assigns appropriate DRGs according to the information provided for each episode of care" (Johns 2007, 276). Transcription companies developed early versions of voice recognition technology, such as Kurzweil VoiceMED, for doctor dictation so that transcription was digitized directly into the computer systems. The development of similar software was partly responsible for the movement to outsource transcription tasks. A lack of qualified transcriptionists also made outsourcing attractive to many facilities. However, technology was at the foundation of the outsourcing trend because the basis of outsourcing is simply communicating data in a digital format, regardless of the physical location of the original source.

Release of Information (ROI)

Release of information (**ROI**) was another area within the HIM field that was sometimes outsourced. Software vendors developed applications for their own use, and outside companies used their own staff to operate within ROI areas of healthcare facilities. Companies would agree to perform the ROI functions of a HIM department for a certain percentage of the profits gained from the revenue collected in the functions of the ROI tasks. Using an outside vendor and that company's personnel, a facility could save salary dollars by not paying their own staff to perform ROI functions. In return, the ROI outsourcing company would have the appropriate number of staff for the facility's workload available on-site to perform the daily ROI tasks and would assume the responsibility for all tasks within the ROI realm. This was a common arrangement until the Health Information Portability and Accountability Act (HIPAA) mandates of 2001 came into effect, after which many facilities thought that they needed to resume responsibility over ROI because of the strict mandates of HIPAA; those facilities restored control of their ROI functions within their departments. However, not all facilities were compelled to respond because the outsourcing companies trained their employees in all HIPAA statutes of the particular state in which they worked. In any case, since 2001, it is left to a facility to choose how it will handle the ROI function.

Abstracting

The abstracting function remained basically unchanged until the 1980s, when software developers created programs that allowed much of the required data to be preloaded from other program screens into the HIM programs. With the new software, for example, much of the patient demographic data that are collected upon patient admission—whether this occurs in the emergency department or in the admissions office—is captured within the computer system and maintained within the mainframe system. Thus, the HIM technician abstracting data does not have to duplicate work by reentering patient demographics. The technician would only need to abstract or input new data. Most of the data that are abstracted is clinical data. For example, diagnoses of cancer that have been coded and staged by cancer registrars would be data that would be abstracted. Thus, the abstracting function is sometimes a function dual to that of an analyst.

Chart Analysis

Within the HIM department the chart analyst continued to use software applications specifically designed for managing physician deficiency of records. In the 1980s, the software packages developed for HIM departments were designed to serve several functional areas so that the department could purchase one software package from a single vendor to support many types of services. These packages could be designed by a department director and customized to meet the department's specific needs. The director could compile a list of the applications needed for the department. This list might include:

- A coding application, to include an encoder and DRG grouper

- An abstracting application for reporting

- A physician deficiency application for chart analysis and tracking or location

- An MPI application, which would be used by everyone within the department

- A transcription application

- An ROI application

- A statistical application for the director's reporting purposes

Networking

During the 1990s, networking among hospital departments became more common, and computers and other digital means helped facilities share data more quickly and with greater ease. In this decade, data entry was performed using technologies such as barcoding of data, voice recognition, touch screens, light pens, and microphones. Hospital departments—such as admissions, business offices, quality improvement offices, and utilization management offices—that worked closely with the HIM departments were networked so that data were shared and less time was spent rekeying data. This obviously made these departments more efficient, and data sharing within hospitals became popularized.

Because the facility computer systems connected many of these departments, data were shared only with those personnel that had a need (and the appropriate permissions) to view patient data. HIPAA mandates clearly defined the federal regulations, and each facility then wrote its own policies and procedures to determine who among the staff and physicians could view patient care data contained within the facility's health records. Although HIM professionals have, since the inception of the profession, strived to follow privacy regulations regarding health data, the HIPAA mandates enhanced the security of confidentiality of health data, both electronically and for patient care in all situations.

Technology's Effect on the HIM Profession

Technology changes and advancements seen in the 1990s were instrumental to the HIM profession. As Medicare and Medicaid billing transitioned to an electronic format, the technicians in the billing and compliance realms of the profession were viewed as experts in the area. Certified coders reviewed the facility's charge description master (CDR), or chargemaster, on the hospital mainframe for coding updates in ICD-9-CM and CPT codes. This review ensured the hospital's proper reimbursement of payment from Medicare and Medicaid for the next year. Without expert advice from experienced coders regarding codes in the chargemaster review, the facility could risk losing thousands of dollars in a single year.

Advances in networked systems in hospitals allowed communication between the admissions department and the utilization review department for preadmission of patients. Standards set by reimbursement entities such as the Centers for Medicare and Medicaid Services (CMS) and other third-party insurance payers required certification and authorization of patients prior to admission. Without proper authorization documenting that individual patients met medical necessity standards for admission, hospitals stood to lose money on patients admitted unnecessarily. In the same way, patients already admitted and staying in the hospital longer than necessary also presented a potential reason for insurance payers to forego payment to the facility. The PPS or DRG assignment from the patient's primary final diagnosis at discharge was a determining factor in reimbursement, and the utilization review personnel needed networked data to achieve fast communication with admissions or the emergency department as well as physician offices, which were often networked within a hospital's computer system. The data used by the utilization review personnel was transmitted electronically to the reimbursement entities because the data were required to verify that the patient's stay was medically necessary. Before these departments were networked, all of these transactions were slow, methodical, tedious, and labor-intensive tasks that required a large number of utilization review staff working long hours to complete. Hospital systems of networked computers saved time and money and reduced the number of employees needed (thereby saving salary dollars); in many cases the utilization review employees were either cross-trained or trained for other departments.

Impact of Computers

The healthcare industry continues to grow in size and in complexity. Without computers to aid in this tremendous expansion of patient data, the American healthcare industry would be comparable to third-world countries. The increased knowledge and advancements in computer technology in the use of data to enhance patient care, research, education, and public health, and to address reimbursement issues, has led to significant changes.

Patient Care

Patients now more than ever also understand medical data and are communicating with healthcare professionals about their health status. Patients use the Internet to read about health issues, and there is more medical knowledge currently available to the general public through the Web. The Internet is a worldwide network linked for exchange of communication that no person, organization, or country controls (White 2008, 312). The Web is the **World Wide Web (WWW)**, which is a confederation of Internet servers that support documents formatted in a computer language that has been written in Hypertext Markup language (HTML) (White 2008, 313). Patients have computers in their homes and at work to build and maintain personal health records (PHRs). Patients are familiar with computers and have 'grown up' with them, unlike previous generations. Computers are considered a safe place to privately house numerous data; with the use of flash drives and other portable devices, data can be made portable if necessary.

The patient health record is the primary source of data. Whether the health record is in a paper or electronic format, the patient record is the center element of data. The patient record can hold information for a physician office visit, emergency visit, clinic visit, outpatient surgery visit, or an inpatient hospital admission. The information contained within this record is centrally the same; it answers key questions about the patient as to the nature of the visit, what treatment or services were provided, when the visit occurred and for how long, and the outcome of the visit. The patient health record has been the source of documentation of a patient visit since the start of the HIM profession and is the core of the profession because the data remain the same whether captured on paper or electronically. The data is used by healthcare professionals to treat the patients during the visit and is analyzed by various agencies after the visit. The patient health record serves as the basis for all healthcare providers to document information in a central location about the patient visit. The patient record also helps facilitate continuity of care during and after a patient's visit for retrospective reviews by various areas such as compliance, credentialing, administration, and quality and utilization management departments. The health record also serves as the legal document of the patient's stay. All of the documentation entered during the course of a patient's stay is considered as the official record and the legal entry of each healthcare practitioner treating the patient. The episode of care is documented and can be used in court, if needed, and for reimbursement issues based on the documentation provided therein.

Finance and Reimbursement

Like other industries, the healthcare industry began using financial software applications in the early 1960s. Financial applications then were easy to support and run on computers. In the late 1960s, computers were integrated circuits used by business for small calculations (White 2008, p. 7). During this time, hospitals saw reimbursement as a fee-for-service from most payers because the prospective payment system (PPS) or what is known as diagnostic-related groups (DRGs) did not come about until 1985 for Medicare patients. Because DRGs were the driving force for inpatient Medicare payment, ambulatory patient classifications (APCs) were developed shortly afterward for outpatient

Medicare payments. Because of the increasing costs of providing medical care, third-party payers began using payment types similar to Medicare and Medicaid programs for the health services provided. These third-party payers included insurance companies, health maintenance organizations, preferred provider organizations and/or associations, point of service plans, and integrated delivery systems. Fiscal intermediaries (FIs) are those agencies contracted by CMS to process the claims for that particular area or state. The era of DRGs changed the payment system from that of fee-for-service to a PPS. The DRG cost is calculated based on a case mix of patients or the average of the hospital's typical mix of patient types and the number of patients treated at the hospital. This cost is figured on a relative weight based on the geographical area of the country in which that particular hospital is located. The relative weights are updated by CMS based on the U.S. economy and distributed twice annually by CMS to all participating Medicare hospitals. Reimbursement to healthcare facilities continued to other types of facilities, with Medicare PPS being used with skilled nursing facilities, outpatient settings using outpatient prospective payment system (OPPS), ambulatory patient classification groups using APCs, home health (HH) settings using HH PPS, and inpatient rehabilitation facilities (IRF) using IRF PPS.

Without the use of computerization throughout the schema of reimbursement of healthcare, finance of payment to hospitals and healthcare facilities would be set back decades. The role of the HIM practitioner and coder has been instrumental with the use of computerization with the encoder and DRG grouper since the implementation of DRGs in 1985. This advancement has almost single-handedly brought the HIM profession into the national spotlight. Formerly thought of as a department of cost, the HIM department is now recognized as keeping the hospital's doors open for all patients. The use of encoders has also decreased coding errors in reimbursement as well as patient care. Software development has improved the use of edit checks; currently, the computer program will notify the coder so that various codes cannot be used with other codes in certain situations. Such edit checks on computer software are done in areas of demographics, diagnosis and procedure codes, and procedure dates with admission and discharge dates. Computerization has aided the reimbursement aspect with the correct DRG for the final diagnosis, and it also helps improve the quality of the data submitted in the coding and data abstracted within the patient's record.

Public Health and Epidemiology

Patient health records are abstracted, and the data submitted into the computer networks of hospitals and healthcare systems are used for many purposes. Public health and research have a great need for these data. Abstracted data taken from patient records can be used as secondary data in databases, such as data within a registry. Secondary data are any data "derived from the primary patient record, such as an index or a database" (Johns 2007, 992). Examples of registries that work closely with hospital patient data include cancer, diabetes, acquired immunodeficiency syndrome (AIDS), human immunodeficiency virus (HIV), cardiac, trauma, and eye injury registries. Registrars use ICD codes to search diagnoses and/or procedures needed from computer databases at healthcare facilities. If a person from such a registry does not work at the healthcare facility, a request is made for specific research data in the HIM department under HIPAA guidelines. It is of utmost importance that research is continued and data requests are fulfilled for these agencies. The goal of these agencies and registries is to collect and analyze data as a continued effort toward fighting these diseases, and the HIM community should assist in every way possible. The public health department battles the same war. The data that serve research efforts also can assist public health endeavors. The health department of a particular county analyzes data to track trends of various types when apprehensive data are suspected.

Scenario: An example of this might be one county that reports two cases of *Klebsiella* to the county health department and an adjacent county reports three cases of the same *Klebsiella* infection. The state health department tracks the county health department cases using water samples, reporting data that have been submitted and finding that these cases originated in a contaminated water drain. The health department then dispatches the local fire department to shut off the water drain until the state health department team can arrive for further testing at the site.

Epidemiology is also closely related to public health and research in that data are collected and analyzed in specific or dedicated computer systems. Epidemiology is the study of disease and its origin in relation to the health of the general population. Data used by epidemiologists can be helpful in tracking disease when trends are studied. Because a primary focus in epidemiology is prevention of disease, the data collected and analyzed by healthcare facilities are of utmost importance to the study of epidemiology.

Research

Clinical trials and studies are based on evidence found in data collected from patient records. Governmental agencies use research studies at national levels, such as the National Institutes of Health (NIH) and the Centers for Disease Control and Prevention (CDC), and other agencies also sponsor research based on data collected from patient records. Institutional review boards (IRBs) are the overseers at larger health facilities that perform clinical research to ensure that patient data are collected confidentially and that patients are treated with respect during the study. To handle the volume of data of clinical trials and studies performed by larger research institutions, computerization is vital to the process. Some of the trials and studies take years to complete and the data increase tremendously. Without computers to handle such a voluminous task, collection of patient data would be a monumental undertaking for a small institution, much less a large research facility. It is imperative that databases are used for research for healthcare facilities performing large volumes of clinical research.

Education

Information in the patient record is used to educate those in the healthcare industry. Healthcare practitioners must learn their skills from an experienced educator and from hands-on practice. Computers have been used in the classroom setting for educational purposes in the healthcare field for the past 30 years. Advanced uses of computers for teaching in the past 20 years include distance education, teleconferencing, videoconferencing, simulation using computer software, and the Internet for worldwide connection to databases such as Medline and the Cumulative Index to Nursing and Allied Health Literature (CINAHL) and medical libraries for student research. The HIM profession has used computers in the classroom since the mid 1980s for transcription and other word-processing tasks. Encoders and DRG groupers for the classroom soon followed as schools were able to budget for these packages from vendors. Other software packages available for educational purposes included cancer registry software, MPI chart location and chart tracking software, and release of information software. After learning the theories behind these various software packages, HIM students receive hands-on experience in the classroom using computers and the relevant software applications. This has become such an important component in the education of HIM practitioners that the Commission on Accreditation for Health Informatics and Information Management Education (CAHIIM) has developed this into one of the standards for HIM students.

Check Your Understanding 1.1

1. The first computers in healthcare were basically processors that used _____.

   A. microchips
   B. integrated circuits
   C. vacuum tubes
   D. dummy terminals

2. Patients use this tool to read about health issues and gain more medical knowledge on their health.

   A. specialized software
   B. dummy terminals
   C. World Wide Web
   D. personal health records

3. DRGs were implemented in what year?

   A. 1985
   B. 1987
   C. 1990
   D. 1995

4. What is considered the "brain" of the standard PC?

   A. dummy terminal
   B. vacuum tubes
   C. microchips
   D. hard drive

Hardware

The first of the two basic parts of a computer or PC is the hardware. The second, software, is discussed in a later section.

The hardware of a computer is defined as physically anything that a person can touch—such as the hard drive, monitor, mouse, keyboard, printer, scanner—and the **central processing unit (CPU)**. The CPU is the computer's brain or the circuits that make the electrical parts function. The CPU operates with speed that is measured in **megahertz (MHz)** and additionally determined by its memory capacity. The temporary memory is **cache memory** (temporary memory) and the long-term memory is **random access memory RAM memory** (a common unit of how memory is measured in a computer). Types of memory will be discussed in detail later. When a PC is purchased, it is important that speed and memory are purchased according to the user's current and anticipated needs. The PC is considered to be a microcomputer in size. Hospitals may use larger computers or **mainframe computers**, which can handle thousands of users or many networks of users simultaneously. Other popular sizes of computers are the thin client computers, which can be a slim or thin **laptop computer** or a handheld device called a **personal digital assistant (PDA)**. The PDA is very popular in the healthcare setting because it is small and can be carried in a pocket. Most PDAs use a special instrument for input rather than a keyboard, and must use a receiving component or dock to a computer daily for data transfer. As technology increases, so also will the capabilities of PDAs.

Hardware can also be in the form of peripherals, which includes anything that is added to a PC to expand its abilities. Most peripherals are optional; however, most peripherals are vital to everyday tasks. Some of the most common peripherals are the keyboard, mouse,

Table 1.1.   Common peripheral devices

Storage	Input	Output
CD-ROM	Trackball	Printer
CD-RW	Mouse	Plotter
CD-R	Keyboard	Braille embosser
DVD-ROM	Joystick	Sound
DVD-RW	Touch screen	Computer speech synthesis
DVD-R	Gamepad	Sound card
Blu-Ray disc	Power cord/transformer	Speakers
USB flash drive	Microphone	Digital camera
Tape drive	Brain-computer interface	Graphics card
Punch card	Image scanner	Braille display
Floppy disk	Computer terminal	Network card
Disk drive	Computer speech recognition	Modem
	Webcam	Scanner
	Digitizing tablet	
	Barcode reader	
	Docking station	
	Light pen	
	Touch screens	
	Scanner	

printer, scanner, monitor, speakers, modem, flash drive, microphone, webcams, compact disc (CD), digital video (DVD), and Blu-Ray disc. Table 1.1 lists some common peripherals and the general categories into which they fall.

Flash drives, "sometimes referred to as a jump drive, is a small, lightweight, removable data storage device to which data can be written {and} inserted into a USB port, a flash drive offers a dense form of storage that is impervious to scratches and dust" (McWay 2008, 314). **Compact discs (CDs)** are plastic encased discs that use a finely focused laser beam to write and read data. There are two types of CDs, those that record only and cannot be erased or changed are called CD-Recordable (CD-R) and those which allow multiple reuse similar to a floppy or flash drive are called CD-ReWritable (CD-RW) (White 2008, 185). The **DVD or Digital Video Disc** is similar to a CD except these hold more data. Whereas the CD holds up to 700 MB of information, the DVD holds up to 8.6 GB of information (White 2008, 185). The **Blu-Ray disc** is even larger than the DVD capacity as these hold between 23 GB and 27 GB of data (White 2008, 185). Capacity of **megabytes** and **gigabytes** are detailed in table 1.2.

Much advancement has been made in PC hardware over the past 25 years, as evidenced by the size of the hard drives from the large box or tower case that holds the brain of the computer, to the powerful PDAs that can be used at the patient's bedside.

Common Input Devices

There are various methods of inputting data to the system. Table 1.1 lists several devices that can be utilized. The two most common input devices are the keyboard and the mouse.

Keyboard

The **keyboard** is a major input device found on most microcomputers and laptop devices. Only the smallest devices, such as palmtops and PDAs, use pointing device instruments or a **stylus** rather than a keyboard because the keypad and instrumentation panel would be too small for human fingertips. The keyboard contains the layout from the typewriter and most have a numeric keypad on the side of the alpha keys. Usually located at the top of the keyboard are 12 **function keys** (F1, F2, and so on.). These function keys perform various tasks within the computer and with certain software. The function keys are not used as much, since the addition of the mouse and drop-down selection boxes.

Table 1.2.   **Units used to measure memory size**

Bit	1 number (either 0 or 1)
Byte	8 bits
Kilobyte	1,000 bytes
Megabyte	1,000 kilobytes
Gigabyte	1,000 megabytes
Terabyte	1,000 gigabytes

Source: McWay 2008, 317

Common Key Functions

A very commonly used key is the **Shift key**, which capitalizes letters when held down while striking a letter key. Similarly, if the Caps Lock key is held down or locked, entire sentences can be capitalized, eliminating the need to manually hold down the Shift key.

The **Delete key** is used to eliminate any text or characters to the right of the cursor's position. The Delete key will delete characters or spaces one stroke at a time; if held down, many characters can be deleted quickly. The **Backspace key** is used to delete any character that is to the left of the cursor. The **Enter key** is a primary key that is used to signal to the computer the end of a paragraph and the end of any command. Within many programs or installations, directions for computers will instruct the user to press the Enter key. The **Insert key** is a toggle switch key in many programs. It can insert and replace text if it is toggled between an on/off mode. For example, if the mouse is moved down one page to insert a sentence, the Insert key can be toggled on, the sentence can be inserted at the location of the cursor, and the Insert key can be toggled off. The user can then return to the original place within the document. The **Tab key** is preset at defined intervals within a word processing program for spacing purposes. One example is for paragraph indentation. If the tabs need to be set to a different width than the preset interval, this can be done within the page set up function as a drop-down box in most word processing software.

The Escape or **ESC key** is used when the user wants to move a step back within a screen or program or quit a screen or program entirely. The **Print Screen key** is either used alone or with the Alt key so that the contents of the monitor's screen can be printed onto the clipboard. Once the information is on the clipboard, it then can be copied and pasted into an application program to be printed or saved. The Page Up and Page Down keys as well as the Home and End keys are used to move quickly through a document. **Page Up and Page Down keys** enable movement through a document one page at a time. Using the **Home and End keys** with the Control (or Ctrl) key pressed takes the user to the very beginning (Home) or the very end of the document. If the text being worked on is extremely long, these keys come in quite handy! The four **Arrow keys** move the cursor in the direction of the arrows. Within some games on the computer, these arrows are used to move the targets left and right. A combination of keys that should be familiar to every computer user is Ctrl, Alt, and Delete. This combination should be used as a last resort, when no other solution works and if the Help Desk cannot be reached. There are times when computers will get "hung up" or "freeze" in a loop and there is nothing that can be done except to press the Ctrl, Alt, and Delete keys simultaneously. However, it is warned that each time this function is used—especially if the keystrokes are repeated before the operating system responds, there is a chance that the data in use could be lost, causing harm to the computer system and the circuits inside.

Mouse

The mouse is a peripheral input device that is used by pointing the hand to correspond with movement on the computer screen. The concept was first developed as a pointing device and due to the device's size and tail-like cable, it was named for the mouse (White 2008, 203). The mouse functions with a trackball on the bottom that rolls and sends signals to the software to indicate directions (White 2008, 206). The modern mouse uses a laser beam instead of a trackball to signal direction. The **mouse** has a wheel that protrudes on top between the left and right buttons so that as the wheel is moved forward or backward, the software is signaled to scroll the screen up or down (White 2008, 206). Keep in mind that not all versions of the mouse are equipped with a scroll wheel. The left and right buttons have functions as well. Clicking the left button wherever the user places the mouse pointer on the screen instantly moves the cursor to that location. Clicking the right button brings up an onscreen message window that informs the user of various functions available in the software at that time. By default, most mice are set up for right-handed users, but the functionality of the right and left mouse buttons can be reversed to accommodate left-handed use. A mouse may be connected by a cord to its host PC, or it may be a wireless optical mouse. An optical mouse uses a digital signal processor to communicate with its host PC so that a USB cable is not needed for connection (White 2008, 207). USB ports are standard on most PCs today because, as discussed earlier in this chapter, many peripheral input and storage devices use USB connections.

Other Input Devices

There are several other input devices or methods of inputting data to the computer system. This section explores several common input devices that are used with the personal computer.

Light Pen

As an input device, light pens are used like a pencil. A **light pen** basically emits an electronic signal and an image on the screen at the exact spot where the pen point touches (Joos et al. 2006, 22). Light pens do not work on LCD screens or plasma screens. An electronic pen uses direct entry, such as a signature, on a special pad that then enters the signature into the computer as a digital entry (Joos et al. 2006, p. 22). Light screens have been used for years and were first popularized on the television game show, *Jeopardy!*, for contestants to write in their answers.

Touch Screens

Another input mechanism, the **touch screen**, is similar to the light pen in that it works by touch of the fingertip onto the monitor screen. As the screen projects images or data, the user simply touches the image or data and the computer recognizes the touch as input for the preprogrammed data of each image to be performed, calculated, or completed. A **graphical user interface (GUI)** is used to present the images or data to the user. In addition to fingertip touch, touch screens also use a stylus, which is similar to a pen or pencil, for touch with some of the smaller devices such as a PDA. Touch screens are easy to operate and are very popular in the business and commercial markets.

Scanner

A **scanner** is both an input and an output device. In this section it will be addressed as an input device. When used as an input device, a scanner converts characters and text to digital data (Joos et al. 2006, 22). Scanners can be as simple as home or personal scanners or as sophisticated as those that can scan barcodes for businesses such as department or grocery stores, and in hospitals for sterile equipment, medical records, and employee identification badges. Scanners are also used as security measures because biometric data such as voice, fingerprints, and retinal scans can be used. Scanners are currently used for numerous purposes and tasks in industry and healthcare. The scanner enables the input of data that is not normally coded for computer use. This machine digitizes data so that it can be read, analyzed, and stored, if necessary, by a computer. Scanners are versatile and can be used to input text, images, and numerical and graphical data.

Digital Camera and Video

Digital cameras are used to take still pictures that are then converted to a digital format. When the pictures are uploaded, the images can be read by the computer. Most pictures are able to be viewed as a .jpg file. Once a picture is digitized, it can be saved on the computer's hard drive or any secondary storage device such as a flash drive, CD, or DVD. Pictures can also be uploaded to the Internet and shared via e-mail as attachment files. Many pictures are saved on CDs at film developing stores for customers. The memory card is removed from the digital camera so that the film developing store can make the CD for the customer. Of course, there is a charge for the service, but the store does the work rather than the customer and the turnaround time is usually fast.

Recording digital video is similar to using a digital camera except a digital video camera records motion rather than a still picture. Digital video recording replaced the old reel-to-reel film that was used on a projection machine. Contemporary video cameras are easy to operate. They digitize the motion of an event similar to the "old movies," but the quality is much better and the files are digitized in the same manner as a still picture. Any film with a long running time can be recorded and uploaded to a computer and saved to the hard drive or a secondary storage device. However, because of the running time of some films, it is best to use DVDs for storage because DVD recording time is longer and more minutes of film can be stored. The content of the DVDs can also be uploaded to the Internet and shared; however, some films may be too long to send in an e-mail. Many people use a Web site to load their film for viewing. A popular, free, and contemporary social Web site is MySpace.com. It can be personalized to an individual's name once it is designed by the user.

A **webcam**—as an input device used to capture and send video images—is very similar to a video camera. The webcam is a small camera "used to send video images as e-mail attachments, to make video telephone calls (video conferencing), and to post live, real-time images to a web server" (Joos et al. 2006, 22).

Microphone

The **microphone** enables a user to input voice directly into the computer. This is a great avenue for instructors who want to add narration to PowerPoint presentations, for people with disabilities, and for users who are not proficient with typing on the computer. The microphone enhances voice recognition systems in certain situations when being hands free is a necessity (such as for a physician performing dictation while doing surgery). **Headphones** are optional with a microphone system and are good if the user will be talking for a long period of time, enabling the user's hands to be free while narrating.

Docking Station

A **docking station** is a device that smaller computer devices such as PDAs or palmtops will rest in as the data are uploaded into the workstation PC. Because a smaller computer is easy to carry during the day and can be filled with data, the data need to be transferred to a larger storage computer daily so the PDA or palmtop can be used again the next day or so. Again, as technology improves the capacity of these smaller devices will also improve; the more data these devices can hold, the less frequently that data will need to be uploaded. Because the docking station is not carried with a person at all times it is less likely to be lost or stolen; data uploaded from the docking station to the workstation PC can be securely backed up into a mainframe system. Thus, data is not carried in the docking station each day and is less of a risk management issue if the smaller device should be lost or stolen.

Optical Character Recognition

Optical character recognition (OCR) is known as 'barcoding'. This process is used to index documents scanned within an optical disc imaging system. Many systems use OCR as an efficient method to expedite data entry into the system. In health information management departments, records are barcoded for quick data entry for scanning processes. Other hospital departments also use OCR technology in computer systems, such as radiology departments for x-ray records, the sterile supply department for materials and supply inventories, and the pharmacy for supplies inventory as well.

Check Your Understanding 1.2

1. Computer speed is measured in _____ and long-term memory is measured in _____.

   A. MHz, RAM
   B. ROM, MHz
   C. MHz, ROM
   D. RAM, MHz

2. All of the following are hardware EXCEPT:

   A. Monitor
   B. Mouse
   C. Printer
   D. Database

3. What device would a stylus be used in conjunction with?

   A. Digital camera
   B. Microphone
   C. PDA
   D. Scanner

4. The use of barcoding falls under the category of what type of input device?

   A. Docking station
   B. Printer
   C. Scanner
   D. Touch screen

Hardware within the Computer

Within the **personal computer**, there are three main parts: the CPU, the memory, and the storage devices of the system. In the PC, the CPU is often called the processor or central processor. Processor speeds are usually measured in gigahertz (GHz). The CPU is often referred to as "the brain" of the computer. It is basically a system board where the circuitry chips or semiconductor chips are located. This is often referred to as the **motherboard**. The chips are actually tiny pieces of silicon that conduct electricity, called semiconductors. The job of the CPU chips is to make the computer work or process functions.

Memory chips contain only memory for storage capacity. In the CPU area of the computer, there are two parts. The two areas of the CPU are the control area and the arithmetic/logic area. In the control area, all of the computer's activities, such as the instructions for the machine to process functions, are received, analyzed, and interpreted. All of the mathematical functions (addition, subtraction, multiplication, and division) are located in the arithmetic and logic area. The logic area functions as a 'determiner' of data, deciding if given data are equal or greater or less than other data. As PCs become faster and greater in their capacity, manufacturers name the versions as letters in a series. The original naming of each version of microcomputer generation was by the processor speed of that version, that is, Pentium 386, Pentium 486, and so on.

Memory

Within the microcomputer, there are several types of memory. As mentioned earlier, the temporary memory needed by the computer at startup and backup is RAM, a common unit of how memory is measured within a computer. RAM is needed so that a computer can function and perform the tasks needed. RAM can be dynamic or volatile, which means that it is constantly swapping memory between the smaller memory cells to ensure that the functions are covered during a process. If the computer takes on even more functions, there may not be enough RAM to support the work process and this is why computers seem to "slow down" to handle the workload. Either a user would need to be patient or have more memory installed to help speed up the processing functions. RAM memory is accessed randomly and was originally named as the computer had to randomly search for data that was stored in different locations in the electronic chips in this area. RAM memory can be both read and written to.

Read-Only Memory (ROM) is memory that has been programmed onto a chip at the factory and cannot be changed. When a user purchases ROM memory, it is purchased at a certain predetermined amount. No instructions or data can be changed in the memory in ROM. The computer start-up instructions are in the ROM memory. A computer cannot write new information to ROM memory.

Cache, another type of memory, is a temporary memory within the computer. Within a PC, this cache memory is basically used when the computer needs to borrow memory temporarily; this keeps the computer from using the computer's main memory. In this manner, the computer keeps its processing speed constant and does not slow down when it must borrow memory during any time of processing. Cache memory is used when speed is needed by the computer. Cache memory is located on the CPU and can also be on a part of the processor. Thus when data is copied from RAM it is placed into the cache memory and can be retrieved faster from the cache memory than from the RAM (White 2008, 50).

System Files

System files are small disk files that contain software codes that are instructions for the computer and are the first files that a computer reads when "booting up" (the term used for when a computer is turned on and the functions needed to have all the components working and the operating system fully loaded are performed; the operating system is discussed later). System files are loaded first after the hardware is booted so that the remainder of the operating system can load properly.

Ports

There are several types of ports for microcomputers. Basically a port serves as a communication device for the computer to talk to peripheral devices such as printers, monitor, keyboard, flash drive, and anything else that can be plugged into a computer. To put this in simple terms, the port is a hole on the computer's hard drive that wires (or devices, such as a flash drive) are plugged in or connected to.

Ports have various shapes and sizes because of their various functions. Most PCs have a serial port, a parallel port, and a universal serial bus (USB) port. The **serial port** and **parallel port** are not used as much with computers today when compared to the faster and more common ports such as the USB port. The serial port arranges data to travel in serial form or one bit at a time (Joos et al. 2006, 26). For two-way communication using the serial port, one piece of data at a time must travel from the external device to the computer; then, to reverse the data flow the information then travels from the computer back to the external devices (Joos et al. 2006, 26).

Parallel ports are "unidirectional ports set up to send parallel data" (Joos et al. 2006, 26). Within parallel ports, data may travel in groups of eight bits or a byte of information (Joos et al. 2006, 26).

USB ports are used for connecting devices such as flash drives, digital cameras, and iPods. The USB ports are built on the outside of computers, usually on the front, where access is easy for the user so that peripheral devices can easily be connected without interrupting any other resources in the computer. A mouse can be used in a mouse port, or in a USB port if a wireless type mouse is used with a device through the USB plug-in. The keyboard port is on the back of the computer and looks similar to a mouse port; however, on newer computers, keyboard ports can also be used with the USB port on the front.

Most computers still have serial and parallel ports, but with the growing popularity and ease of use of the USB ports on the front of computers, these ports are all but obsolete.

Other ports located on the computer tower are the printer port and modem. The printer port is a slot to allow the wiring for a peripheral printing device. The **modem** is a port to allow the wiring of the PC to a phone line so that the computer can connect to the Internet and for facsimile purposes.

Another special port is the **FireWire port**, which is similar to a USB port in that several devices can be attached to it (Joos et al. 2006, 26). These ports can handle 63 devices and are typically used for camcorders, DVD players, and digital audio equipment plug-ins (Joos et al. 2006, 26).

The **Infrared Data Association (IrDA) port** is used to transmit data by infrared light waves (Joos et al. 2006, 27). By having an infrared port on a device such as a laptop and a workstation PC, files can be transferred without the use of wires. If a notebook computer has an infrared port and a printer also has this type of port, then the user can print by using the IrDA rather than the use of wires. The user must simply make sure that the IrDA ports are in total alignment with each other on each computer or device so that the two ports can communicate without the wires, making this a totally wireless network.

Another port that is currently popular is Bluetooth. It is very similar to the IrDA except rather than using infrared waves the **Bluetooth port** uses radio waves as its signals. Bluetooth technology is often used in cell phone technology and in hands-free cell phone use in vehicles. Because Bluetooth technology uses radio waves, there is no need for a direct line of sight between devices as in the infrared light wave technology (Joos et al. 2006, 27). Bluetooth uses Wireless Application Protocol, or WAP technology. WAP basically sends the instructions on tiny screens over the cell connections on a card. A single message contains many WAP cards and this reduces downloading by a computer. The WAP uses **Wireless Markup Language (WML)**. This is similar to **Hypertext Markup Language (HTML),** the language used on the Internet, but with WML there is no need for a keyboard or a mouse for input because the WAP cards are used as the input data. The card type is encoded and is read by the WML and sent, so the computer instructions are read by the WAP technology. The browser displays the data (using WML technology) to the user as the output.

Other Hardware in the Computer

Video Card

The **video card** is needed to translate images or pictures from electrical currents onto the monitor or screen.

Sound Card

The **sound card** enables the computer to reproduce sound from electrical currents for speakers, headphones, the microphone, and input from peripheral devices. The sound card connections are external jacks to allow the peripheral devices to be plugged in, such as headphones or a microphone for data input or output.

Fan

A microcomputer produces a large amount of heat from the processors and the mechanics of the electrical components within the hard drive. A fan is needed to cool the air within the tower itself to prevent overheating of the circuits.

Expansion Slots

Most microcomputers have unused slots where the user can plug in circuit boards and hardware to add features to a computer. This is where the name "expansion" comes from, as it enables the owner to add more 'bells and whistles' to a PC in order to upgrade a computer at a later date. Most PCs currently are personal computer interface (PCI) or the latest generation, the **PCI-Express (PCI-E)**. This interface allows data to move more quickly. The PCI-E is a bus architecture that can route data at greater than 8 gigabytes per second in each direction within the bandwidth (White 2008, 29). This greater bandwidth is used for applications such as streaming video and photo editing, which place huge demands on the data lines because of the number of pixels or characters that need to flow through the lines per second (White 2008, 29).

Bus

Within the PC, there are several types of buses that send data within the computer. A bus is basically defined as a connection between two devices connected to the computer for communication. A bus allows a CPU to talk to the memory card or a sound card, for example, within the computer. All microcomputers have an internal bus and an external bus.

The **internal bus** permits the communication inside the computer's components; that is, within the memory. The **external bus** allows communication with external devices such as a printer or scanner. The bus speed is always measured in megabytes per second (MBps). Also within the PC, there is an **address bus** that contains the lines or unique address of the data's destination. The data bus also is located within a PC. The **data bus** is a bank of electrical bits; basically, these are the actual data.

A bus is like a traffic cop within the computer, directing the electrical traffic so that it does not stop or slow down. The more buses that are used to direct traffic flow, the faster the data flow within the computer. Most PCs use two or more buses that are specialized to perform certain functions within the computer. The first bus used was the Industry Standard Architecture (ISA) around 1982 and was rated at 9 megabytes per second (9 MBps) (White 2008, 201). It is rarely seen now, except on older computers as a bridge. It was used until the 1990s when the Peripheral Component Interconnect (PCI) bus was developed at 132 MBps (White 2008, 201).

With the PCI bus, there could be more than one bus on a computer simultaneously. Also, the megahertz increased with the processor speeds from 8 MHz up to 33 MHz with the PCI bus. The bus speed increased dramatically when the Windows 95 version supported **"Plug and Play" (PnP)** (White 2008, 42). The PnP technology by Microsoft changed the bus technology and has pushed it to its limits. The next step in bus technology could be PCI-Express (PCI-E), **HyperTransport**, or **Accelerated Graphics Port (AGP)**, which flows at 2.1 gigabytes per second, but no speculation can be made on the future of bus technology (White 2008, 28). The PnP technology is almost at its limits and manufacturers are looking into new technology for bus technology.

Surge Protectors

A surge protector (also called a power strip or surge suppressor) acts as an extension cord to an AC outlet for a computer, but also adds protection against bursts of current of electricity. Electricity is provided through wall sockets in voltage, and it is not always flowing evenly. A surge occurs when there are current spikes in voltage. The surge protector acts as a buffer between the electrical outlet and the computer and other electrical devices that are plugged into it. Most surge protectors have several plugs, so that many devices can be plugged into it all at once. It is recommended that the user purchase a surge protector that is powerful enough for computers and other electrical devices. Manufacturers of surge protectors document voltage level capacity on each box and the type of devices for which the surge protector is made, so that the user can make the appropriate purchase.

Output Devices

Monitor

Another example of technology advancement is the computer **monitor**. Monitors were once as large as television screens and resembled them in many ways because the resolution of a monitor is quite similar to that of a television set. **Resolution** of monitors is measured in dpi or dots per inch. The greater the number of dpi for a resolution, the better the quality of the picture on the computer screen. This is because the pixels are closer together within a 1-inch square. A **pixel** is actually a combination of two words that stands for 'picture element' and denotes the smallest piece of information in a digital image. Pixels are arranged in dots or squares and typically contain three or four colors, such as some combination of red, green, blue, magenta, yellow, and black. Pixels also are used with digital cameras as a measure for resolution purposes. Common measures might include 2,400 pixels per inch (ppi), 640 pixels per line (ppl), a color ink jet printer with 200 ppi, or 720 dpi for an ink jet printer. For pixel examples on a monitor screen, early monitors used a standard of 640 by 480 pixel display for a video graphics array (VGA) display (meaning 640 pixels from each side across and 480 pixels from the top down for a total of 307,200 pixels or 0.3 megapixels). The VGA display monitors were some of the earliest monitors and were first introduced around 1987. This type of monitor used a basic standard of pixels, which has now been replaced by digital technology. A standard pixel is made up of three primary colors in a look-up table sent by the PC, according to White (2008, 244). As White states, "in a normal Video Graphics Array (VGA) adapter, the table contains values for 262,144 possible colors, of which 256 values can be stored in the VGA adapter's memory at one time" (White 2008, 244). In the Super VGA (SVGA), there is enough memory for high color or 16 bits of data per pixel or 65,536 colors or 24 bits per pixel or 16,777,216, which is true color (White 2008, 244).

Another example is the liquid crystal display screen or **LCD screen**. These monitor screens have become very commonplace in the market. An LCD screen also uses pixels; however, these are wedged between thin plastic layers of electric current or electrodes, making the pixels translucent and resulting in a bright image (White 2008, 201). LCD screens are seen in computers, but are more popular in television screens. **Plasma screens** are very similar to the LCD screens in how the pixel arrangements are viewed at a distance by the eye. The schematic arrangement of the pixels is how LCD screens differ from plasma screens; the grid arrangement uses what is known as subpixels. The details of the pixel arrangement differences are beyond the scope of this chapter. Here, it is enough to know that pixels can be arranged in various sequences for LCD, for plasma, and for the megapixels used in digital cameras and other technologically advanced equipment in healthcare and industry.

A **megapixel** is one million pixels. Standard digital cameras currently use approximately 8 to 10 megapixels (which is a very sharp image for the camera sensor and lens) producing a clear picture as the end result. For the current use of the computer with imaging in radiology and ultrasonography, detailed images can be obtained with the use of megapixels. These digital images are used in surgery and in therapeutic and diagnostic tests for patient care. Computerization has made tremendous advances in imaging in patient care. Physicians use digital images in diagnostic testing with computer tomography (CT scans) to see visual markers within the human body more clearly. The use of increased pixels in radiographic and ultrasonographic imaging has improved the radiologist's ability to view the film results, which enhances the patient's care and, possibly, outcome.

Other devices found within the monitor are signals that the computer uses to mark a location on the screen. The **cursor** was originally similar to the underscore "_" and would blink at the user. This would signal to the user where on the screen the cursor was last used. Computers also use the "l" or a vertical line to mark the cursor on the screen. A cursor also can be called a pointer. Within some programs, such as Windows, the cursor changes to an hourglass icon to inform the user that there is a process being performed and will be finished shortly. Also, within Netscape and other browser windows, the cursor may change into a hand icon to inform the user that there is more detailed information within a particular site at a sublevel.

Printers

Printers are peripheral devices that convert the text and images on the screen into text and images on paper sheets. There are two basic types of printers: impact and nonimpact printers. Impact printers are those in which the printing mechanism actually touches the paper to make the impression onto the paper sheet with ink. This includes the **dot-matrix printer**, which was the first type of printer used with computers, and also includes line printers and plotters used in business and industry. The dot-matrix printer is just that, a printing mechanism that makes a series of **dots per inch (DPI),** and these tiny dots would create the text letters or image. Dot-matrix printers were loud because of the noise of the mechanism striking the paper and the carriage of the mechanism returning to position for the next row of dots to be printed. These printers are not used much now because of the noise and the slow printing. Dot-matrix printers were replaced by the ink jet and laser printers in homes and offices.

The nonimpact printers are those in which the printing mechanism does not touch the paper sheet, such as the laser, thermal, and ink jet printers. **Laser printers** use energy from a fast, flashing laser light source to create the images on a special drum; from static electricity, the ink powders (whether black or various colors) are transferred to the sheet of paper. **Thermal printers** use heat to transfer the ink onto the sheet of paper or other medium. Much of the thermal printing is seen in barcoding, done in the industry on large commercial printers. **Ink jet printers** use tiny nozzles to spray the ink (whether black or various colors) onto the sheet of paper.

A multifunction machine is a printer that also functions as a copier, a scanner, and a facsimile machine. Most users classify this multipurpose machine as a printer because most of the time the usage is for routine printing tasks. It also performs these other tasks all in one machine, thus eliminating the need for several separate machines. Other benefits include cutting costs, minimal use of space, and it can communicate with a PC easily.

Speakers

These peripheral devices are for the computer to produce sound for the user. Most computers come with a minimum grade of speaker, with a few PCs offering a midlevel quality speaker that has a subwoofer inside for more bass sound. There is an external knob on the outside of a better-quality speaker for those offering the subwoofer package. Users can upgrade to better quality speakers from many vendors and add speakers to their microcomputers at any time. The speaker ports are all the same for external speakers. Some speakers are mounted onto the monitor screen and have a slide control panel for volume control. Mounting the speakers on the monitor screen helps gain needed space on smaller desks. Many users prefer to wear headphones for optimal sound. This produces a clear sound and also removes background noise. If the user is in a large room with other users, such as a classroom or library setting, the use of headphones is a common courtesy.

Data Projectors

A **data projector** is used to display a presentation on a screen to a large audience or classroom. The projector is connected to a computer and the projector uses the same principle as the LCD display of a laptop. However, the data projector light is brighter to produce a sharper image because the image must travel a greater distance to the screen from the projector. Some projectors are small and portable for travel, others are stationary for use in classrooms or other purposes, and some are mounted from the ceiling.

It has been years since overhead projectors have been used in a classroom; they have been replaced by the data projector. Data projectors are connected to a PC with data input (connected from the PC) and data output (connected to the PC's monitor) cables. The power cord to the data projector plugs into any AC electrical outlet and the data projector is ready for use. When the power is turned on to the projector, the image is shown on the screen; if the angle of the image is projected slightly tilted in any direction, an effect known as **keystoning** can occur. By turning the keystoning knob on the data projector, the angle of the image can be corrected and any distortion eliminated. If the image is out of focus, the lens can be rotated in either direction to sharpen or lessen the resolution, depending on the need of the focus of the image.

Because of the powerful light source within the data projector, a fan is needed to cool the light source at all times. When the projector is turned off, the fan must continue to run in order to cool the light source; if this does not happen, the data projector bulb may need to be replaced. Data projector fans turn off automatically when the light source has cooled properly.

Scanners

As previously stated in this chapter, scanners can be both input and output devices. In this section, scanners are discussed as output devices. There are various types of scanners on the market, each with a different outcome but all with the basic premise of converting text or image to a digital format. When used as output devices, scanners ensure that information is created digitally and then output to a display or printed format (Joos et al. 2006, 33). The first scanner developed was the drum scanner in the 1950s; it is no longer popular because it basically uses a large drum onto which the original document is pasted. A light is passed over the drum and a negative is produced. It is currently used in art museums and for magazines and advertisements. Another scanner that is declining in popularity is the hand scanner, a small, handheld device that usually is swiped across the text or image that is to be scanned. However, because of an unsteady hand or a rapid motion, scans can be blurred easily. The most popular scanner is the flatbed, which is used in most offices and for most home use (on a smaller scale). The flatbed scanner works by placing the document on a glass platform with a light background behind the glass. A light source is passed under the glass to etch the patterns of data that are read by the sensor. The data are converted digitally to the computer where the scan can be transferred to the hard drive and saved, or be sent externally to the computer such as via the Internet or e-mail.

Optical disc

Optical disk technology uses a format that is known as **write once read many (WORM)** technology (Abdelhak et al. 2007, 257). Optical disks are etched by a laser onto a disk platter. Data cannot be altered or misfiled on health records once it has been permanently etched onto a laser disk with WORM technology. Imaging systems using optical disc technology can be costly, but can prove valuable by offering record usage to a multiuser at any given time. However, the system security that a computer system provides with access to authorized persons only is another attractive benefit to the use of optical disc for imaging. One can use optical disc or CD or DVD to store data in imaging systems. Within optical disc storage, the system digitizes documents on laser discs to capture, store, retrieve, process, distribute, and print information. Optical disc systems use a computer, a scanner, a magnetic disc, a file server, optical disc platters, a jukebox, and a printer. Some larger systems may use a jukebox for disc storage but these are rarely used these days. The use of jukeboxes to locate and retrieve the exact platter is a slow process and because of cost, other technology is replacing jukeboxes in many facilities. The documents, which are on paper, are scanned into the system. The data are input into the optical disc from other systems (these could include bedside terminals and voice recognition). User identification controls what a person may access or modify in the system. Advantages to optical disc systems include: quick access to data, multiple users simultaneously, security levels for access for authorized users, documents cannot be lost or misplaced once scanned into the system, and documents cannot be altered once scanned into the system. Whether optical discs, compact discs (CD), or DVD are used, imaging systems are a valuable method of storage.

Wireless Connection

Within the computer peripherals already mentioned, there is the capability to connect laptops or PDAs to the Internet without wires (**Wi-Fi**). Of course, the laptops and PDAs must have a significant battery charge for wireless capabilities. Battery life has increased over the years and continues to increase with technological advances. Many people prefer a wireless connection because of its many advantages. Many of the wireless computers are small and are easily carried to nursing units for patient care at the bedside by healthcare practitioners. This eliminates the need for handwriting notes for entry, and notes can be downloaded later into a computer by docking into a standard size computer at the end of the day.

Many facilities save money by purchasing wireless computers for staff to eliminate the need for wiring departments for computer cables for each workstation, which can be expensive. However, because wireless computers are not stationary, they are easy targets for theft if the opportunity is given. Users of wireless equipment must take great care to protect devices from theft and misuse from unauthorized individuals. Confidentiality applies to wireless computers just as for PCs with password protection.

Computer security, including security and privacy issues associated with portable devices, will be discussed in further detail in chapter 12.

Notebook PC

What are the differences between a workstation PC and a wireless PC? Most of the components of the computers are similar, but these may differ in how they look to the user. The wireless computers or laptops are smaller in size so that they are portable for use. Most laptops, sometimes called **notebook computers** or simply **notebooks**, use a battery power source as well as electricity. The computer's battery is charged by electricity so that a full charge can be held by the battery. The laptop then can be used at any time, powered by the battery for as long as the particular battery charge lasts. Some laptops have a slot to provide space for a second battery to provide even longer battery time for usage. Lithium batteries also stay charged longer than other batteries. It is the batteries that give the laptop computers their weight because the computer itself does not weigh as much as the battery alone. For the electrical charge, the laptop is simply plugged in to any AC outlet for use. An AC adapter is a box on the electrical cord that is attached to the laptop. The AC adapter helps run the laptop and charge the battery.

Rather than a mouse on a workstation PC, a laptop computer usually has a pointing stick in the center of the keyboard that rotates in all directions and acts as the mouse and cursor. A laptop computer can also have a touchpad in the front of the keyboard so that the cursor can be operated with the touch of a fingertip, similar to a mouse. The touchpad is usually located on the shelf provided for wrist support on laptop computers. Notebooks usually have built-in speakers; these smaller computers are limited in size and sound capability, and sometimes the speakers are monophonic. The keyboard on a notebook is sometimes smaller than that of a regular workstation PC and the depression on the key downward is shorter. Again, this is because of the notebook's smaller size. The notebook also has external ports for USB and docking capability. Here, peripherals are attached such as a mouse, an external modem, and docking to a regular workstation PC and printer, as well as to other peripheral devices. Notebooks and laptop computers have floppy drives or external drives to accommodate a CD, DVD, or Blu-Ray disc. Some have one or two bays; if there is only one bay, it is interchangeable and the drive is an attachment device that can be swapped out as needed. Most notebooks also have headphone jacks for better sound quality than the built-in speakers. The modem is also built-in to allow easy connection to the Internet for users. Probably the most noticeable difference between the notebook and the workstation PC is the monitor screen. The LCD screen eliminates the heaviness of a standard desktop monitor and provides the thin screen needed for a small, lightweight, portable device. The monitor screen LCD uses light rays shining through the crystal-colored cells toward the user. LCD screens are the standard on notebooks and laptop computers.

Wireless computers also provide the practitioner with instantaneous bedside access to patient records for data entry, notes, laboratory results, and vital signs. If there are any urgent or emergent alerts about a patient on a particular entry, these can be immediately flagged by e-mail or entry by the practitioner through the computer system. The wireless computers also can provide software programs for the practitioner in their field, such as a formulary for prescriptions carried by the facility, case protocols for treatment for patients, Physician's Desk Reference and drug references, and other reference tools that are particular to that healthcare practitioner. Wireless computers are used for more than data storage; they are tools used for patient care, sending and receiving e-mail, and fax communication. Wireless computers are used to connect to the facility's network and the Internet as well as to reference software for patient care.

Check Your Understanding 1.3

1. The weight of a laptop computer is most attributed to the _____.

   A. LCD screen
   B. AC adapter
   C. keyboard
   D. battery

2. The port that uses infrared waves that are directed between two devices to communicate is known as:

   A. Bluetooth
   B. IrDA
   C. FireWire
   D. USB

3. If you were to purchase a digital camera, which of the following would have the best resolution in pixels on this camera?

   A. 10 pixels
   B. 8 pixels
   C. 1 megapixel
   D. 3 megapixels

4. Monitor resolution is measure in _____.

   A. ROM
   B. GHz
   C. MBps
   D. dpi

Software

The area of software within the PC includes operating systems, software programs or applications, utility programs or functions of the computers (instructions), and programming languages. **Operating systems** are the instructions that direct the computer in its operation, regulate the hardware, and allow several programs to run simultaneously; these are the instructions to make the computer work (White 2008, 9). An operating system also makes any compatible software application run in any microcomputer. All computers must have an operating system. Familiar examples of operating systems include: Windows XP or Vista, UNIX, Solaris, and Mac OS. One of the **free and open source software (FOSS)** operating systems, which is currently popular, is Linux, an alternative to Windows. The computer's operating system instructions allow it to handle several tasks at once. This is called **multitasking**, which involves the computer CPU, or brain, working to timeshare the tasks so that several functions can be done at once, using a share of the computer's time to execute. A connected storage such as a hard drive is accessed for a workstation PC through a **device driver**, a specific type of software that is made to interact with hardware devices. A device driver basically acts as a communication device.

A question frequently asked by novice users is, "My workstation is a PC, so if I have a Mac, what do I have?" Novice users do not understand that the PC and Mac are brands or types of computers, not the software or applications that reside within. Although the software must be compatible to the computer that is purchased, the computers themselves are made by various manufacturers. For example, Mac is short for Macintosh, a brand of computers that specializes in graphics, varying from the IBM-compatible computers (White 2008, 8). Most of the rest of the market share of computers made are IBM-compatible, even though not all are made by the company IBM and could be made by Hewlett-Packard, Dell, Gateway, and hundreds of other manufacturers. The Macs were first made by Apple, Inc. in 1984. These computers had a mouse and a GUI instead of a command line interface. This meant that the user saw pictures of objects on the screen rather than words on a line as instructions. For example, the Delete key did not have to be used any longer. With a Mac computer, the user could click on the picture of a trash can and the document would be deleted. This may sound like a primitive concept now, but in 1984 only the Mac computers had this new technology.

Application programs are designed to help users perform certain types of work. In comparison, software runs a computer and a utility program performs maintenance or tasks. Application software can work with text, numbers, graphs, images, or a combination of these. Some of the applications are very adaptable and are able to work with several application types simultaneously, and some are very powerful—these are called integrated software. Microsoft is a common software vendor that packages several of its applications as a suite, such as Microsoft Office. This package includes applications in word processing (Microsoft Word), spreadsheets (Microsoft Excel), databases (Microsoft Access), and a graphics package (Microsoft PowerPoint). Users find it more economical to purchase a suite of applications than to purchase them individually.

Many companies and facilities also may have their computer departments or information technology (IT) departments create or write software programs for their own use at their facility. Programmers are familiar with the computer languages and instructions needed in order to perform this task and the facility can save costs by having this done in-house. Creating software is advantageous because it is custom-made and has all of the features needed for a particular facility, avoiding the need to pay for unnecessary features. Tailor-made software meets the facility's needs and can include applications for the entire facility or for a single department. The term **enterprise software** is typically used when an application is used for the entire facility, such as applications involving e-mail, network, security issues, and the Internet. Many software applications currently are on the market and are too numerous to list; however, some of the subcategories of common software are listed in table 1.3.

Programming Languages

A computer cannot operate by itself. It must have instructions in order to function. A user does not have to be a computer programmer to operate a computer because these languages are encoded into the computer to instruct on what to do and how to operate. Computers are

Table 1.3.   Subcategories of common software applications

Organizational Software	Information Software	Simulation Software	Educational Software
• Workflow • Database management system (DBSS) • Document management • Geographic information system • Financial • Supply management • Travel expense • Management • IT Helpdesk • E-mail server • Network management • Security management	• Accounting • Task and scheduling • Contact management • Spreadsheet • Personal database • Word processing • Desktop publishing • Diagramming • Presentation/graphic • Statistical • Console games • Video game • Wireless or mobile phone • Computer-aided design (CAD)	• Scientific simulator • Battlefield simulator • Emergency simulator • Flight simulator • Driving simulator • Video editing • Sound editing • Music sequencing • Web development	• Classroom • Educational • Training • Reference • Survey • E-mail • Blog

for the most part user friendly and most operate in a similar manner, with drop-down menus for selections from the user. The computer does the tasks from the instructions that have been preprogrammed into the system from the **programming languages**. These instructions, as previously mentioned, are the operating systems and the applications. However, these are written in a language that can be read by the machine. A computer does not read English or French or a traditional language, but rather in binary numbers, 0 and 1. A basic unit of storage within a computer is called a **bit** (Joos et al. 2006, 15). This is the smallest unit of information known and is either a 0 or a 1 within the computer. When the computer groups a string of 0s and 1s together in certain arrangements or order, it means a certain function to the computer. A string of eight numbers is called a '**byte**' of information (Joos et al. 2006, 15). Memory within a computer is measured in bytes. However, most computers currently are so powerful that they now have gigabytes of memory rather than **kilobytes** and megabytes. Table 1.2 presents a chart to help put these terms and their approximations into perspective.

If the system shown in table 1.2 is viewed as a '2 to the power of 10' system, then each level is basically multiplied by the power of 10 again to get the next level. What comes after **terabyte**? The current generation will probably be retired when the next level in the system is determined, but it should be interesting (as technology advancement always is).

Several earlier programming languages have been around for many years; some still are in use. Examples of these include: **FORTRAN** (formula translator), **COBOL** (Common Business-Oriented Language), **BASIC** (Beginner's All-Purpose Symbolic Instruction Code), and C. Another familiar programming language still in use in the healthcare industry is MUMPS (Massachusetts General Hospital Utility Multi Programming System). This programming language was specifically developed for use in hospitals. Computer languages exist for users to interact with the computer as well as with others on the Internet. Languages are much more complicated now than the early languages previously mentioned. **Java** is a very popular programming language that was developed by Sun Microsystems as an offshoot from the programming languages of C and C++ (White 2008, 96). Java is very popular among programmers because of its versatility; it can be supported on most any operating system platform because of its independence, and is known as a 'write once, compile once, and run it anywhere' program (White 2008, 96).

Several computer languages are used primarily with the Internet. The most commonly used is Hypertext Markup Language (HTML), which allows text to be displayed onto the screen with a browser directly from a computer browser to the Internet (White 2008, 312). HTML uses a '**tag**' as a '**header**' at the beginning of a message to instruct the computer what to do. HTML also uses a tag as a '**footer**' at the end of the message with another instruction for the computer. The term '**markup**' in computer languages simply means this is the way a computer encodes text (White 2008, 356). It also tells the computer how to format or do what it needs to, similar to a blueprint or a map. It is like a printout for the computer for following instructions.

Another computer language used but not as popular as HTML is **Extensible Markup Language (XML)**. One of the primary advantages of XML is that it is text-based on international standards; however, it does have limitations with its use of wordy syntax to the human eye. Although computers are able to read this language, it is an advanced version of HTML (White 2008, 313).

The third computer language that is in common use is **Standard Generalized Markup Language (SGML)**. This was one of the first languages developed and was primarily intended for use in text and database publishing. It was even used in the Oxford English Dictionary, but because of its complexity it has not seen widespread use in the computer industry because of difficult syntax usage. HTML was an offshoot of SGML, but was reformulated to its current design. XML is a subset of SGML, and the design of XML is easier to implement than SGML because it has a more general purpose in its use (McWay 2008, 317).

Check Your Understanding 1.4

1. Apple, Gateway, Hewlett-Packard, and Dell are examples of what within the computer world?

   A. Application software
   B. Computer manufacturers
   C. Internet design
   D. Computer language design

2. What computer language is more commonly used for programming on the Internet?

   A. HTML
   B. SGML
   C. XML
   D. C++

3. The computer's instruction set that governs the entire functions of all processes are known as the:

   A. operating system
   B. device driver
   C. application
   D. programming language

4. What would a utility program BEST perform within a computer?

   A. Maintenance
   B. Word processing
   C. Graphics
   D. E-mail

Communication and Internet Technologies

Networks

PCs that are linked together in a facility need to communicate with each other and to a server (the central hub). The **hub computer** can serve numerous workstation computers at a single site or remotely. Networks are very complicated because these connect to one another and can link internally and externally without the user realizing physically when there is a crossover. Networks are virtual systems that continue to grow. Within facilities, networks continue to grow when computers are added to existing networks—for example, when personnel are added because of staff growth and expansion. In classrooms, computers are added to a computer laboratory. Networks continue to grow in size, and the need for networks within facilities grows as businesses increase. Usually one computer within a network is a controlling computer—that is the hub or central computer. The hub is the device where all the computers on a network connect. If a network does not use a central server or hub, this is referred to as a **peer-to-peer network** and all the computers on this network can perform the duties at the same time (White 2008, 313). Most networks have a **firewall**, which is a security device that controls access from the Internet to a local area network. **Routers** also provide firewall security for networks and route data between networks using Internet Protocol (IP) addresses. The IP address is basically an identifier for a computer on a TCP/IP network as a 32-bit number written as four numbers separated by periods (White 2008, 312). The TCP/IP network is the Transmission Control Protocol/Internet Protocol, which is the method used to connect servers on the Internet to exchange data, and the TCP/IP is a universal standard (White 2008, 313).

Networks are faster than running individual computers alone. The server that hosts the community of computers on this network is sometimes referred to as the host computer.

Larger companies use networks and systems to operate efficiently. Familiar network names of operating systems include Unix, Linux, Novell NetWare, and Windows Server 2003. These large networks that could run hundreds of computers in various counties or states are called **client/server networks**. Within this setup, PCs attached to the host server are called the clients. A fat client is one that uses minimal data from the host server and much of the work comes from its own machine. A thin client or "dumb terminal" is one that uses very little data from its own machine and most from the host server. Some thin clients have no hard drive at all. Dumb terminals, or dummy terminals, can reside within this setup and consist of a monitor, keyboard, and the minimum hardware needed to connect them to the server to perform their functions.

Another network is the **local area network (LAN)**. These computers are located within a local area and are networked to a host server. These are found within a building (White 2008, 312). Networks that are not geographically located near each other are called **wide area networks (WANs)**. These can reach across offices or buildings (White 2008, 313).

Interfaces

Within networks, an **interface** is a connection between a computer and a network. An interface also can be a connection between two or more networks. An interface is what enables applications to communicate with each other so that systems can be integrated. According to Amatayakul, the best example of an interface is Microsoft's "Word, Excel, Access, PowerPoint, Outlook, and other components of the suite [as] they all look the same and exchange data easily (although any power user knows that even in this case the programs do not work 100 percent exactly the same)" (Amatayakul 2007, 241). Vendors now write interface programs and technology, called interface engines. This helps networks communicate with each other, especially when networks are numerous or in large facilities. For example, the importance of a functional interface between a lab information system and an electronic health record (EHR) ensures the accuracy of lab data into the EHR for treatment purposes.

Internet Connections

There are several types of common Internet connections used within networks. Those typically used in cable systems are the Ethernet networks for fiberoptic cables, which are faster network cabling units. Wireless connections are another method that has become very popular. These connections are discussed within this section.

Ethernet

An Ethernet network sends data from one node to another in packets. In a **star network** (discussed under types of networks), switches and hubs turn signals on and off as the data move through the cables to each node or workstation. In the other network configurations, the nodes or workstations check the address data and each determines which data are for a particular computer and which data move down the network line to other workstations (White 2008, 321).

Wireless

Instead of using cable connections, the network uses signals by a router from the Wi-Fi systems from the network (White 2008, 320). No cables are needed at any workstations because of the Wi-Fi setup. Wireless can employ "radio (broadcast, microwave, and satellite) and light waves (infrared) to transmit the data" (Joos et al. 2006, 39).

Fiberoptic

Fiberoptic cables are extremely fast, carrying one billion bits per second through the network (White 2008, 320). Signals are carried through the cables to each node until the message reaches the designated workstation.

Modems

A **modem** is a bridge between digital and analog signals that converts digital data on and off; or, it modulates the frequency of the waves, then it demodulates the analog signals back into digital code. The name "modem" was derived from "MODulate-DEModulate." Most computers have built-in modems, so one does not have to be purchased separately. For older model computers that do not have modem capability, an external modem would be needed for the computer to be used to communicate through the telephone line for Internet (e-mail) use to allow digital conversion of data. An external modem would be a separate box that would sit near the computer and plug in to a port in the back of the computer. There are several types of modem connections for computers.

A **dial-up modem** is used for computers with a telephone connection only and Internet service through the local telephone company. The original modem connections were managing data at 28.8 kilobits per second, but most dial-up modems now use a V.90 rate.

The cable and DSL modems are not really modems because these work with digital signals only. The **cable television modems** connect to a PC and a cable-ready television using the cable television pathway. The **digital subscriber line (DSL) modem** uses the telephone lines but also uses pure digital signals. Both the cable and DSL modems use a **broadband bandwidth**, which has a large capacity, so there is no waiting for signals and accessing the Internet is instant.

Wireless Cards

A **wireless network interface card or simply wireless card** is a device for a plug-in for the PC, laptop, or PDA to communicate to the network. These come in various sizes and shapes depending on the type of computer for which the card will be used. Some wireless cards may look more like a flash drive than a card and simply plug into the computer using a USB port for connectivity. Other wireless cards are the size and shape of a credit card and slide into a bay on the side of a PC or laptop. In all cases, the wireless cards are to function as a communication device so the computer can use a network provider through an antenna technology to connect to the Internet. Many users subscribe through their telephone carriers, and this service also is available in Bluetooth technology.

Types of Networks

There are several ways that networks can be set up or shaped within a LAN. Each of the network types has a shape or purpose in how the information is moved from one computer to the next. Figure 1.1 shows three different types of networks.

Bus Network

In a **bus network** the computers that are networked together are lined up on a single cable. The computers and other devices on this network do not have to be lined up in a single row but they can be all on one single line. Christmas tree lights are used as an example here to help illustrate the bus network. If one tree light bulb is removed along a string of lights, then the lights from below that point where the light was removed do not work. That is the same principle with the bus network. If a computer or printer device is removed from any point in a bus network or the cable line network, then those further down the cable line on this network will not work.

Star Network

A star network is the most common of the network setups for a LAN network. All of the cables that connect to computers at any point connect to the hub or center, which is called the star. A star network is analogous to a bicycle wheel that has many spokes on it where all are outreaching yet all connect to a center hub. Many star networks often connect to a second network, especially in large facilities. Data flow to the center of the circle and are then passed along to a specific computer.

Token Ring Network

The **token ring network** is similar to a ring or circle of cable of computers in the network. There is no beginning or end within this loop. Data flow around this circle until it reaches the exact computer address that it is meant to reach.

Figure 1.1.   Network types

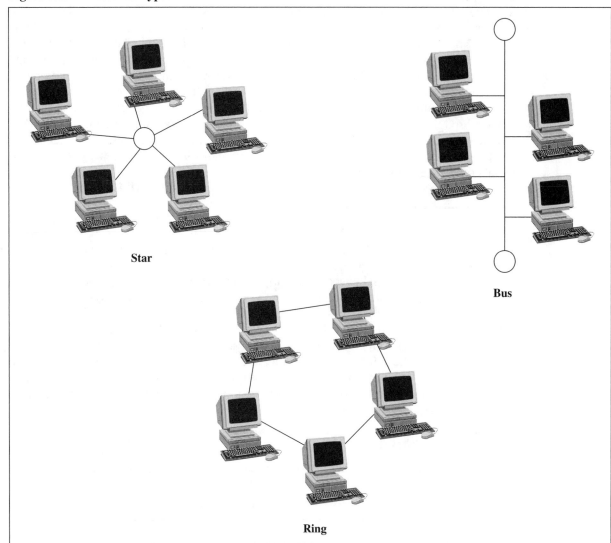

Source: Durkin and Just 2008, 41

Tree Network

The **tree network** is sometimes called a hierarchical network. The main computer is the root or the first level; the next level of computers that are connected is the second level. In the second level of the hierarchy, computers are connected from the second computer in the series. There can be other levels within this network but no other computers can be connected above the central computer or node in the hierarchy. A tree network must have three levels or else it would be a star network.

Hybrid Network

A **hybrid network** would basically be any combination of the above types of network that can work together. Examples of this might include star-bus network, star-tree network, and so on.

Daisy Chain Network

The easiest way to add more computers into a network is by connecting each computer to the next in a series. This is called a **daisy chain network**. Each computer forwards a message down the line to the next until a message reaches the correct computer for which it is intended using a computer's unique address.

Internet Technologies

Internet

The Internet is really hundreds of networks with thousands of computers linked together to share data and information. People from around the world are connected within seconds with a click of a mouse. The Internet is free; however, connecting to the Internet costs each user according to how the connection is made. Some users are connected in their homes privately through an **Internet service provider (ISP)** such as a telephone, cable, or satellite provider in their community. Others are connected through their business accounts, where connections might use fiberoptic or T1 or T3 cables. These are high-speed and broadband bandwidths for heavy use. Networks have been created across the country and the world so that high-speed lines have major highways; so, if Internet traffic is too heavy, communication can be rerouted to another information highway. No single person or agency owns the Internet; however, several organizations have been developed to create standards to ensure that basic architecture and maintenance of the Internet is continued for the world. Some of the more common agencies are the Internet Society (ISOC), Internet Architecture Board (IAB), World Wide Web consortium (W3C), the Internet Corporation for Assigned Names and Numbers (ICANN), and the Internet Assigned Numbers Authority (IANA) (Joos et al. 2006, 275). Under ICANN, IANA works to oversee the distribution and maintenance of domain names and Internet Protocol (IP) addresses; however, ICANN has the overall responsibility for the Internet agencies.

As previously mentioned, the standards for the Internet are the Transmission Control Protocol/Internet Protocol (TCP/IP). This is the communications protocol or set of rules that is the foundation for how computers can talk to each other using the Internet; these rules are used globally. Data are broken into chunks and separated into the transmission (TCP) packet and sent on to the destination computer. When the IP packet reaches the destination computer, the TCP packet then reassembles the packets so the message is in its original form for the receiver.

Intranet

Also within networks, many facilities have a private network that is available for their own employees and authorized persons to gain access; this is called an intranet. The **intranet** is not the same as the Internet. A facility's intranet is based on TCP/IP protocol (of the Internet) but belongs strictly to a particular organization. There is a firewall built around the intranet to prevent unauthorized access to it or restricted parts of the Web site. An intranet of a facility might house particulars to a healthcare facility's mission, vision, and philosophy, give updates on upcoming events, house the bylaws and rules and regulations as well as the policies and procedures of the facility, a directory of employees, a map of the facility, and other items helpful for employees. It can also provide users with a site search engine for items not found in the contents page. An intranet looks like any other Web site because it is built on the same platform as the Web sites of the Internet; however, the firewall security to restrict unauthorized users is what primarily distinguishes it from the Internet.

Extranet

An extranet is an efficient way to share information with people outside of a particular organization. An **extranet** is "an intranet system that allows selected external users limited access to the private networks (McWay 2008, 321). Network space within an organization that is authorized for its users only is considered to be an extranet. The term 'extranet' term is not used as widely as the term 'network' because an extranet is, at its foundation, a network.

Computerized Records

Significant pioneering work has been accomplished over the past four decades in automating patient records. Before the 1950s, punch cards were used as a method of entering data into a computerized system. From the 1960s until the 1990s, departmental-based programs were developed. Large mainframe computers gave way to microcomputers, laptops, and PDAs. There are knowledge-based systems in database operations, and expert systems with artificial intelligence and voice recognition. All of these newer technologies are a part of advancing knowledge of what computers can do in what is called the 'fifth generation' of computers.

In the late 1980s our profession changed from being a medical record department to being a health information management department. Although many departments were still paper-based at that time, our profession began a movement toward the computerized patient record (CPR). To transition to the CPR, the electronic health record (EHR) and the electronic medical record (EMR) began as steps to implement the CPR. These terms basically were used interchangeably among many in the profession because the documentation was on paper and had to be scanned in order to be digitized and entered into the computer system. Many today believe a truly computerized patient record doesn't exist as there will always be some report types that will have to be scanned in under some circumstances (that is, transfer of patients from other facilities to yours).

Johns' definitions of the EHR, the EMR, and the computer-based patient record (CPR) are listed below:

"EHR   a computerized record of health information and associated processes. (see computer-based patient record)"

"EMR   a form of computer-based health record in which information is stored in whole files instead of by individual data elements"

"CPR   an electronic patient record housed in a system designed to provide users with access to complete and accurate data, practitioner alerts and reminders, clinical decision support systems, and links to medical knowledge; See electronic health record" (Johns 2007, 957, 963).

The ultimate goal of the electronic or computerized health record is that technology affect the delivery of healthcare, and the HIM professional's attention should be focused on the needs of its users. There are several workgroups and agencies collaborating on the standards for data exchange and vocabulary for the EHR. A widespread communication technology is needed in healthcare for the delivery of quality information to the end user. Healthcare is in the process of standardization of the computerized patient record.

The entire patient record must be computerized. The factors for a computerized record are generally considered to be the following:

- Must provide for instant access

- Must allow for automatic transfer of data

- Must have 100% availability—no down time

- Must interface with all other hospital systems—HL-7 (HIPAA initiative)

- Must be user friendly

- Must have secure security semantics

- Must provide confidentiality—the control of user rights (passwords, for example)

- Integrity of system—The information is changed only in a specified and authorized manner, and the computer resources operate correctly without risk of material breakdown

Again, the computerized health record is totally generated by computer key entries; at no time is paper a part of the process. The advantages of using a computerized patient record (CPR) are numerous; a few benefits are given here:

- Improved access to education resources

- Decreased clinical errors (with alerts and reminders)

- Reduced redundant data entry
- Reduced duplicate testing (costly)
- Improved data analysis (more information to compare)
- Improved record accessibility
- Increased accountability for accurate and complete records (auditing)
- Improved patient confidentiality and record security
- Consistent data presentation
- Increased patient healthcare communications
- Increased efficiency
- Reduced operating costs
- Frees up space for document storage
- Reduction in lost or misfiled documents
- Improved workflow
- Increased reimbursement turnaround time
- Ensured backup and disaster recovery

Check Your Understanding 1.5

1. The linking of components within a geographically contained area is called a:
   A. daisy chain
   B. LAN
   C. WAN
   D. star network

2. Advantages to using a CPR or EHR include all of the following EXCEPT
   A. Decrease data and testing redundancy
   B. Working from home
   C. All records are immediately accessible
   D. Reduced operating costs

3. The reasons why networks are used in organizations include all of the following EXCEPT:
   A. Application programs can be shared
   B. Peripheral hardware can be shared
   C. Databases can be shared
   D. System security is easier to control

4. The network topography that will allow users to access portions of the network when one section is down is the:
   A. bus network
   B. star network
   C. ring network
   D. tree network

References

Abdelhak, M., S. Grostick, M.A. Hanken, and E. Jacobs. 2007. *Health information: Management of a Strategic Resource*, 3rd ed. St. Louis, MO: Saunders/Elsevier.

Amatayakul, M.K. 2007. *Electronic Health Records: A Practical Guide for Professionals and Organizations*, 3rd ed. Chicago: AHIMA.

Durkin, S. and B. Just. 2008. An IT primer for health information exchange. *Journal of AHIMA* 79(1):38–42.

Johns, M.J., ed. 2007. *Health Information Management Technology: An Applied Approach*, 2nd ed. Chicago: AHIMA.

Joos, I., N.I. Whitman, M.J. Smith, and R. Nelson. 2006. *Introduction to Computers for Healthcare Professionals*, 4th ed. Sudbury, MA: Jones & Bartlett, Publishers.

McWay, D.C. 2008. *Today's Health Information Management: An Integrated Approach*. Clifton Park, NY: Thomson/Delmar Learning.

White, R. *How Computers Work*, 9th ed. 2008. Indianapolis, IN: QUE, Publishing.

Chapter 2
Common Software Applications

Objectives

- Discuss common software applications for the personal computer and the operating system environment.

- Differentiate between word processing software applications and desktop publishing.

- Give examples of common software used, including word processing, spreadsheets, databases, scheduling, presentations, project management, and e-mail software applications.

- Illustrate how spreadsheet software can perform statistical calculations and graphical capabilities within the same utility.

- Identify three common examples of database usage within the healthcare facility.

- Develop a patient case scenario where a software application would be used to help in the caregiving of a patient to speed delivery of care and increase the quality of the level of care provided.

- Summarize what you have done in your HIM clinical experiences to date with software that has been used to directly or indirectly improve patient care in the facility.

Key Terms

.bmp
.jpg
.tif
American National Standards
   Institute (ANSI)
Asynchronous
Bitmaps
Boolean search
Broadband
Browser

Cable
Database management system
   (DBMS)
Desktop publishing
Domain name
DSL
Encryption
End-User License Agreement
   (EULA)
Fiberoptic

Field
File Transfer Protocol (FTP)
Gantt chart
Graphical user interface (GUI)
Hierarchical model
Hypertext
Hypertext Markup Language
   (HTML)
Hypertext Transfer Protocol
   (HTTP)

Internet Protocol (IP) address
Internet service provider (ISP)
Junk e-mail
Listserv
Modem
Object-oriented model
Project management software
Query
Relational model
Rich text format

Satellite
Scheduling software
Search engine
Software licensure
Software piracy
Spam filter
Standards development
    organization (SDO)
Synchronous
T1 line

Third-party license
Transmission Control Protocol/
    Internet Protocol (TCP/IP)
Uniform Resource Locator
    (URL)
Web page
What you see is what you get
    (WYSIWYG)
World Wide Web
Zip

Introduction

Although software is not thought of as a recipe, it matches the definition of one. A recipe is a basic set of instructions in a step-by-step format on how to execute and complete a process. Software is similar in that it is a recorded set of instructions that control the actions of a computer. Data are a collection of raw facts and are a common element to all software. A computer translates all data into numbers of 0 and 1, the binary digits, and manipulates those digits into strands of 8 bits of numbers coded into a language the computer can use and understand. Software transcribes the strands of numbers from the binary strings of data into results that have meaning to the user. The different software types process data in different ways. This chapter will explore the various kinds of software and the ways that the computer uses the data in healthcare for common software applications.

Development of Software

There are thousands of software applications available for the functions of computers in word processing, databases, spreadsheets, and graphics applications. So, where does software come from? Should the software be purchased from a vendor or should the information systems department at the facility develop it? These are excellent questions that should be explored and answered before any decisions are made.

The development of software internally by a facility's information systems department is a great undertaking that requires much thought. The costs to develop software in-house are probably lower than purchasing software from an outside vendor, but in-house software development is labor-intensive and time-consuming. A thorough cost analysis, benefits analysis, and project plan proposal should be completed to help make a full and informed decision. Would the time spent by the programmers be equal to or exceed that of what the cost would have been if software had been purchased from a vendor? A needs assessment should be completed to assess the needs and purpose for the software. What functions are needed? What is required of the output/end result of the software? A great deal of specificity is needed so that the information systems department can accurately estimate the work hours needed to determine staffing costs. The facility must then decide if internal software development would be more cost effective than outsourcing the project to a vendor.

For software applications that already exist or have been developed by external vendors, the market is extremely open. The specifications range from simple to complex as well as inexpensive to overpriced, with the capabilities of the software ranging from plain to elaborate. The advantage for the user is that the application software is already developed and ready to use, so access is easy. The user only needs to purchase and install the application onto the current computer system or network. Most applications are developed so that interfacing with computers and networks is not problematic; this adaptability is a major selling point with vendors and adds to their products' marketability. The drawback to purchasing an application developed by external vendors is that it can either lack or exceed certain provisions that might be needed for a specific user or facility. This is when in-house software development may be the better choice, because a programmer can customize functions needed by a user or facility. The level of specificity or customization may or may not be attainable with predeveloped software.

Software Licensing

Software purchased by an outside vendor is subject to restrictions in licensure and use; software developed by the vendor has been copyrighted by the manufacturer. **Third-party licenses** can be involved with **software licensure**, which means that an additional licensure is required between the user and the vendor. Licenses are usually handled by a separate agreement or an addendum to the original licensure contract by the vendor. Licensure of software is provided to a user for a specified amount of time as agreed upon between the user facility and the manufacturer of the software. The system license is negotiated by a contract where the terms of agreement are negotiated between the vendor and the buyer. The software license is granted as agreed upon with the key issues being: identification of products and services, license grant, delivery terms, installation, warranties, remedies [liability], acceptance and testing, price and payments, terms and termination, and support and maintenance (Abdlehak et al. 2007, 352). Licensure is also awarded by the number of users, either by the number of seats (users) or the number of concurrent licenses (Abdelhak et al. 2007, 352). **Software piracy** occurs when unauthorized copying or use of copyrighted software happens outside the terms of the agreement (Joos et al. 2006, 381). Licensure of software not only safeguards the vendor in protecting their copyrighted property, but also gives the user protection in the warranty of the merchandise that has been bought for the period of the licensure term.

Word Processing

Word processing is a computer software program that provides text usage and other special options in addition to being a spelling and grammar editor. The term 'word processing' gives the exact definition of what the software specifically was created to do, and that is to build and develop text documents. The software can perform other functions such as create tables, insert clip art, and insert templates of preprogrammed forms or graphs onto a blank document; thus, the text document can become an endless information- and image-filled document. Word processing has the capability to enable the user to turn on or turn off a markup with the click of a mouse so that editing can be shown (or not shown) on the screen (this is especially valuable when several people are working on a document). Computer instructions typically not seen by the user can be viewed with the markup function turned on in most word processing software. This visual showing of paragraph marks and space indents to the user can make marked-up text hard to read. Most users do not show markup on the screen for this reason. When the markup is not shown, it is called "**WYSIWYG**" or "what you see is what you get" (pronounced "wizzywig"). The screen mimics the output of the printer, so the user can see what the final output of the document will be.

Basic Elements of Word Processing Software

Most word processing programs contain the same types of commands, although ways to access those commands may vary. Most programs almost always have file handling commands, including commands to Load, Save, Save As, and Print. Typical features of word processing software include characteristics such as printing and formatting text as the primary responsibilities. Other key functions include deletion and replacement of text by a "copy and paste" task with a few clicks of the mouse. Word processing software also includes margin justifications, preset tabs with user-adjustable tabs, merging of words or files from other documents into word processing (or other types of documents such as spreadsheets or images into word processing), and headers or footers. Many word processing applications have built-in spelling and grammar checking programs and many other specialized features. As word processing applications become more expert, they are then called desktop publishing applications (discussed in further detail later in the chapter).

Uses of Word Processing in Healthcare

Word processing software applications are used for various purposes in healthcare. In the HIM department alone, this software will be used for creating text and graphs for purposes such as administrative reporting, financial reporting, statistical documents, employee performance evaluations, quality monitoring of performance of employees, credentialing reports, public health reporting, writing goals, objectives, job descriptions, policies and procedures, as well as minutes and agendas for committee meetings to name a few. Other health information professionals who work in healthcare facilities such as physician offices, clinics, surgery settings, long-term care, rehabilitation, behavioral health, and drug and alcohol centers have duties similar to those who work in acute care facilities. Those professionals working in specialty facilities may have to complete various reports and also may have additional reporting duties for other agencies according to their discipline.

Common Word Processing Software

Many types of word processing software are currently on the market. Microsoft Word is probably the most common word processing software available. If purchased by a user in the Microsoft Suite, Word is packaged with other Microsoft applications including spreadsheet (Excel), database (Access), and the graphics/presentation software (PowerPoint). Other word processing software programs include Corel's WordPerfect, Microsoft Works, and a host of others that can be categorized as free and open source software (FOSS), commercial software, and freeware or shared software. The future of word processing software involves applications that are available both online and offline so that data are stored in the user's PC and then can later be docked with the online application when the user is back online. There are three major word processor applications currently on the market that have spreadsheet, database, and graphics packages and other applications within a suite that are online software. The top three competitors are Zoho, Thinkfree, and Google Docs. It is advised that users with personal digital assistants (PDAs) and iPhones keep the current platforms until the online word processing software applications and office suites are more advanced. The Zoho Web site FAQ states that some (but not all) of Zoho's applications do work on PDAs (AdventNet 2008).

A complete discussion of each of the word processing software applications currently available to the user is beyond the scope of this book; thus, the discussion will focus on the two most common word processing applications in the United States, Microsoft Word and Corel WordPerfect.

Microsoft Word

Microsoft Word is used daily for various duties at work and correspondence at home and to friends; however, Microsoft Word has not been around as long as computers have been in existence. The "trade name of '*Microsoft*' [was] registered with the Office of the Secretary of the state of New Mexico in 1976" (White 2008, 84).

Corel WordPerfect

The history of Corel WordPerfect is similar to that of Microsoft Word. Corel debuted WordPerfect in 1996 (Corel Corporation 2008). Like Microsoft, Corel continued to add other software applications to their suite of software to package the word processing software as a bundle to be sold to users. Both Corel and Microsoft have international sales with their WordPerfect and Word software applications.

Desktop Publishing: A Step above Word Processing

A **desktop publishing** application is professional software that is highly specialized word processing software. This software performs many other features in addition to the basic features of word processing. Desktop publishing gives the user more control over moving text and images in a document and is a general-purpose design tool for projects such as greeting cards, banners, calendars, and other flyers that are of value to business and to the home user. Some common examples of desktop publishing software include PageMaker, QuarkXPress, and Adobe InDesign. These are dedicated applications whereas word processors also offer some features of desktop publishing, such as Microsoft Publisher. (Fuller and Larson 2008, 213).

RTF—Language Used by All Word Processing Software

Rich text format (RTF) is a "format for text and graphics interchange that is used with different output devices, operating environments, and operating systems" (Microsoft Company 2008). RTF uses the "American National Standards Institute (ANSI), PC-8, Macintosh, or IBM PC character set to control the representation and formatting of a document, both on the screen and in print" (Microsoft Company 2008). With these specifications and standards, documents can easily be transferred between software applications operating under these systems and applications. When using specific formats, such as MS Word 2007, Word saves a document with a ".docx" extension to the name. However, if using RTF with this same document, a user "can save a document in a different format such as a Web page, a plain text file, a rich text format, or an earlier version of Word" and MS Word 2007 can still read the file (Rutkosky et al. 2008c, 22). Rich text format, developed by Microsoft, is meant to be a universal format so that it can be read on the Internet, as plain text and by earlier versions of Word as well as most other operating systems.

Web Pages and Word Processing

A **Web page** is the text written on a Web site and displayed on the Internet or **World Wide Web**. To post a Web page on the Internet, a user must first develop a Web page, usually in a word processing software application that may also include other applications such as images and clip art, videos, or animated graphics. As discussed in chapter 1 of this text, most languages used on the Internet are written in HTML, XML, or SGML. Web pages are then stored on the server as a text file in **Hypertext Markup Language (HTML)**, which is a collection of formatted codes that the computer reads (White 2008, 370). As a user searches the Internet for a particular Web site and comes to a Web page, the browser reassembles the cache memory on the Web page for the user onscreen to place the hidden HTML codes of text, graphics, videos, and other codes before the user (White 2008, 371). Because not all portions of the Web page arrive at the PC at the same time, some parts of the Web site appear onscreen before others; usually the text that is the simplest to send arrives first, followed by still and animated graphics, sounds, music, and videos (White 2008, 371). For users with high-speed capability this process is not noticeable, but sometimes those users with dial-up modems can see this loading taking place and can understand this process better. Word processing is the text that makes it happen when the user is first developing a Web site, before it is uploaded to the Internet.

Spreadsheets

Spreadsheets are software application programs that "manipulate numbers in a format of rows and columns and contain special functions for adding and computing statistical and financial formulas" (Joos et al. 2006, 42). Years ago, calculating numbers by hand for financial statistics was a tedious job for hospitals and industry financial officers. Some reports of finance would take chief financial officers (CFOs) many weeks to complete when having to calculate reports of statistics by hand, before computers with spreadsheets were developed. One of the first software applications for finance was VisiCalc, which was developed for the Apple II computer for accountants, bankers, and financial officers (White 2008, 121). The development of this software boosted spreadsheet development by other software developers, and many manufacturers began their own versions of spreadsheet applications. The early electronic spreadsheets were also important in another way in that these represented the first **graphical user interface (GUI)** to display programs (White 2008, 122). GUI was a basic display for spreadsheets, but Windows and Macintosh systems further developed this program for graphical icon display (White 2008, 122).

Uses of Spreadsheets in Healthcare

Spreadsheets have a variety of uses in business, in industry, and in healthcare. Within the HIM department, spreadsheet applications are used for calculations, budgets, and reporting for various department functions to administration. These include productivity charting, inventory of supplies, compliance and reimbursement statistics, quality outcomes and monthly reporting, quality control, credentialing statistics, vital statistics and reportable diseases, revenue cycle data, professional development information on credentialed staff, denials and bill holdings reports, cost benefit analysis reporting, and other employee statistical reporting among many others. Department directors must also report to various agencies, such as The Joint Commission for quality, medical staff, and credentialing data; local and state health departments for mandated reporting; and other state and federal agencies as needed. Spreadsheets are the easiest way to "number-crunch" statistical data, as HIM departments are the data collection centers of the facility. The spreadsheet is a vital tool for reporting the data to various persons and agencies when the reporting is needed and the data collection must be transmitted from the department to the requesting party.

Common Spreadsheet Software

Spreadsheet application software may be purchased separately or as a suite, meaning it is bundled as a package with other software from the manufacturer. The most popular spreadsheet application is Microsoft Excel; other available programs include Lotus 1-2-3 and Corel Quattro Pro (Fuller and Larson 2008, 214). Lotus 1-2-3 was the first spreadsheet vendor to introduce naming cells, cell ranges, and spreadsheet macros (Power 2004). Excel was one of the first spreadsheets to use a graphical interface with pull-down menus and a point and click capability using a mouse pointing device (Power 2004). Corel's Quattro Pro is the spreadsheet application that is packaged as part of the suite of products along with WordPerfect and their other software applications, but not as a stand-alone product. There are other spreadsheet application software that are web-hosted, meaning they have "the capability to upload files to an online site so they can be viewed and edited from another location" (Coyle 2009, 201). Two examples of web-hosted technology for spreadsheets are Windows Office Live and Google Docs. These offer mostly free services, but you do need to create an account and sign in before use (Coyle 2009, 201). Spreadsheets that can be viewed and used via the Internet offer the usual features such as formulas, functions, and chars, but offer these to users in real time. For healthcare and other industries, the Internet technology allows spreadsheets to be collaboratively shared for financial calculations, budgets, shipping, and ordering across the country and the world.

Basic Elements of Spreadsheet Software

A spreadsheet consists of a grid of rows and columns. Rows are numbered horizontally across the page or user's screen, and columns are vertical and are represented by letters of the alphabet. Each box in this sample grid below of a spreadsheet is called a cell. Figure 2.1 represents a typical spreadsheet.

Each cell of the grid can be referred to in terms of its column and row label. For example, a cell can be referred to as "A1, B3, and AC342 each representing an individual cell in column A, row 1; column B, row 3; and column AC, row 342, respectively" (Coyle 2009, 226). The

Figure 2.1. **Basic spreadsheet display**

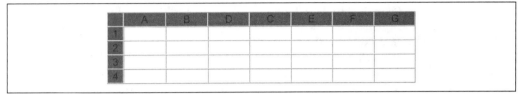

basic function of any spreadsheet application is to calculate numbers. Within the toolbar of the software, the user enters the formula, which is the instruction to tell the spreadsheet application which mathematical function to perform. Because spreadsheets are number-crunching and statistical packages, various symbols are used to represent mathematical functions.

In addition to the basic mathematical operators, a variety of special mathematical functions are usually available, including:

- ABS(A1) the absolute value of the number in A1

- AVERAGE(A1:A5) calculates the mean average of the data

- COS(A1) the cosine of the angle in cell A1 (Excel works *in* radians)

- INT(A1) the integer part of the value in cell A1

- MAX(A1:A10) the maximum value in the cells A1 to A10

- MIN(A1:A10) the minimum value in the cells A1 to A10

- SIN(A1) the sine of the angle in cell A1 (Excel works *in* radians)

- SQRT(A1) the square root of the value in A1

- SUM(A1:A10) the sum total of cells A1 to A10

- TAN(A1) the tangent of the angle in cell A1 (Excel works *in* radians)

- ^ the power function; for example, A1^3 means the cube of A1.

Formulas refer to the contents within a particular cell in the spreadsheet. If there are several cells involved within a formula, then the formula includes those cells in the formula within the toolbar.

A complete discussion of all the available spreadsheet software applications to the user is beyond the scope of this book; thus, the remainder of the spreadsheet discussion will focus on the most common spreadsheet application in the United States, Microsoft Excel.

Microsoft Excel

Scenario: A user wants to add together two cells of a spreadsheet. The two cells to be added are B5 and D5 whose values equal 8 and 10, respectively. The formula is entered into the cell where the user wants the total of the calculation to display, cell F5. Figure 2.2 illustrates this scenario using Microsoft Excel.

In this scenario, the user simply selects the desired cells, B5 and D5, and enters the values into each cell. Cell F5 is then selected to calculate and display the total value from cells B5 and D5. Microsoft Excel systematically recognizes an equation first by the initial use of the equal symbol (=) entered into the cell, followed by a formula enclosed in parentheses. Because this is an addition calculation, the formula to be entered is "B5+D5." So, the complete formula entered into the F5 cell would be entered as "=(B5+D5)". Once the formula is entered, the user presses the Enter key on the keyboard to execute the formula.

The parentheses will briefly bold (similar to a flash), notifying the user the formula was accepted. The total value will display in cell F5. An entire column could have easily been done by changing the cells and the rows on each. Once formulas are set up, the calculations then are completed by the spreadsheet application. Formulas can be extremely complicated, much more so than the example shown here. For a formula involving multiplication, the asterisk (*) is used to denote this function and for division, the slash (/) symbol. Formulas can be entered by clicking the mouse for ease of use and faster data entry by the user. Tricky calculations such as those that may involve multiplication, addition, and percentage in the same formula are no problem for spreadsheet applications once the formula has been correctly entered into the cell of the spreadsheet. The average function works out the mean average of the numbers within the cells. For example, if the cells to be averaged are in the rows of B1 through B10, the formula for this would be written in the toolbar as:

=AVERAGE(B1:B10)

This formula then would calculate the mean of the numbers or values within these cells. If this formula would have been in another worksheet, spreadsheets can be instructed within the formula to look in another worksheet to calculate them. The formula for this same calculation as given above would be written as:

=AVERAGE(Sheet1!B1:B10)

The exclamation point (!) is the instruction that gives the address to cross reference the formula to the worksheet. As noted in figure 2.2, remember to always use the equal (=) sign before a formula, or the spreadsheet will not recognize it as a formula but rather as

Figure 2.2.   Screenshot of spreadsheet software example

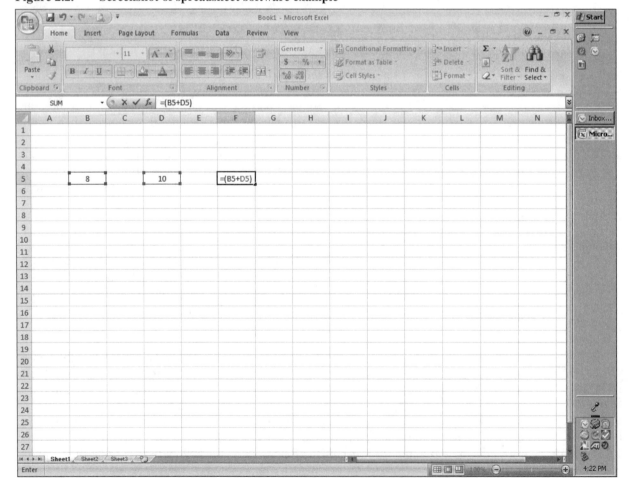

plain text. A space should never be placed between the function and the first parenthesis. If these errors occur, a user will certainly receive an error message and the calculation will not happen.

If a user wanted to perform statistics such as total counts with large volumes of data, this is again easily done with spreadsheet software. To acquire the total or a tally count of data as in a frequency distribution, spreadsheets also are capable of producing graphs from the data entered into the cells. Once the data have been entered, the cells that are to be counted or totaled are highlighted by the user with the Shift key pressed down and the mouse highlighting all the cells to be tallied. Within the cell that the total is to be placed, the user enters the formula for the frequency. The frequency formula is FREQUENCY(C5:C10,D5:D10). If the cells are highlighted in E5 to E10, the total of these two rows would then be placed in the row beneath these. This is the main quality of spreadsheet software: every cell can have an entry of a number, text, or a formula. The user can specify the numbers to the decimal place desired, the text can be labeled to describe data, and all formulas can be from the very simple to the utmost complex. This is done usually within most spreadsheets via drop-down boxes from the menus at the top of the screen. Many options are provided to the user from these menus, allowing for customizable spreadsheets to provide the appearance and functionality needed.

A great feature in spreadsheet application software is the ability to sort data in different orders. Spreadsheets can automatically sort volumes of data that would take many work hours if done manually. This can be easily done by clicking on the appropriate icon. Microsoft Excel and most other spreadsheets allow for sorting to be done from the top down or vice versa. Microsoft Excel includes the standard toolbar, as shown in figure 2.3 (Rutkosky 2008a, 84).

Figure 2.3.   Excel spreadsheet with toolbar across top of screen

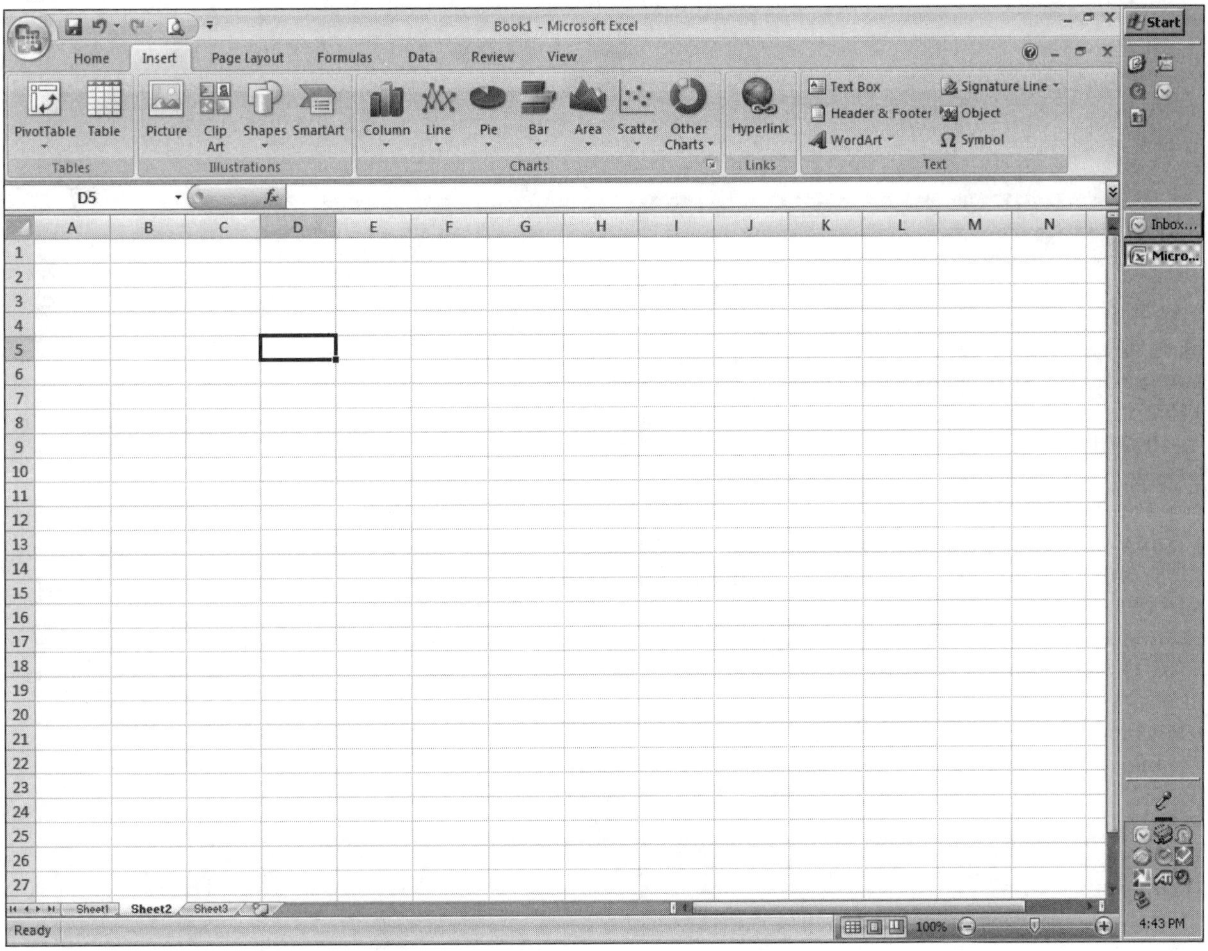

Graphing in Excel

Creating a graph in Excel is a value-added feature and is simple to use. Once data have been entered into the spreadsheet, graphing is simplified with the use of Microsoft Excel 2007. Each cell containing data to be graphed should be highlighted using the mouse or keyboard so that it becomes shaded or selected. The user then chooses the Insert Tab located at the top of the screen and chooses which type of graph or chart (from the Charts section located toward the center of the screen) best suits the data for display. See figure 2.4 for the example of graph selections.

The user selects the desired graph type by clicking the mouse on the graph. The software automatically takes the highlighted data and places it into the graph selected, and displays it. The user must still move and/or resize the data display as needed, as well as add any titles and/or legends as needed. If there are any other optional designs the user wishes to add or customize, these may be added as additional selections (such as subtitles or 3-D shading, etc.). All charts can be adjusted in size. By clicking and dragging the mouse simultaneously from any corner of the graph, the user can adjust the size as needed.

Graphs are a different way to convey meanings. It is up to the user to select the best graph for the appropriate data. Spreadsheet software can perform the task of creating and building the graphs; however, it is up to the user to understand what type of data is entered and the most optimal method for it to be communicated.

Figure 2.4.   Example of Excel for graphing

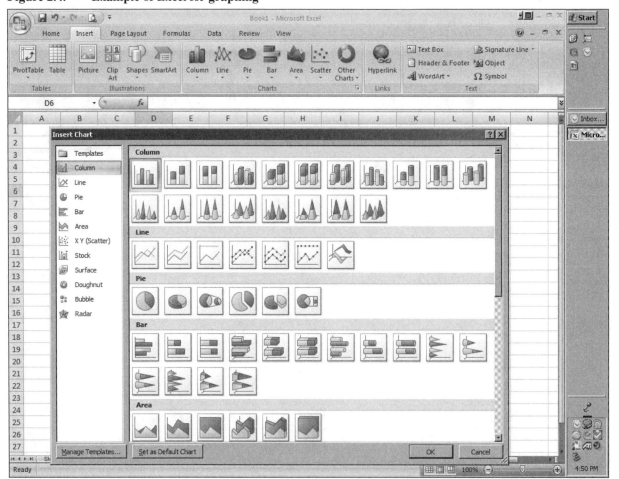

Check Your Understanding 2.1

1. The first consideration in choosing the right spreadsheet software application should always be _____:

   A. formulas used
   B. graphs used
   C. needs of the user
   D. functionality of the application

2. Online word processing software applications that can be shared so that two or more persons can work on a document together via the Internet is a fast-growing market. Which of the following software applications is not online word processing software as mentioned?

   A. Zoho
   B. Show
   C. Google Docs
   D. Thinkfree

3. A document language format that is developed in either plain text or in formatted text of ASCII characters so that other computers can read the language besides its own Windows applications format is called:

   A. Microsoft
   B. GUI
   C. HTML
   D. RTF

4. If a user enters an "=" before entering a formula, what do most spreadsheet software applications think the user wants the application to do next?

   A. Add the items and get a total
   B. Sum the formula
   C. Enter text
   D. Cross reference to another worksheet

Databases

Data are everywhere and can be seen as numbers, text, and in computers; however, some data are unseen. According to McWay, a database is "a structured storage or collection of data on multiple entities and their relationships" (McWay 2008, 169). Business, industry, and healthcare collect and manipulate data daily. The handling of data and information by technology software is called database management. There are several types of databases or models, most of which emerged with the evolution of technology.

History of Databases

A database program is a data collection system that organizes data in one of two methods. A database can be a simple flat file that is a collection of records of data—for example, Microsoft Excel or most other spreadsheet programs (Coyle 2009, 467). The second type of database is a database management system, which manages multiple files or tables—for example, Microsoft Access (Coyle 2009, 467). The flat file database systems are not as easy to link to other systems, but they are easier to use and less expensive (Coyle 2009, 467). Around 1970, E. Codd, a mathematician employed by IBM, gave a lecture at a symposium on how databases (at that time) stored large amounts of data in **hierarchical** structure that was difficult to navigate and not flexible (Rob and Coronel 2009, 3). From this research, he eventually convinced IBM to develop the SQL and DB2 databases; however, an audience member, Chamberlin, first created and brought the SQL to the market (Rob and Coronel 2009, 3). The SQL is a "language used by nonprogrammers to retrieve information contained in relational databases" (McWay 2008, 171). In the mid-1980s, the object-oriented databases (OODM) were the model to support complex data using data warehouses (Rob and Coronel 2009, 35). Some of these examples include Versant, FastObjects.Net, Objectivity/DB, DB/2 UDB, and Oracle 11g (Rob and Coronel 2009, 35). These models were known as semantic models because they indicated meaning based on the facts within the object (Rob and Coronel 2009, 43). At this same time personal computers were becoming more widespread and a popular database for use was Microsoft Access. Other programs used at this time included Approach and Paradox (Fuller and Larson 2008, 217). Also at this time, a client/server model for very large companies using a front-end query database system was developed in software such as Oracle from Oracle Corporation, DB2 from IBM, and SQL Server from Microsoft (Rob and Coronel 2009, 469). Today, the relational model has joined with the **object-oriented model** to become the current database model known as the "extended relational data model (ERDM) (Rob and Coronel 2009, 53). Many of these use the Internet with customers during the query process, such as credit card usage. The future of online databases increases with the evolution of the Internet; databases now reach terabytes as a standard. Knowledge and data are increasing at the speed of light.

Uses of Databases in Healthcare

Databases are used in a variety of ways in business and industry as well as healthcare. Databases help organize data once it is collected, so that a user can easily query to find a small amount of data from an extremely large amount of information with very little effort. Healthcare facilities also use databases in research, education, statistics (trending and tracking purposes), and for individual statistics of hospital admissions and discharges, which are reported both monthly and annually. Other statistical information kept in databases includes information on physicians, procedures, surgeries performed, anesthesia, pathological and laboratory specimens, complications, infections, deaths, and births.

All data must be collected, maintained, updated, and tracked, and this is done easily with database software. Data are in a central place, and the information is easily accessed. Control and security of the data is easily maintained in that only those authorized may access the database, and the database can have a "view only" or "make changes/add data" function for each authorized user. Databases decrease the number of errors because the data within the file are consistent when select users enter data according to set rules; it is less likely that data will be duplicated when this method is used as compared with other systems. There are many departments within a facility that can benefit from using a database. The next section will discuss several of those departments.

One department is the personnel or human resource department. This department uses databases as a method for tracking personnel data, annual evaluation data, scheduling, and other employee-related information. Large facilities that have many employees must use a database in order to keep track of hire dates and anniversary dates for annual screenings and merit raises. Documentation that is mandated to be done annually for all staff must be tracked within the personnel file, and the database is the method used for facilities to perform these duties.

Similar to personnel tracking is the inventory department. This department orders and receives from outside vendors the supplies needed for the facility and the sterile supplies and equipment needed for the operating room. Because of the volume of shipments and the items within each shipment, a database must be used to track the order placement, dates received, and items returned. Inventory on existing stock must be done from the database on items within the stockroom and supply room before reorders are placed, and the database can easily be queried before the next order is placed.

Another department within the healthcare facility that uses databases extensively is the quality or performance improvement department. This area works with data on each patient while in-house as well as performing retrospective and preadmission reviews. Each patient has many diagnoses and with hundreds of reviews going on simultaneously by several clinicians, a database must be used so that clinicians can share data among themselves and review the data of all the patients for a team approach to quality of care. Performance review is an ongoing effort by this department, and the clinicians must be able to review all patient data at any time against the preestablished criteria of the facility as well as the mandated state and federal standards. The database makes this process possible for this department.

Within the HIM department, databases are used for several purposes. Prior to the implementation of computer databases, many paper-based statistical reports were created from logs and indices. However, with the use of databases, there is no need for bulky logbooks or heavy index binders; computers can easily run standard reports of physician admissions, discharges, or operations that are accessible to authorized personnel at all times.

In hospital facilities, the master patient index (MPI) is a database that is a central repository of data of patient information that includes names, patient record numbers, patient demographic information, history, surgical information, and other needed information on finances and administrative issues. The MPI is used many times a day when looking for health information regarding a particular patient. The MPI is the key to locating a certain patient; without a database, it would surely be an impossible task. The cancer registry, whether housed separately or within the HIM department, is a database of cancer patients. All information contained in this database is strictly about the patient's cancer diagnosis and treatment. The registrar is dependent on the database for accurate information and also enters information into the database for inclusion as part of cancer research efforts and reporting. Research is closely tied into the cancer area. Although not all research is cancer-related, research efforts require a database to help in the search of patients with a particular diagnosis as well.

Electronic Health Record as a Database

The electronic health record (EHR) is a collection of data within a system. Data can be linked together when they are housed in a database. This is actually a **relational database model** that will be discussed later in this section. Relational databases are one of the greatest advantages of the EHR. A **database management system (DBMS)** is a program that "enables users to work with electronic databases to permit data to be stored, modified, and retrieved from the database" (Joos et al. 2006, 246). The DBMS can retrieve data that are searched and queried by the user. Electronic records are housed within computers and servers so that users of the DBMS can easily search and locate data as well as sort and print data in report form as needed. Any data within a patient record, including clinical data, financial data, and administrative data, can be used in this manner.

Types of Data in a Database

Within database software, the commonality is that "data is stored in tables with relationships among the tables" (Abdelhak et al. 2007, 276). This commonality is found in most applications regardless of the vendor. The descriptions of the types of data available in most database software include: text or characters, numbers, alphanumeric (a combination of text and numbers), currency or money, dates and times, greater than (>), less than (<), or equal to (=), and various fields that may differ among the vendor applications. Within the structure of the database, a hierarchy must be used in order for the computer to recognize the database structure. The lowest level (smallest) is the **field**. The field is one attribute. The user would enter patient data into each field of a patient record. For example, to enter a patient's name of John Lee Doe, would require three fields. For a date of birth, one would enter the month, day, and year as three fields as well. Most fields, such as numbers, usually have a drop-down box; for example, days of the month would have a selection from 1 to 31 days. The months of the year may have a drop-down box as well from January to December. For fields that have a common known start and stop reference point, drop-down boxes are frequently used to speed data entry.

The patient's record is created as all fields are completed within the patient's record for a particular healthcare visit. The record is the second level of the hierarchy. All entries have been entered and documented electronically within this patient record. Data within this record can be typed into the fields, and data entered into this record in other ways that were mentioned earlier (chapter 1) are secured in the patient record and are now confidential.

If this particular patient were to have many other visits, additional records would be created similarly and also stored electronically. As those records are created, they are linked electronically and a patient's file is created. The file is the third level of the hierarchy. The file functions so that if a physician or other practitioner wanted to view the entire file of this patient, then every record or the entire file could be assimilated from the database on the screen for the user. The highest level of the hierarchy is the database. A database makes the electronic data captured easy to organize, sort, gather, print, store, retrieve, and run reports from. The days and endless hours of manpower wasted trying to sort and gather paper charts and data for research and other purposes are no longer necessary because of databases. The electronic health record is now part of the database. Patient information can be tracked and trends easily recognized for quality and utilization reviews, and this can help patients manage their care upon discharge.

Common Database Software

There are two categories of database software, flat file and database management system. These were previously discussed in the History of Database section. For the desktop database application software, as stated previously, Microsoft Access and MySQL are popular software as database management systems applications and for flat file, Microsoft Excel or any spreadsheet application software (Coyle 2009, 467). Other popular desktop database software includes Access, DB2, FileMaker Pro, MySQL, Oracle 11g, Paradox, R:Base 7.6, SQL Server, and Visual FoxPro (Coyle 2009, 467). The other category of database software is server database application software. Server databases power enormous files for huge companies with tremendous needs for data. These server databases also may have multiple users as opposed to the desktop databases that generally reside on a single desktop computer. Several of the more common server databases are Microsoft SQL Server, Oracle 11g, and IBM DB2 (Rob and Coronel 2009, 35). Database software are discussed in detail in chapter 4 of this text.

Graphics Presentation Software

Graphics presentation software is an application that combines word processing with desktop design so a user can create an audiovisual presentation. Presentations can include handouts, flyers, bulletins, posters, slide shows, onscreen presentations, or a colorful picture gallery. There are several popular software applications that are used for the desktop PC; PowerPoint is probably the most common (Center for Faculty Excellence and ITS Teaching and Learning 2008). However, all presentation software applications have one thing in common: the graphical user interface (GUI), which was discussed in chapter 1.

GUI technology was invented by Microsoft. It gives users the ability to see images and graphics on the screen. GUI was first developed by Microsoft for the Windows and Macintosh systems for graphical icon display (White 2008, 122). Graphics software can use a variety of small extensions or **bitmaps** that signal to the computer that the data are a graphical piece of information. Familiar types of bitmaps include extensions such as **.bmp, .tif,** and **.jpg**, which are usual extensions for files that are pictures or artwork. The extensions are a signal to the computer that the file is an image in pixels. The computer then "determines the parameters of the graphic file and reads the bytes of data of the image as a pattern of bits as the simplest bitmapped image has only black-and-white pixels" (White 2008, 132). The more complex the image, the more complex are the pixels. A color bitmap could contain up to 256 colors for an 8-bit or single pixel, or 24-bit color can contain up to 16 million possible colors (White 2008, 133). It is easy to see how graphical images can become so large and why images take up a lot of space in the computer.

The GUI technology allows images and graphics to be viewed on the screen. The Windows technology allows many views of data or data screens to be displayed at once (Amatayakul 2007, 384). This function is particularly valuable within the electronic patient record where the user may display patient demographics on one screen and also pull up a second screen about a particular visit to view insurance or clinical data. Another scenario might be where a physician may be viewing a patient's x-ray online within the patient record and use the toolbar features to enlarge the screen to zoom in on the x-ray or to darken the image for better visibility. All of these functions can be done using GUI technology, which is part of graphics presentation software.

Presentation software, such as Microsoft PowerPoint, is a powerful tool that is used to communicate to an audience. PowerPoint can be used to make presentations on large display screens with a computer data projector or create flyers, posters, bulletins, slide shows, handouts, and other printed material with artwork and/or illustrations. PowerPoint can also deliver sound messages within a slide show or presentation. Sound can be recorded with the show and provided with each slide to create a professional presentation.

Although creating fancy presentations and printed materials is an art in itself, the user must realize when too much of a good thing is not always a good thing. Overuse of artwork, colors, sound effects, and other special effects can be distracting, and cause the message of the presentation to be lost. It is best to always keep slide shows simple and plain, so that the message remains clear. Simple and plain is particularly important when it comes to health records, where slide shows are used to convey HIM messages to keep your audience's focus.

Uses of Presentation Software in Healthcare

Graphics presentation software in healthcare is mainly used for presentations (for example, for training and education) and visual graphics displays (for example, for posters and graphs). For this reason, presentation software has become a popular vehicle among speakers in healthcare when delivering presentations and talks during continuing education seminars and workshops. PowerPoint is commonly used to deliver these messages. The same software also may be used for facility meetings among the medical staff, governing board, hospital committee members, or administration staff. PowerPoint also can be used to enhance training programs such as new staff or faculty orientation, regular staff training for Occupational Safety and Health Administration updates and fire safety, and student education. The HIM department may use a PowerPoint presentation at various meetings to give committee reports. Using the "picture is worth a thousand words" metaphor, graphs and charts show physicians and administrators involved with hospital and medical committees the trends from previous quarters and the previous year of hospital data. (An HIM director would be smart to use PowerPoint to illustrate trends in data with the use of presentation software by providing the numbers as well as showing the data on graphs and charts. Not only is the message better conveyed to the audience, but the message is made clear to those who are auditory and visual learners.)

Common Graphics Presentation Software

There are several popular graphics presentation software packages on the market for the PC user; as stated earlier, Microsoft PowerPoint is the most common. Other common presentation software packages include Harvard Graphics, Corel Draw, and Keynote, as well as online software programs such as KPresenter, GoogleDocs, MagicPoint, OpenOffice.org

Impress, ZoHo, and Beamer (LaTeX) (Center for Faculty Excellence and ITS Teaching and Learning. 2008). Other programs may be used with presentation software, such as Adobe when photos are created in other programs. The graphics are created in Adobe Photoshop or Adobe Illustrator and then may be imported into presentation software such as Power-Point (Center for Faculty Excellence and ITS Teaching and Learning. 2008).

Basic Elements of Presentation Software

Most presentation software are similar in function. Their primary function is to create visual displays using illustrations to communicate a message to an audience. Presentation software is built on a slide platform or template; that is, all text, graphics, images, and illustrations are posted or created on slides within this type of software. Each slide is then horizontally read by the software so the message is conveyed from start to finish. The user can easily add or delete text or objects by adding a slide within the lineup of slides. For example, if there were 100 slides in the slide show and the user wanted to rearrange two slides, the user would simply click and drag that slide into its new position. The slide format is universal in presentation software. Text, images, movies, and illustrations may be posted or created onto each slide until a slide show is complete. The user may view the completed slide show and make changes in the arrangement of the slides until satisfied. The arrangement is then saved. Presentation software is ideal for clip art images, illustrations, cartoons, and text. These elements can be easily combined to create a presentation.

Graphic presentation software is also very user friendly; most applications have icons for the user. These options can be easily used to create the presentation. However, not all of the selections to create a presentation or slide show are located on the icons displayed on the menu bar. Some of the options are inside drop-down boxes that can be selected by the user.

Microsoft PowerPoint

PowerPoint offers the user a method to create, customize, and personalize a presentation or visual graphic display to their needs. PowerPoint users can create a presentation using a blank template, they can create their own template, or they can choose from a large variety of pre-designed templates built into the software. A user can also search the Internet for pre-built templates by other users for specific themes and purposes. PowerPoint also offers various template layouts for slides that contain tables, graphs, pictures, only text, or a combination of each.

PowerPoint customization choices range from simple to complex. One example of an easy customization is slide transition. PowerPoint offers many options for a smooth transition between slides. This can be done for one or all of the slides in the presentation. Slides can also be set to transition automatically with a set timer or manually by the user. The more complex choices will involve sound, animation, and visual effects (for example, flashing or rotating objects), which PowerPoint also tries to simplify for users.

One helpful tool for the user is the insertion of notes, or "cues," to the presentation. If the speaker wants to add these, it can be easily done without the audience being able to see the notes. Many guest speakers and lecturers use speaker notes to help them during professional engagements. However, it is not a good idea to type out every word or the audience will see the speaker reading the notes. Just a few key words as reminders or prompts are the best idea for use here. Users should also always remember to preview the entire slide show to ensure the presentation works properly and looks exactly the way the user wants it to be viewed by the audience.

Remember, PowerPoint is a tool for communication of a message to an audience. The software application, regardless of the vendor, is a wonderful product and it is in the user's hands to be effective as a messenger to convey information to the listener. PowerPoint can be used for onscreen presentations and lectures. Handouts can also be made for these presentations by printing out the slides. As shown in figure 2.5, the text can be printed as the entire screen per page (slide view), handouts as black and white or color, and as many per page as a choice of 1, 2, 3, 4, 6, or 9 per sheet (handout view, notes page view, or outline view).

Figure 2.5.   Example PowerPoint handouts: 6 per page

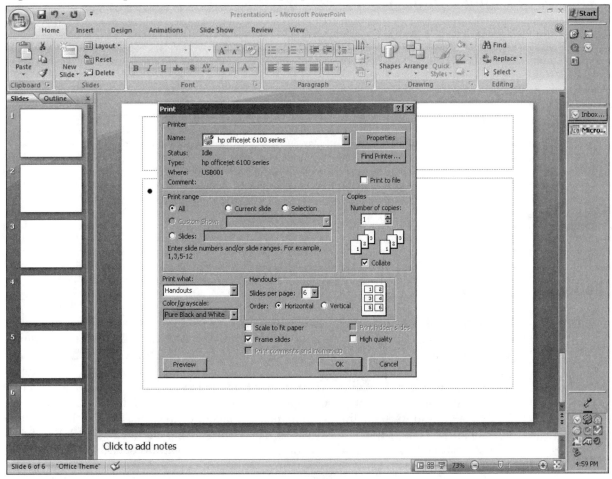

Having such an array of choices for printing gives PowerPoint the ability to make flyers, posters, brochures, and other colorful printed documents in addition to the slides and presentations. This is a powerful graphics presentation software application. By using the software and its capabilities, the HIM director and others in healthcare are using a tool for effective communication with patients, physicians, staff, and healthcare practitioners.

Check Your Understanding 2.2

1. The computer-based patient record is an example of which database model?

   A. Relational model
   B. Object-oriented model
   C. Hierarchical model
   D. Network model

2. When referring to data in a database, which level of data is a file referred to as?

   A. First
   B. Second
   C. Third
   D. Fourth

(continued on next page)

Check Your Understanding 2.2 (continued)

3. Graphics presentation software have one thing in common in all applications. This would be that all have _____.

    A. graphing capability
    B. GUI
    C. drop-down menus
    D. user friendliness

4. File extensions that signal to the computer an image is to be displayed include all of the following EXCEPT:

    A. .docx
    B. .bmp
    C. .tif
    D. .jpg

Scheduling Software

Scheduling software is an application for administrative processes that includes "electronic scheduling systems for hospital admissions, inpatient and outpatient procedures, and identifying eligible or potential eligible patients for clinical trials" (Thakkar and Davis 2006, 10). Scheduling software is used in healthcare for various types of appointment scheduling such as patient clinic visits, return trips, follow-up, surgical visits, ambulatory visits, physician office visits, and diagnostic testing visits. Scheduling systems are also used for administrative functions to help manage data in various areas of healthcare's daily functions; for example, activities such as the staffing of nursing units, scheduling hours for vacations and holidays, human resource functions for overtime scheduling of flexpool, temporary hires, and other types of part-time staff.

Scheduling software can range from the simplest application of keeping track of patient appointments in, for example, a tickler file to the most complex scheduling of benefits eligibility inquiry with direct data entry functions with Health Information Portability and Accountability Act (HIPAA) carriers (Amatayakul 2007, 408). Scheduling software applications commonly are connected with the registration and check-in of patients for a healthcare visit completed prior to the appointment; however, some also use scheduling software during the checkout process to schedule follow-up visits or return appointments.

Various Types of Scheduling

Scheduling for the inpatient for one of the largest commercial vendors, Sunrise, combines "financial and clinical operations so important patient information can be captured and validated once and communicated electronically throughout each stage of the patient visit" (Eclipsys Corporation 2008). This process allows the hospital to collect and manage patient information more efficiently and accurately with scheduling software. Also, Eclipsys can "check for medical necessity and insurance eligibility verification" (Eclipsys Corporation 2008).

Hospitals also use scheduling applications to coordinate within clinics many activities for busy physicians and keep track of many patients, examination rooms, treatment rooms, and diagnostic testing facilities. All of these may be housed within a single building and may share a scheduling system. The appointment system can handle many physicians seeing many patients, including walk-in appointments. This software can even handle physician meetings such as conferences and staff meetings, and can track duplicate appointments. From large outpatient clinic settings to a one-person physician office, scheduling software is an effective manager of resources for healthcare practitioners. Hospitals may provide patients with the ability to schedule appointments within the scheduling or registration system. However, the facility must ensure security measures so that confidentiality is not compromised. An example of a facility that offers this type of secure Internet access is Geisinger Health System. "Using one module within the organization's clinical information system, patients can access their medical information, e-mail their physicians, request appointments, and renew prescriptions" (Friedman 2005, 42).

Surgery schedules may also be used for inpatients or outpatients with this type of scheduling software. Software applications can be customized for most any type of situation and can be networked into the healthcare facility for all settings.

Uses of Scheduling Software in Healthcare

Scheduling software is used at many places within the healthcare facility. The scheduling systems within the hospital may operate on a stand-alone basis, or these systems may operate within a network capacity so the system can interface with other scheduling systems on the healthcare network.

Besides for the purposes of the patient (that is, appointments, registration), one of the areas in the facility that may use the scheduling software would include the finance area. The applications might be tied to the personnel and attendance records for hours worked or for scheduling shifts for work. The scheduling systems may also be used for calculation of total hours worked for benefits and holidays as well as vacation and sick time accrual. The payroll and accounting departments use these hour accumulations to calculate pay and employee's benefits packages for end-of-the year totals to determine salary and wages packages, and for Internal Revenue Service reporting. The human resources department is closely tied to these scheduling systems for the employees in keeping track of employee's hours, hours of vacation taken, sick time, holiday pay, and so on. Time accrual that is automated for scheduling is easily calculated by these systems with the swipe of an employee's identification badge into a reader that uses a barcode (chapter 1). Accurate data can be collected, maintained, and stored daily for each employee at the facility for the fiscal year. A review of time and attendance data from this system makes the supervisor's job easy at the time of the employee's annual performance evaluation. Scheduling systems are also used to make call lists for shift work for nurses, emergency department staff, and other healthcare practitioners who work around the clock in shifts, especially when there is a need for extra help in certain areas.

Common Scheduling Software

As previously mentioned, one of the large commercial vendors is Sunrise by Eclipsys. This product is available for scheduling software for healthcare facilities and has been used for four decades (Eclipsys Corporation 2008). Another vendor of scheduling software similar to Sunrise is Cadence Enterprise, made by Epic systems. Their system has two separate entities; the ADT/Prelude Enterprise is for inpatient registration, and the Prelude Enterprise registration is for ambulatory access (Epic Systems Corporation 2008).

Basic Elements of Scheduling Software

Scheduling software applications provide hospital and clinical staff easy access to patient health record data. This is the primary means for scheduling patients for future appointments within the networked systems after hospital discharge, for follow-up visits with clinic appointments, and for routine physician office visits. All patient demographics are available within the scheduling software, providing easy access for healthcare staff and authorized practitioners.

For the patient registration process—upon check-in, when a patient arrives for a scheduled appointment, and afterward when scheduling a follow-up appointment—the software is a very effective and efficient tool. The scheduling software contains an electronic calendar for both short-term and long-term patient visits, for follow-up and for long-term patient tracking. It is preferable to follow cancer registry patients for life; therefore, scheduling software that is used within the networked facility helps other departments (such as the cancer registry and many others) to stay current and follow up on their reporting and research. Scheduling software "provides tailored workflows, wizards, and extensive error checking to help users complete registration swiftly and accurately, while addressing verification and HIPAA-compliant electronic eligibility queries to help ensure accurate billing" (Epic Systems Corporation 2008).

Scheduling applications software also may be used for productivity statistics in many areas of the hospital, for time and effort studies, attendance reporting, and trending with data across departments. Physicians, administrators, and other healthcare practitioners within the facility must have access to the scheduling software for the scheduling of patients across the continuum to work accordingly. If everyone on the staff is trained properly and the software is used correctly, the scheduling software is a wonderful tool for organizing the flow of patient appointments for outpatients, clinics, hospital admissions, and the scheduling of surgeries. It is also useful for scheduling meetings and conferences of the healthcare facility.

Project Management Software

Project management software is an application used within a management task that helps bring a particular project to its desired outcome. Project management by definition uses the "basic management principles of planning, organizing, directing, and controlling (with an emphasis on planning) to bring a project to a successful conclusion" (Abdelhak et al. 2007, 629). There are many ways that a director or supervisor may lead a team in a project, and there are also various methods of supervision; thus, the uses of problem-solving skills during a crisis in healthcare will vary. Project management software is aimed at providing a supervisor with direction in both short-term and long-term projects. The software guides the project manager in entering data such as timelines and personnel tasks into the software. Tools within the software—such as graphs and charts, calendars, e-mail, discussion tools, and task management tools—also help in the process. Used in combination with each other, these tools can be very helpful to a manager when used with department staff or project team in the planning function. Project management software focuses on managing the tasks and in planning by the leader; however, the manager of the department or project must have some foundation principles and leadership skills.

Uses of Project Management Software in Healthcare

Project management software applications do not direct the project or provide the assignments to the team; the software guides the manager to create the guidelines for the project, plan its scope and outline, and assign tasks to the members on the team. It facilitates keeping the project on target throughout the life of the project.

Project management software is used in many scenarios within healthcare. Some examples include the construction of a new facility or remodeling of an existing facility, the implementation of a new information system, or the implementation of a privacy and security program. A project timeline is needed for planning any project. Project management software is used to help keep the project timeline on schedule. The software stores and maintains all the project details and data including issues, resolution, and changes throughout its lifecycle to ensure the outcome, which is to meet the project goal or deadline. The same software can also be used for meeting hospital strategic plans and long-term goals. Strategic plans and goals of the hospital are all part of the administrative planning process where project management software easily can aid in meeting short-term goals by showing how time constraints, resources, and communication place demands on healthcare goals. The use of a Gantt chart is a common method of plotting planned activities on a timeline within a larger timeline, and is an optional tool in the software. A 'Gantt chart' is used to illustrate project tasks, phases, and milestones, and their start, end, and completion dates" (Amatayakul 2007, 84).

Administrators are frequent users of project management software because of the overwhelming number of projects and tasks that must be overseen by the hospital administration staff. Other departments that might use project management software applications include quality and utilization departments. These areas use this type of software, such as the Gantt chart, for large-scale projects over time. Another quality tool within the software that can be used is the Project Evaluation and Review Technique (PERT) chart, which "helps to evaluate the entire schedule and to make adjustments based on dependencies, criticality of tasks, and minimum, maximum, and average duration time of tasks" (Amatayakul 2007, 84).

Also because some of these software applications are online, it is very easy to share software among departments, and the data can be easily shared via the network or the Internet. This promotes discussion between departments and planning intradepartmentally directly into the software application. Performance indicators and other instruments of measurement in quality are examples of data that can be entered into the software by department heads or responsible parties. Productivity data and team work data are other examples of quality data that are entered by other departments for their own quality reporting data. Because every department in healthcare must monitor and report quality data, data sharing is easy with the project management software that is networked within a facility.

Common Project Management Software

Any manager who needs to use a project management software application can find several common software packages for the PC. The most common is Microsoft Project. However, most of the common applications will have the basic component of a Gantt chart within the software (Amatayakul 2007, 84). Other common project management software applications for the PC are EnterPlicity, OPM creator, Intellis Project, Milestone, and MinuteMan, as well as online project management software such as OpenMind, Project KickStar, and Fast Trac Schedule. Whether the software applications is networked within a facility or online, healthcare practitioners may use the functions to work together to plan and organize the pieces of the project so that the team functions as a unit and the desired outcome and/or deadline is met.

Basic Elements of Project Management Software

Project management software comprises an application software package that allows the project manager to keep everyone on the team or in the department on the same page and delegate tasks accordingly. It allows the manager to guide a long-term project by breaking a larger project into smaller pieces and placing it on a timeline, usually a Gantt chart. Other useful tools in the software include calendar function with reminders, e-mail to employees or team members, a discussion page, and a task manager (similar to a to-do list or a tracking sheet). Project management software can also track the progress of each task on a timeline throughout the project, keep the lines of communication open, schedule deadlines for smaller tasks, keep track of the project's budget, prioritize the tasks on the timeline, and provide support when questions arise during the process.

Every project management software application must provide a method for communication among all team members. Communication is the key to any project and its success. Without communication, the team does not function, and even the best project management software will not be able to keep the project from failing. Some members may be in another facility, county, or state, so networking or communication via the Internet must be an option. It is also important that members on the team be able to provide feedback on the task assignments so that there is two-way communication at all times. Resource monitoring must be ensured with the project management software. The open format of the communication with e-mail and discussion in the networked project management software allows the team to discuss any problems as they arise.

Some project management software have the capability of using "balanced scorecards, key performance indicators, and dashboards" (Amatayakul 2007, 84). Besides the quality improvement tools such as the Gantt and Pert charts (discussed in chapter 3), project management software will also provide a basic graphing capability so that tracking and illustration of trends can be done during the project. Additionally, most common applications have a basic budget package with a method for tracking expenses and calculating costs for the project.

E-mail Software

Electronic mail, or e-mail, software is an application used within a networked environment. E-mail is a typed message that is created and "sent over a computer network to a person or many people who have an electronic mail address" (Joos et al. 2006, 323). E-mail is an easy way to correspond with anyone connected to a computer. All it takes is a computer, the e-mail software of the receiver and the sender, and the transmission connections. Whether the distance is the next room or across the world, the e-mail function only takes a few seconds to a few minutes to send a typed message across the network or the Internet. This is the communication method that people use in the business world and the social world for transmitting personal messages and for sending business memos and correspondence and attachments. Anything that is created on a computer can be sent by e-mail. This includes text, images and pictures, spreadsheets, videos, files, and audio files. It is more difficult to send larger files because they are slower to transmit and sometimes a recipient's mailbox may not be large enough to receive the file once it has been sent. If this is the case, a sender can compress or "**zip**" the files, or it "uses a process to remove redundant data so that a file is smaller" (White 2008, 151). When the data is **unzipped by the recipient**, the files are restored to the original size by the receiver so the data are recovered in the original state.

In the world of fast and must have it now mentality, e-mail is a growing commodity. E-mail is seen everywhere in business transactions, banking, schools, and now in healthcare. How can e-mail benefit the healthcare industry, and how much can it be used to help patients? The next sections will explore these questions further.

Uses of E-mail Software in Healthcare

Electronic mail is used daily in healthcare. E-mail can be used to answer simple patient questions by healthcare staff and practitioners. Increasingly, the general public is more comfortable in using online services for Internet research now than ever before. Information and data such as drug books, medical dictionaries, and other medical reference aids are easily accessible online to the general consumer. Thus, if a patient has a question about anything found online, he or she can now simply e-mail their physician or nurse. Patients will have fewer in-person encounters and more direct access through e-mail to providers. "Medicare is currently considering reimbursement for such services. As an example of this application, Partners Healthcare in Boston is participating in a demonstration project that uses laptop computers issued to breast cancer patients for postoperative monitoring at home" (Wing and Langlier 2004, 16). In a study done in England, e-mail was used as a strategy to encourage patients to come to their healthcare facility for routine and follow-up visits. The study was done after reading current literature to improve patient response in seeking care. Their study cited that the "Institute of Medicine encourages flexible consulting as a key strategy for improving the quality of health care as it notes that access to care should be provided over the Internet, by telephone, and by other means in addition to in-person visits . . . instead of a $65 office visit and a half-day off work, a 2-minute e-mail communication could meet many patients' needs more responsively and at lower cost" (Car and Sheikh 2004a, 435).

E-mail is used to deliver reminders for visits and for other contact with patients. Many practices and clinics also use e-mail to allow patients to schedule their own appointments. Patients can be authorized to access the appointment scheduling area within a hospital or clinic system. This would allow the patient direct access to the scheduling system to make an appointment into the system when there is an opening. The patient could select the name of the provider and the date, type in the patient's name, and the appointment would be entered. Access would be read-only; thus, a patient could only add or change his or her own data. Using e-mail, the patient requests an appointment with a practitioner. The practitioner would make the appointment and then return the appointment date with an e-mail message to the patient. This works because e-mail is **asynchronous**, meaning "not involved on the computer at the same time", but at whatever point the other person reads the e-mail message (Joos et al. 2006, 326). This has become a common routine with clinics and physician practices across the country.

Another popular patient use of e-mail in healthcare is to handle prescription refills for pharmacy items. Sending in a patient refill request from a physician by e-mail is quite common now. It is certainly easier for the patient to submit a refill request by e-mail than to call a physician's office and be put on hold or to have to navigate a series of telephone prompts in order to leave a message for a nurse or physician. E-mail is simple because it can be accessed at home or anywhere there is an Internet connection at any time. Information about the medication that needs to be refilled, such as the name of the medication, the milligrams of dosage, the date to be refilled, and the prescription refill number, is on the label of the medicine bottle.

All of this information can be typed into an e-mail message and sent to the physician very quickly. Unless the patient needs to be seen by the physician, the refill can then be sent to the pharmacy by the physician. If the patient needs to be seen, the physician can send an e-mail asking the patient to set up an appointment for a visit before the medication will be refilled. So, if this is such an easy system, why isn't every person with a computer in America doing this? Because of confidentiality and privacy issues, e-mail has not been established as a secure medium of data transfer. Because e-mail uses the Internet, the basic premise is that unless the data are encrypted, they are prone to be seen by hackers and the data can be compromised.

> **Encryption** is a method of coding software that creates two keys, public and private. The public key encryption creates a digital signature or hash value that contains a mathematical algorithm that is encrypted with the private key. The recipient uses the sender's public key to decrypt the hash value and runs it through the algorithm of the sender. If these match and did indeed come from who it claimed to have come from, it will match and the file can be read. But if any piece has been changed in any way, either it will not match or the sender is impersonating someone else and the document will not open up (White 2008, 396–397).

Confidentiality and privacy are addressed by federal and state mandates such as HIPAA and continue to be issues with federal laws. In the 2008 U.S. Department of Health and Human Services' Office of the National Coordinator for Health Information Technology (ONCHIT) publication, the "Patient–Provider Secure Messaging Detailed Use Case" states that "secure messaging tools should address security needs in the disposition of all patient and clinician communications. Use of standard electronic mail is not considered adequately secure, and users of electronic mail should consider not include[ing] personal health data in this type of communication" (ONCHIT 2008, 13). Further privacy and security-related issues and topics will be covered in chapter 12.

In the second part of the British study by Car and Sheikh, it was noted that standardizing "specific communications (use of customised templates or protocols) to meet the needs of various specialties and tasks (such as repeat prescriptions) may make communication easier and increase quality and safety" (Car and Sheikh 2004b, 440).

E-mail can create a dilemma in healthcare. On one hand, HIM professionals must be watchful and take care not to violate patient rights and concerns by sending unencrypted, sensitive data through the Internet by personal e-mail to various healthcare providers. On the other hand, the use of e-mail and templates for standard or common prescription refills may speed communication and improve quality of care for both the physician and the patient. There is a happy medium here in that healthcare personnel must know and use the E-prescribing guidelines and HIPAA guidelines when protected health information is involved, and encryption devices must be in place to include electronic mail. For the use of prescription refills, the template or protocol system should be in place for quality purposes and to efficiently use the system to decrease the wait time for the patient. There is always room for improvement for every process, and as technology improves, the quality of each process should also improve.

One final area in which e-mail has been used for patients in healthcare is the provider-to-provider consultation. A provider or practitioner may have a unique patient case, and e-mail can be used to contact another expert practitioner in the field across the country regarding this patient's case. E-mail saves time, can minimize expenses, and eliminates the need for busy physicians to make phone calls. E-mail can be convenient for both the sending and receiving physician; each physician can send and respond to e-mails at times when it is best for them. Technology has changed the world, and e-mail is now a part of this change.

HIM professionals should be familiar with AHIMA's practice brief, "E-Mail as a Provider-Patient Electronic Communication Medium and Its Impact on the Electronic Health Record" (see Appendix A) and share it with all healthcare staff who manage patient documents. It is an absolute necessity that everyone working in healthcare and with patient confidentiality issues know that e-mail documents must be treated as a legal health record just as the paper record and that computerized records are legal documents (Nunn 2008, 54).

Common E-mail Software

E-mail is one of the best and most common ways to communicate with others in the electronic age. The software program that allows the computer to do this is e-mail software or an e-mail application. There are e-mail programs for Windows-based computers, Macintosh computers, and networked computers such as Linux or Unix. Network computer systems often have an e-mail software application already installed.

There are many types of computer e-mail applications available, and one of these software tools will work with the PC. No one owns the Internet and no single entity is in charge of the Internet. There are people and companies who control pieces of it, and agencies that oversee the governance of the Internet, but this is why it works so well for everyone. Several companies have started their own service to allow the general public access to the Internet for a fee—these include America Online, CompuServe, Microsoft Network, and Prodigy (White 2008, 333).

Another company, more commonly known to the public, Microsoft, offers two types of email software, Outlook Express and Outlook. Within the Microsoft Vista application, Windows Mail replaced Outlook Express. Both were developed by Microsoft and have a similar appearance. Both of these applications are client based; however the "full" Outlook application is part of the Microsoft Office Suite package (Coyle 2009, 71).

Table 2.1 describes several common e-mail and other Internet services.

Free e-mail services are also available that usually include the user connection by a browser interface. The user subscribes to a free e-mail Web site and after logging on, the user can send and receive free e-mails (Fuller and Larson 2008, 306). Services can be provided to users for these free e-mail subscriptions as these companies derive their income from advertising and these users must read through the advertisements to get to their e-mails. The advantage to these primarily is the cost, but also a user is not locked into any contract with an Internet service provider (ISP), and if any type of situation or problem arises, the user can close the account immediately (Fuller and Larson 2008, 306).

Basic Elements of E-mail Software

E-mail is created by typing a message using a software application and then sending it through a network or the Internet to a recipient(s). The sender creates a message similar

Table 2.1.   Commonly used Internet & e-mail services

Service	Client	Web-based	Comments
E-mail			
AOL Mail	X	X	Available with AOL Desktop installation or as Web-based service
Google Gmail		X	
Microsoft Outlook	X		Part of the Microsoft Office suite
Microsoft Windows Mail	X		Replaced Outlook Express in Windows Vista
Mozilla Thunderbird	X		Coordinates with Mozilla Firefox
Windows Live Hotmail		X	Replaced MSN Hotmail
Yahoo! Mail		X	
Instant Message			
AOL AIM	X	X	Available with AOL Desktop installation or as Web-based service
Google Talk	X	X	Available for download or as Web-based service
meebo.com		X	Users can access other IM clients on the meebo site
ICQ	X	X	Available for download or as Web-based service
Yahoo! Messenger		X	
Windows Live Messenger		X	Formerly MSN Messenger
Internet Relay Chat (IRC)			
mIRC	X		
Mozilla ChatZilla	X		Runs only in a Mozilla Firefox browser
Trillian	X		Also supports instant message clients
Plug-ins			
Adobe Reader	X		Viewer for Adobe PDF files
Adobe Flash Player	X		Viewer for Web animation (Flash) files
Apple QuickTime Player	X		Used for animation, music, MIDI, audio, and video files
RealPlayer	X		Used for streaming audio, video, animations, and multimedia presentations
Windows Media Player	X		Used for MP3 and WAV files, live audio, movies, and live video broadcasts

Source: Adapted from Coyle 2009, 71

to a memo format in that most e-mail software uses a "To or Receiver Name" line. Most software applications also give the user choices of sending to multiple recipients), a "From or Sender" line, a "Cc or Copy line" (which can be to multiple recipients), a "Bcc or blind copy" line (which can be to multiple recipients), a "Subject or Header" line, and a "Date" line. It is important to understand that all e-mail addresses entered into the "Cc or copy" line can be seen by the recipient and all e-mail addresses entered into the "Bcc or blind copy" line cannot be seen by the recipient. There may also be an "Attachment" line, if the sender chooses to attach a document to the e-mail message. If a document is not attached to an e-mail, this may not be seen as a line in the heading format of the e-mail. E-mail software also offers the option of sending any e-mail high or low priority, which is helpful for those e-mails needing a quick or urgent response. All of this basic information is standard within most common e-mail software applications.

The body of the e-mail is a blank text box in which the user types or creates the message or text desired. The user clicks a "Send" button when the message has been completed so the e-mail can be forwarded or sent to the recipient. Similar to that of a word processing application, most e-mail software also provides for spelling and grammar check. The user must know the recipient's exact e-mail address; otherwise, the e-mail will not be sent and will be returned as an error message to the sender. E-mail addresses are discussed later in the Internet address section.

Transmission Types

The communication channels that computers use to send messages may vary across networks or the Internet. These channels can include telephone lines, fiberoptic cables, cable lines, digital subscriber lines (DSL), and broadband (White 2008,325). The telephone lines are analog, or what is called dial-up. Not many dial-up or modem lines are in use now; however, these are generally about 56 K. This means the transfer rate is 33,600 bits per second (White 2008, 326). Figure 2.6 describes various standard transmission rates.

The term "**modem**" was defined in chapter 1 as MODulating-DEModulating," which means converting the analog signal into digital and back again (White 2008, 325). The remaining types of channels listed are all modems; these also use digital signals that offer a fast response for Internet connection to the user because of the bandwidth (White 2008, 325). The **fiberoptic** cables connect directly to a network or the Internet and are small hairlike fibers covered by silica glass covered by cladding with light pulses that carry the data along the wires (White 2008, 320). **Cable** is the coaxial cable within the television network where a copper wire is used that is shielded by plastic and braided copper (White 2008, 320). The **DSL** line is a coaxial line but uses a twisted set of wiring comprising four pairs of insulated wires to help with noise reduction (White 2008, 320). DSL uses a phone line so that would probably tie up a phone line for incoming phone calls, but it doesn't do that! Actually DSL uses the twisted copper wires that the signals are carried within. With DSL, the user does not dial in; the DSL connection is always connected. This is why a phone and a computer can be used at the same time on the same line. A "splitter next to the DSL modem combines the low-frequency voice signals and the higher-frequency data signals" and it allows the user to talk on the phone and use the computer at the same time (White 2008, 328). **Broadband** means the bandwidth is a certain capacity to carry large amounts of data. This term means "high speed, high capacity Internet and data connections" (White 2008, 311). Broadband includes DSL, satellite, and cable. **Satellite** also offers a connection that can send broadband anywhere

Figure 2.6.   Transmission communication rates

Type	Bits per Second
Analog:	
Dial-up telephone lines	33,600 bps
Digital:	
Coaxial cable (i.e., television)	6 Mhz
Fiberoptic cables	1B bps
Digital Subscriber Line (DSL)	
RADSL (rate adaptive DSL)	8 Kbps–1 Mbps
G-Lite or universal DSL	1.5 Mbps
ADSL (asynchronous DSL)	6–8 Mbps
VDSL (very high DSL)	10–26 Mbps
T1 Line	1.5 Mbps
T3 Line	45 Mbps

Source: White 2008, 320–330

(White 2008, 325). Another type of transmission that carries point-to-point digital communication circuits with 25 channels, each of which carries 64,000 bits per second, is the **T1 line** (White 2008, 313). The T1 line channels can be used for data and are extremely powerful to carry large chunks of data. Thus, communication can be quickly sent and received virtually anywhere in the world within minutes with these types of transmission devices.

Internet Service Providers

To connect to the Internet, every computer must connect to a network that connects to the Internet; companies may use this method or the computer may connect directly to the Internet using an **Internet service provider (ISP)**. An ISP, sometimes referred to as an Internet provider or IP, is a computer company system that provides access to the Internet, or they supply a gateway to the Internet (White 2008, 312). Some ISP companies provide local service, and others provide national coverage and offer packages that vary with coverage that is optional for a monthly fee. All ISP companies provide access to e-mail and the World Wide Web, and usually offer their own individual services such as discussion areas, address book utility, chat areas, and information areas. These can vary according to the individual provider. As discussed in chapter 1, no single entity owns the Internet; it is called the information superhighway. As also mentioned in Chapter 1, the organizations that have influenced the maintenance and overseeing of the Internet are the Internet Society (ISOC), Internet Architecture Board (IAB), Internet Engineering Task Force, (IETF), World Wide Web Consortium (W3C), Internet Assignment Numbers Authority (IANA) and Internet Network Information Center (InterNIC) (Joos et al. 2006, 275). As discussed previously in this section, the TCP/IP are the protocols for the network communications that make the Internet function. All of the ISP providers must adhere to these protocols and the above agencies' standards to ensure service to each of their users when providing Internet service to the customer.

E-mail Messages

E-mail is analogous to a post office box; when a message is read, it can be replied to, forwarded to another person, or deleted. Messages can even be stored in separate folders as to not take up space in a user's mailbox. E-mail usually doesn't get lost on the Internet. If an e-mail address has been typed incorrectly, it will usually come back to the sender as an error message and the user will need to verify the address. It only takes one letter, period, comma, or underscore to be omitted or out of place for an e-mail to be returned. E-mail addresses are also case sensitive, thus it is best to verify that a new e-mail address has any capital or lowercase letters because this makes a huge difference in the e-mail address itself. Once e-mail is used for a few weeks, "junk e-mail" will begin to appear in the Inbox folder. **Junk e-mail** is unwanted and unsolicited mail that is similar to the junk mail that comes to a person's home mailbox. Most ISPs have a **spam filter** that can be used to send the junk mail to the ISP, so that the amount of junk mail can be filtered and decreased. Will all junk mail be deleted? Probably not, but much of it will stop coming after a few weeks as each piece of junk mail is flagged and sent to the ISP.

Listservs

A **listserv** is a professional mailing list organized by an association for its members or interested persons. Anyone may join a listserv by contacting an agency that maintains a listserv, as these are typically nonprofit agencies. The user's e-mail address is added to the mailing list and group mailings are sent to all members. Also, the user may join in by posting a message on the listserv for conversations on topics that are of interest on the listserv at any time. E-mail has become a popular communications tool in the electronic age.

Check Your Understanding 2.3

1. A tool for organizing the flow of patient appointments for outpatients, clinics, hospital admissions is:

   A. project management software
   B. scheduling software
   C. presentation software
   D. productivity software

2. One of the common elements of project management software is:

   A. Gantt chart
   B. Budget plan
   C. Strategic plan
   D. Tracking plan

3. The largest channels of transmission that carry point-to-point digital communication are the:

   A. DSL lines
   B. cable
   C. T1 lines
   D. fiberoptic lines

4. If an e-mail has been sent on the Internet incorrectly, the message will then be _____ _____.

   A. deleted
   B. returned to sender unopened
   C. classified as Junk Mail
   D. returned to sender as Error Message

Internet and Web Browsers

As discussed earlier, every computer has a unique identifier address. When connecting to the Internet, this identifier allows the computer to send and receive data from around the world to this particular computer. The software that resides within the ISP so that a computer may connect to the Internet may use a browser. A **browser** is a PC program that displays information from the Internet (White 2008, 311). The user's computer (client) communicates with the server whenever an Internet connection is needed. The software used on the server is a Web browser application.

Most Common Browsers

There are many Web browsers to access the Internet; some of the most common are Microsoft's Internet Explorer, Netscape's Navigator, Apple's Safari, and Mozilla's Firefox. A Web browser allows the user to display a Web site from the World Wide Web (WWW). The World Wide Web part of the Internet is the "graphical portion that stores electronic files, called Web pages, on servers that are accessed from a computer" (Joos et al. 2006, 277). A Web browser allows the user to view text, images, audio, and video on any Web site or local area network. Text on Web sites and the WWW are formatted in HTML for display; however, browsers allow easy display of the Web site of both text and images. Browsers are available free of charge for computer users and often are updated with newer versions at each of the manufacturer's Web sites. Many Web pages also contain hyperlinks to other Web sites. A hyperlink is a navigation element that is embedded within a document or Web page that when clicked on will automatically take the user to another Web site or deeper within that main Web site for further information. A hypertext link is "an embedded object within the Web page that enables direct access to another related Web page" (Abdelhak et al. 2007, 282). Usually hypertext will change in form when the user places the cursor over a hypertext word(s) and the cursor will change to a hand icon or some other symbol or form to indicate that it is a hypertext.

Internet Address

A computer has its own unique address on the Internet so that messages from around the world can be sent from it and received to it. The Internet address uses an Internet Protocol (IP) address with a unique identification number. An Internet Protocol (IP) address is "an identifier for a computer or a device on a TCP/IP network" (White 2008, 312). A **domain name** is also assigned to this **IP address** as users are better with text than a string of numbers, unlike computers. Domain names are registered by one of the official Internet agencies and assigned by those who have been given rights under that domain name. Sub-categories can then be issued to users under that domain name within businesses, agencies, schools, and organizations. The domain name is the last ending on the right, that is, ".com". The common address extensions (from the IANA Web site) are as follows:

.aero	Air and aerospace industry
.com	Commercial business
.edu	Educational institutions
.gov	Governmental agencies
.info	Informational sites
.jobs	Employment-related sites
.mil	Military
.net	Networks and ISP (commercial) providers
.org	Nonprofit organizations
.pro	Professional/licensed persons

Internet addresses will search the Web site and can find an exact computer, much as with an e-mail address. However, to locate an exact document on a Web site, a URL is needed. A **URL** is a Web site address that will take the Web browser directly to the document located on a Web page. To do this, a URL address is actually broken down into several segments, and it uses the domain name of the user. Most URLs begin with "http://" as it signals to the Web browser that the computer language that will be used for all text that follows that lead-in will be HTML.

What follows the "http://" is the remainder of the URL address, which must be written in HTML language. This is why it may look strange to new computer users at first, because of the periods and slashes located throughout the address. The next portion of the URL address is commonly seen as "www," which stands for World Wide Web. This is when the user is going to search for a Web site (such as for a reference) or to look for something specific on the Internet. Most browsers do not have to use the "www", but can find the Web site without it. The next portion of the URL is the user's domain address. This will vary according to the user's address. After the address is entered, the domain is then entered last in the user's address portion. At the end of the domain address, a forward slash (/) is used to indicate to the Web browser that the next portion of the URL address will be the Web path to the file. The user would need to know where the document is located—that is, on a computer's hard drive in a folder named ComputerClass, for example. After the path information is entered by the user, another forward slash (/) is entered in the Web address to indicate again that this portion is completed and that the last piece of information to be entered would be the exact name of the document. For example, if the name of the document was "data storage," then the user would enter this information into the Web browser. To signal to the browser that this is the end of the information, a period and html is the last entry on the Web browser's line that is made, such as ".html". To put this example together, it would look like this:

http://www.acme.college.edu/computerclass/datastorage.html

Indicates HTML	Server and Domain Address	Path to the Document	Document name	End

Although this is a fictitious Web site, it is used here to show the components of a typical URL address. Remember, URLs are case sensitive. Care should be taken when writing these addresses down. It is best to copy and paste these addresses from a secondary source whenever possible to alleviate any chances of missing letters or misspelling any portions of a URL. It only takes one letter or space to be entered improperly to cause error and not be able to find the Web site!

Searches

If certain information is being sought on the Internet, it can be overwhelming. There is a vast library of networks and data throughout the WWW readily available, so where and how does one start? The easiest way to start is with a search engine. **Search engines** are programs on the Internet that search for key words or phrases entered by a user browsing the Internet. A search engine functions in a certain order. It first crawls through Web sites or follows every link it sees. Next it indexes through Web sites, which means the data within a Web site is 'tagged' as relevant to be a match to the user's query. A **query** is a "search for data that meets specified criteria to allow you to retrieve certain subsets of the data" (White 2008, 121). And finally, the search engine performs a thorough search. This means it uses the best matches from the search criteria and the user's query and provides the user with a listing of matches or hits. Most search engines use a **Boolean search** process that is an advanced search feature where the user can specify to add descriptive terms to the search such as "and, or, and not" to the search to help limit the search fields.

Common Search Engines

Using a search engine, a user usually performs a Boolean search process as described in the above section and does a query of either a key word or a key phrase in the search process. Search engines vary in how the data are organized within each, but these are ranked and organized by topic of the data. Search engines are powerful tools and use enormous databases to store and link to other enormous databases that within seconds can "sweep" volumes of data during a query process. A search engine does not really search every document on the Internet, but uses "spiders" to go out and feel for potential links that are in place on the databases. This is what is termed "Web crawlers" (University of California, Berkeley, Library Web site 2008). The spider stores this so it can be indexed next. The "program identifies the text, links, and other content in the page and stores it in the search engine database's files so that the database can be searched by keyword and whatever more advanced approaches are offered, and the page will be found if your search matches its content" (University of California, Berkeley, Library Web site 2008). Google has one of the largest databases of Web pages, including many other types of Web documents (blog posts, wiki pages, group discussion threads) and document formats (for example, PDFs, Word or Excel documents, PowerPoint) (University of California, Berkeley, Library Web site 2008). Other common search engines include Google, Yahoo!, Ask.Com, Dogpile, MSN Search, and Lycos.

Other Communication Within the Internet

Chat Rooms

Within the Internet, chat rooms have developed for users to have a place to communicate and have social interaction with other users. Because of the user's communications via computer, for years it was thought this was a safe harbor to meet new people. However, in the past decade it has been found that chat rooms can be one way to invite danger into one's personal life if too much information is inadvertently given over the Internet. Many users know their friends before talking to them in a chat room and only meet them there for a synchronous visit—**synchronous** meaning "involved on the computer at the same time" (Joos et al. 2006, 326). This works well for students in classroom settings and for coworkers to discuss business projects.

Online Courses

Many schools offer courses online using the Internet. Courses may be strictly posted on the Internet using software applications on a school's restricted Web site for its students. Courses can also be online using the Web site with other types of media along with the Internet, such as video and audio applications. Videoconferencing would include videotaping to appear on the monitor via the Internet within a course, as would audio or sound of a course. Students could also use just an audio conference via the Internet without video capability for classes along with PowerPoint slides. The combination of media for online classes is endless with technology and the Internet.

Instant Messaging

One modality of electronic communication is instant messaging (IM). This is a service that "permits the user to send real-time messages via a private chat room to other individuals who are online" (Joos et al. 2006, 323). However, instant messaging requires that all users use the same system or software or the communication will fail. Instant messaging is a great technology tool for use with health networking and is gaining popularity (Goldstein et al. 2007, 331). It is important to understand that IM is not a proven secure method of transmission, so any PHI transmitted via IM is at risk. IM should only be used according to organizational policy, if at all.

Online Meetings

Many conferences now are being held online in order to save time and money for their company. Having virtual meetings by conference calls seemed sufficient several years ago, however with the electronic addition of online media, visual presentations, audio, and video are now added so the entire meeting can be held online.

Online meetings, sometimes called webinars or video conferences, are electronically delivered. A videoconference uses a computer, videocamera, microphone, and speakers, so that along with the audio, the images that appear in front of the videocamera are delivered to the participant's monitor (Joos et al. 2006, 326). Webinars also involve PowerPoint slides with audio by the speaker. Online meetings "can involve just two participants or multiple ones in a 'virtual' conference" (Joos et al. 2006, 326). Today, with the Internet and networks converging, "patients can have voice discussions with physicians and simultaneously examine information on a corresponding Web site" (Johns 2007, 839).

Wiki

"Wiki" is a term that was originally developed by Ward Cunningham "on March 25, 1995 when he started his Web site Cunningham & Cunningham using the software WikiWiki-Web, developed by himself" (Harris and Zeng 2008, 1). "Wiki" is a Hawaiian word meaning "quick," and the developer of the software bearing this name wanted a term to denote something fast for the Internet. The wiki is used as a collaborative tool by many users on the Internet to edit Web pages. Many wikis have been developed, and anyone with a Web browser connection can edit a document on a wiki server (Harris and Zeng 2008, 1). There are many corporate organizations that use wikis as a method of online sharing to perform open editing of documents that are posted on the wiki server software online (Harris and Zeng 2008, 1). Healthcare professionals are realizing it pays to share knowledge and resources inside organizations and across organizational boundaries (Goldstein et al. 2007, 332). Wikis allow online editing to increase knowledge transfer internally as well as internationally.

Standards and Protocols

As previously discussed in chapter 1, networks are constructed in different ways for various purposes. Some of the networks covered in chapter 1 were local area networks (LANs), wide area networks (WANs), and types of private networks such as intranets, extranets, and the Internet (which is a public network). In private networks, governance and control is easily overseen and maintained. With the Internet, control over a public network that no entity has ownership over is not always a straightforward issue. There are many agencies and entities with interests in the Internet who have supported its emergence from its early beginnings. As the Internet grew, so did the need for rules of maintaining the architecture of the network. Those agencies and entities began developing standards and protocols that have developed into those standards of the Internet summarized below.

Transmission Control Protocol/Internet Protocol

The **Transmission Control Protocol/Internet Protocol (TCP/IP)** is a universal standard for connecting to the Internet that includes a collection of methods used to connect servers on the Internet and to exchange data (White 2008, 313). Within the TCP/IP protocols are several familiar protocols, among them File Transfer Protocol and Hypertext Transfer Protocol (FTP and HTTP). **FTP** is used within a Web site address immediately before the slashes to signify that it is a plain text listing of a file that is available for downloading from the World Wide Web (White 2008, 368). **HTTP** is used within a Web site address to signify the Web site as one on the World Wide Web that uses HTML (White 2008, 368).

Electronic Data Interchange

The Electronic Data Interchange (EDI) is a standard transmission format that uses strings of data for business information that is communicated among computer systems of independent organizations (Giannangelo 2006, 302). Within healthcare facilities across the country and the world, there must be standards that are shared but at the same time understandable between all systems and networks so that data can be sent and received between organizations. Within the private sector **standards development organizations (SDOs)** are accredited by the **American National Standards Institute (ANSI)**, which are the primary developers of data exchange standards (Giannangelo 2006, 255). There are many standards and protocols that are classified as data exchange with these organizations. These include HIPAA with electronic transaction standards, Accredited Standards Committee (ASC X12), Health Level Seven (HL7) for clinical data, National Council for Prescription Drug Programs (NCPDP) for prescription data, Digital Imaging Communications in Medicine (DICOM) for medical images, and Institute of Electrical and Electronics Engineers Standards Organization-(IEEE 1073) for medical devices (Giannangelo 2006, 257–266).

Health Level 7

HL7 is an SDO that develops data exchange standards for clinical data. It is accepted globally for healthcare information within healthcare facilities and outside the facility (Giannangelo 2006, 258). The most commonly used standards for developing electronic, clinical, and administrative datasets were established by the HL7 of ANSI (Abdelhak et al. 2007, 38). These standards are "focused on the exchange, management, and integration of electronic healthcare information for healthcare organizations" (Abdelhak et al. 2007, 38). It is the basis of these data exchange standards that can use point-of-care systems within healthcare facilities to exchange data quickly and make patient care fast and safe in this country—and globally as other countries become more technology-oriented. HL7 is an accredited SDO by ANSI, a body that oversees and accredits private SDOs in the United States and coordinates with international bodies (Abdelhak et al. 2007, 215). There are several versions of HL7, where each version updates the previous version of interfaces of various systems that send or receive data (Giannangelo 2006, 259). HL7 versions vary with each update as each one focuses on the context, terminology, models, and definitions, rather than by trying to support any certain type of system architecture (Giannangelo 2006, 259). HL7 data exchange standards are about clinical data; this includes the electronic health record and patient data on computers.

Check Your Understanding 2.4

1. Within the Internet, this space is reserved for synchronous discussions between two or more parties.

   A. E-mail
   B. Listserv
   C. Chat Room
   D. World Wide Web

2. In the following Internet address, http://www.acmesolar.edu, what does the "www.acmesolar" mean?

   A. The HTML address
   B. The file name
   C. The path name of the document
   D. The server and domain name

3. A private network within the Internet that is meant for authorized users only is known as

   _____.

   A. intranet
   B. extranet
   C. domain
   D. IP address

4. The HL7 messaging standard is the accepted protocol for communicating

   _____.

   A. administrative data
   B. medical device data
   C. prescription data
   D. clinical data

References

Abdelhak, M., S. Grostick, M.A. Hanken, and E. Jacobs. 2007. *Health information: Management of a Strategic Resource*, 3rd ed. St. Louis, MO: Saunders/Elsevier.

AdventNet, Inc. 2008. Zoho FAQ. www.zoho.com/zoho_faq.html.

Amatayakul, M.K. 2007. *Electronic Health Records: A Practical Guide for Professionals and Organizations*, 3rd ed. Chicago: AHIMA.

Car, J. and A. Sheikh. 2004a. E-mail consultations in health care: 1—scope and effectiveness. *BMJ*. 329(7463):435–438. http://www.bmj.com/cgi/reprint/329/7463/435.

Car, J. and A. Sheikh. Aug 2004b. E-mail consultations in health care: 2—acceptability and safe application. *BMJ*. 329(7463):439–442. http://www.bmj.com/cgi/content/full/329/7463/439.

Center for Faculty Excellence and ITS Teaching and Learning. 2008. IT Connections: An online sourcebook for teaching with technology. http://itconnections.unc.edu/presenting.html. University of North Carolina at Chapel Hill.

Corel Corporation. 2008. Our History. www.corel.com/servlet/Satellite/us/en/Content/1208981227678.

Coyle, D.M. *Computers Are Your Future*, 10th ed. 2009. Upper Saddle River, NJ: Pearson Education, Inc.

Degoulet, P. and M. Fieschi M. 1997. *Introduction to Clinical Informatics*. 1997. New York, NY: Springer-Verlag Publishers.

Eclipsys Corporation. 2008. "About Us." http://www.eclipsys.com/aboutus/.

Epic Systems Corporation. 2008. "Software." http://www.epicsystems.com/software-access.php.

Friedman, B. 2005. Health records get personal: A technology outlook for consumer access to personal health information. *Journal of AHIMA* 76(1):42–45.

Fuller, F. and B. Larson. 2008. *Computers: Understanding Technology*, 3rd ed. St. Paul, MN: Paradigm Publishing, Inc.

Giannangelo, K., ed. 2006. *Healthcare Code Sets, Clinical Terminologies, and Classification Systems.* Chicago: AHIMA.

Goldstein, D., P. Groen, S. Ponkshe, and M. Wine. 2007. *Medical Informatics 20/20: Quality and Electronic Health Records Through Collaboration, Open Solutions, and Innovation.* Sudbury, MA: Jones and Bartlett Publishers.

Harris, S.T. and X. Zeng. 2008. Using Wiki in an online record documentation systems course. *Perspectives in Health Information Management.* 5(1):1–16.

Johns, M.L., ed. 2007. *Health Information Management Technology: An Applied Approach,* 2nd ed. Chicago: AHIMA.

Joos, I., N.I. Whitman, M.J Smith, and R. Nelson. 2006. *Introduction to Computers for Healthcare Professionals*, 4th ed. Sudbury, MA: Jones and Bartlett Publishers.

McWay, D.C. 2008. *Today's Health Information Management: An Integrated Approach.* Clifton Park, NY: Thomson/Delmar Learning.

Microsoft Company. 2008. Word 2007: Rich Text Format (RTF) Specification, version 1.9.1. http://www.microsoft.com/downloads/details.aspx?familyid=dd422b8d-ff06-4207-b476-6b5396a18a2b&displaylang=en #RelatedLinks.

Office of the National Coordinator for Health Information Technology. 2008. The Patient–Provider Secure Messaging Detailed Use Case. 1–44.

Nunn, S. 2008. Managing e-mail as records. *Journal of AHIMA* 79(9):54–55.

Power, D.J. 2004. A Brief History of Spreadsheets. http://dssresources.com/history/sshistory.html.

Rob, R. and C. Coronel. 2009. *Database Systems: Design, Implementation, and Management*, 8th ed. Boston, MA: Course Technology/Cengage Learning.

Rutkosky, N., D. Seguin, and A. Rutkosky. 2008a. *Marquee Series: Microsoft Excel 2007.* St. Paul, MN: Paradigm Publishing, Inc.

Rutkosky, N., D. Seguin, and A. Rutkosky, A. 2008b. *Marquee Series: Microsoft PowerPoint 2007.* St. Paul, MN: Paradigm Publishing, Inc.

Rutkosky, N., D. Seguin, and A. Rutkosky. 2008c. *Marquee Series: Microsoft Word 2007.* St. Paul, MN: Paradigm Publishing, Inc.

Thakkar, M. and D.C. Davis. 2006. Risks, barriers, and benefits of EHR systems: A comparative study based on size of hospital. *Perspectives in Health Information Management.* 13(5):10.

University of California, Berkeley, Library. 2008. Recommended Search Engines. http://www.lib.berkeley.edu/TeachingLib/Guides/Internet/SearchEngines.html.

White, R. 2008. *How Computers Work*, 9th ed. Indianapolis, IN: QUE Publishing.

Wing, P. and M. Langlier. 2004. "Data for Decisions: The HIM Workforce and Workplace—Recommendations to the AHIMA Board of Directors from the Center for Health Workforce Studies Based on the HIM Workforce Research Study." Chicago: AHIMA.

Chapter 3
Data Quality

Objectives

- Describe the difference between raw facts and information as given within the healthcare setting.

- Identify the various data sources that populate the electronic health record.

- Explain the Nationwide Health Information Network (NHIN) and the health information exchanges (HIEs) and how these affect the future of the national health information superhighway.

- Describe the differences between the Health Level 7 (HL7) format and the ASC X12 format languages.

- Identify the common data sets for reporting to the various agencies by most healthcare facilities that are under the Medicare and Medicaid mandates.

- List and give an example of each of the AHIMA Data Quality Model characteristics.

- Discuss the importance of data quality charts and graphs and why these can be effective instruments.

Key Terms

AHIMA Data Quality Model
American National Standards Institute (ANSI)
ASC X12 format
Centers for Medicare and Medicaid Services (CMS)
Clinical data repository (CDR)
Data accuracy
Data collection
Data content standards
Data Elements for Emergency Department Systems (DEEDS)
Data integrity
Data mining

Data reliability
Data set
Data sources
Data warehouse
Department of Health and Human Services (DHHS)
Edit check
Essential Medical Data Set (EMDS)
Flowchart
Gantt chart
Health information exchanges (HIEs)
Health Plan Employer Data and Information Set (HEDIS)

HL7 format
Hot spot
Master patient index (MPI)
Minimum Data Set for Long Term Care (MDS LTC)
National Committee on Vital and Health Statistics (NCVHS)
National Health Information Infrastructure (NHII)
Nationwide Health Information Network (NHIN)
Office of the National Coordinator for Health Information Technology (ONC)
ORYX

Outcomes and Assessment
   Information Set (OASIS)
Peer review
Physician advisor (PA)
Project Evaluation and Review
   Technique (PERT)
Qualitative analysis

Quantitative analysis
Regional health information
   organizations (RHIOs)
Standards Development
   Organizations (SDOs)
Subjective data

Uniform Ambulatory Care Data
   Set (UACDS)
Uniform Hospital Discharge
   Data Set (UHDDS)
Workgroup for Electronic Data
   Interchange (WEDI)

Importance of Data Quality

Patient history has been recorded for centuries on paper; even back to the Middle Ages, there have been written records of treating the sick. Although these records are not what currently might be thought of as quality records, these records provide proof that written records exist of documenting healthcare given to those in need of treatment. The history of healthcare and the importance of recording written data are a part of the foundation that has been expanded into the complex healthcare delivery systems currently in place. The importance of data quality cannot be overstressed or understated. Every piece of information from the patient record is vital to patient care. The practitioner must read, review, analyze, and compare the patient's record to similar cases so a judgment can be made and treatment administered accordingly. Therefore, it is critical that all information is timely, accurate, and complete.

Raw Data vs. Information

The legal health record serves several purposes: it provides documentation of services for continuing patient care by all practitioners who treat the patient; it serves as evidence in legal proceedings; it serves to assess the effectiveness of healthcare services provided to a patient; it contains documented healthcare services provided for reimbursement claims submitted for third-party payment; and it serves to supply information for administrative planning and decision making, research, education, and public health, and for accreditation purposes of the facility (Abdelhak et al. 2007, 44). The data contained within the record by itself would be raw data or figures; however, when these data are organized and presented to produce meaning, this results in information (Abdelhak et al. 2007, 44). Healthcare users must rely on information so that patient care can be provided at its highest level. The patient chart containing only raw data is a record that is full of numbers and useless data that have no meaning to anyone. These data must have meaning attached to them; once this occurs, these data become useful information that can be used by the practitioners to treat the patient.

> **Example of Raw Data vs. Information:** A routine laboratory report contains a list of test results for a patient. The normal range scale for each test is listed next to the results, thus giving it meaning and translating it into information. If the normal range scale is not listed and there is no knowledge of where the normal ranges fall, it remains raw data as the numbers have no meaning.

Most health records are documented with the best intentions and are done so appropriately by practitioners. Hospital personnel are trained properly on how to document appropriately within patient records and how to use computerized records and databases accordingly. However, errors can still be made when charting, computer problems can transpire, or other data mishaps can occur. Because of the possibility of errors related to data, the quality of information must be a priority in healthcare.

Data Sources

Information that populates the computerized health record comes from many **data sources**. The primary source is the patient. The highest quality of care will always come from the primary source, the patient. The history of the present illness is recorded within the history and physical form in the current record. Previous history about the patient on subsequent visits or past medical history may be obtained at this time and be recorded as past medical history within the health record. The patient will always supply the history of the illness.

The patient's primary care physician will also be an excellent source of information. From the physician's office, data can be obtained on the patient's history, along with laboratory, radiology, and other data. Any information about the patient contained at the physician's office may be useful in the patient's care. This information can be used as part of the history if it is sent as part of the admission paperwork by the admitting physician within the time limitations of the date of admission.

Other sources of data may include laboratories and radiology treatment facilities. Patients often have diagnostic testing performed on an outpatient basis by their primary care physician at these facilities, and many times these healthcare facilities may send healthcare data to hospitals as part of the patient's care upon admittance. Pharmacies are another possible data source once a patient is admitted to a healthcare facility. When a computerized record is online, the electronic data sources are much more accessible and data can easily be transmitted across networks so that patient care is uninterrupted and the quality of care for the patient is optimal.

Data Collection Initiatives

As a result of computers, networks and databases, there are more and more data being collected. **Data collection** is used for many purposes in healthcare such as research, education, accreditation, decision making in administrative functions, billing and claims reimbursement, public health and epidemiology, legal and legislative issues, quality and utilization issues, patient care and treatment issues. Data collection processes are imperative to ensure that healthcare is safer, of the highest quality, and more efficient than ever before.

Data collection is not a simple task. There are many challenges to be faced including cost factors related to the purchase and implementation of software systems, privacy and security concerns regarding patient data in transit and at rest, and a lack of standards to regulate the electronic realm across healthcare. For efficient and quality collection of data, the healthcare workforce must be educated on its processes and significant role in healthcare. The right equipment and software must be available.

Data collection must be performed within databases and networked within facilities across the country as mandated in legislative standards such as the creation of the **Office of the National Coordinator for Health Information Technology (ONC)** in 2004, which oversees the widespread model of a health information exchange (HIE) network. Another mandatory compliance issue was the creation of the nine HIEs in the country. These may also be known as **regional health information organizations (RHIOs)**, introduced in 2007. Data are being collected at the regional level and will soon progress to the national level.

The ONC is "advancing the NHIN as a 'network of networks,' built out of state and regional **health information exchanges (HIEs)** and other networks so as to support the exchange of health information by connecting these networks and the systems they, in turn, connect" (NHIN 2008). The **Nationwide Health Information Network (NHIN)** is part of the government's **Department of Health and Human Services (DHHS)** division, as is the ONC. The NHIN is responsible for providing the infrastructure for health information that is secure and that will operate nationally for everyone involved in healthcare. This means that providers, practitioners, and consumers may be confident that all patient data will be secure, private, and safeguarded in the maintenance and transmission of healthcare data across the country. The NHIN will enable health information to follow the consumer, be available for clinical decision making, and support appropriate use of healthcare information beyond direct patient care to improve health. The NHIN's goals are listed in figure 3.1.

Figure 3.1.   NHIN goals

- Developing capabilities for standards-based, secure data exchange nationally
- Improving the coordination of care information among hospitals, laboratories, physicians' offices, pharmacies, and other providers
- Ensuring appropriate information is available at the time and place of care
- Ensuring that consumers' health information is secure and confidential
- Giving consumers new capabilities for managing and controlling their personal health records as well as providing access to their health information from EHRs and other sources
- Reducing risks from medical errors and supporting the delivery of appropriate, evidence-based medical care
- Lowering healthcare costs resulting from inefficiencies, medical errors, and incomplete patient information
- Promoting a more effective marketplace, greater competition, and increased choice through accessibility to accurate information on healthcare costs, quality, and outcomes

Source: NHIN 2008

NHIN began the first trial implementations of the DHHS Awards Cooperative Agreements with six healthcare facilities and/or networks. In 2007, the governmental agency increased the number from six to nine trial HIEs for the second year. All of this is part of the legislation enacted in 2004 to meet President Bush's goal of having access to electronic health records by 2014 (NHIN 2008). These HIEs that are in the trial implementation phases with the NHIN are under contract and are reviewed by the following measures:

1. Patient lookup and information retrieval

2. Secure information routing and delivery (including but not limited to a defined summary patient record)

3. Provision of data for population uses

4. Consumer-managed access to appropriate information (NHIN 2008)

The trial implementation of HIEs is moving forward with testing of a national infrastructure for an electronic health record. Due to the complexity of standard implementation, the agencies are continuing to work on improving the processes.

Data Standards

Within DHHS, there are subdepartments that collect and work with data for various purposes. Electronic data are easily collected for statistical purposes at the national level concerning issues on health. One advisory committee to the DHHS is the **National Committee on Vital and Health Statistics (NCVHS)**. Their major purpose and role is to advise and recommend guidelines for the electronic health record in all activities, including standards, data sets, and terminologies. The NCVHS is a public advisory agency to DHHS that supports the HL7 standard as the standard for the **National Health Information Infrastructure (NHII)** (McWay 2008, 175). The NHII may also be called NHIN, as discussed earlier.

The architecture that will transmit data across the country must ensure confidentiality and security of data while ensuring usability for patient healthcare. The standards in data communication are of utmost importance. The transmission of data must be uniform across the architecture, and the electronic data interchange (EDI) is the rules or protocols for how information is transmitted between networks. The **standards development organizations (SDOs)** in the United States are the efforts of two organizations, the **American National Standards Institute (ANSI)** and the **Workgroup for Electronic Data Interchange (WEDI)** (McWay 2008, 173). The ANSI is a voluntary organization that accredits groups in the private sector for data standards. The WEDI group is a formal organization under DHHS that serves to "identify ways of increasing the use of electronic billing to reduce administrative costs" (McWay 2008, 174). In order for data to be understood from one network to another, the data must be equal to one another by definition. These organizations serve to ensure data elements and data sets are defined and equal so that information can be transmitted.

Figure 3.2.   UHDDS criteria list examples as data content standards

Sex	Male = 1
	Female = 2
Ethnicity	Caucasian = 1
	Asian = 2
	African = 3
	Pacific Islander = 4
	Latin American = 5
Disposition	Home = 1
	Nursing facility = 2
	AMA = 3
	Died = 4
	Nursing facility = 5
	Home health care = 6

Source: Abdelhak et al. 2007, 130

To communicate data, two messaging format languages are used. Health Level 7 (HL7) and ASC X12 have been through the SDOs for approval to ensure communication between networks. The **HL7 format** is used for communicating mainly clinical content whereas the **ASC X12 format** is used primarily for processing of financial data, such as claims billing (McWay 2008, 174). All data processed are based on the foundation that electronic data must be in a universal architectural format.

Data content standards is defined as the "clear guidelines for the acceptable values for specified data fields" (Fenton et al. 2007). Data content standards achieve user friendliness because they explain the details of the data contained within the database of the facility. These standards are similar to a legend or a key on a table; users see data content standards daily and probably do not recognize that they are being utilized. Examples of such standards might be those used from the **Uniform Hospital Discharge Data Set (UHDDS)** list, shown in figure 3.2.

Check Your Understanding 3.1

1. Health information exchanges (HIEs) are also called _____.

   A. SDOs
   B. NHII
   C. RHIOs
   D. NHIN

2. The public advisory agency that supports the DHHS in standards development is the

   _____.

   A. NHIN
   B. ONC
   C. WEDI
   D. NCVHS

3. The data standards group that has been approved by SDO and operates under the DHHS is:

   _____.

   A. WEDI
   B. ANSI
   C. EDI
   D. NHII

Data Collection

Data collection results when data elements are captured in a central area. Databases are typically used for the collection of data within healthcare facilities. As the healthcare staff collects data items from the patient and other primary sources (as previously discussed), the health record becomes the primary source of data. When the health record is electronic, the data source serves as an electronic database and it is a matter of organizing the data into useful information for its user.

A common electronic means of collecting data within healthcare is the **clinical data repository (CDR)**. By definition, the CDR is a large database within a healthcare facility that is the "master holder of all the enterprise's clinical information; it allows multiple disparate systems to populate the data into the CDR" (McCoy et al. 2006). Data can be stored within the CDR, making access easy. Organization for reporting is quick, and data are integrated so analysis by the user can be completed at any networked computer. Healthcare facilities can then interface the clinical data repositories that house patient clinical information with other databases, such as administrative and financial, to form what is known as a **data warehouse**.

The systems housed in a facility's data warehouse may or may not be physically separate; the key factor is that these networked systems be interconnected so the computer architecture can communicate, allowing queries to be made on many levels and from various departments within the facility. Warehouses provide a network of clinical, financial, and administrative information about patients that is comprehensive, provides easy access, is secure and confidential, and enables all users to have a network of knowledge to maintain, analyze, and report on information. The term '**data mining**' describes a process used by some analysts when working with data within data warehouses to improve decision making. Data mining is the "process of extracting information from a database and then quantifying and filtering discrete, structured data" (Amatayakul 2007, 460).

Data Sets

Within data collection and data standards are the basic data elements to be collected as part of the DHHS. A **data set** is defined as "a list of recommended data elements with uniform definitions" (Johns 2007, 160). Healthcare facilities collect data for various agencies now more than ever before. Data collection purposes for the government and for other agencies include research, statistical data collection, public health, epidemiological issues, legal and legislative health issues, and state and local health issues, and these are just a few examples of why data collection is performed.

The basic data elements collected are uniform across many common data sets for various agencies so that duplicate data collection efforts are not performed. With electronic data collection, the process of collecting data and extracting it for reporting to various agencies is common practice. The common data sets for reporting by most healthcare facilities under the Medicare and Medicaid mandates are as shown in figure 3.3.

Figure 3.3.   Common data sets for reporting

UHDDS	Uniform Hospital Discharge Data Set	by NCVHS
UACDS	Uniform Ambulatory Care Data Set	by NCVHS
DEEDS	Data Elements for Emergency Department Systems	by CDC
EMDS	Essential Medical Data Set—part of NHI infrastructure	
OASIS	Outcomes and Assessment Information Set	by CMS
MDS LTC	Minimum Data Set for Long Term Care	by NCVHS
HEDIS	Health Plan Employer Data and Information Set	by NCQA
ORYX	--------- by the Joint Commission (JC)	by JC

Source: Johns 2007, 162–172

The common data sets shown in figure 3.3 are a part of standard data definitions by various agencies. A health record practitioner should know these basic data sets and the agencies that require these data elements. Table 3.1 describes each data set and its purpose in more detail.

Data Definitions

All data within the patient health record, whether paper or electronic, must have meaning assigned to each data element. As stated earlier, data not associated with information or knowledge is useless. Users of data must know what it means universally—whether text, abbreviations, or numbers. For example, legends may be used to identify numbers

Table 3.1.   Purpose of common data sets

Data Set	Purpose
UHDDS	The **Uniform Hospital Discharge Data Set (UHDDS)** is required by the Department of Health and Human Services (DHHS) through the National Committee on Vital and Health Statistics (NCVHS). These data elements are collected to capture a minimum amount of demographic and admission-specific information on all inpatient discharges (LaTour and Eichenwald Maki 2006, 150). The UHDDS is required by this agency as a hospital inpatient standard by federal and state agencies (Giannangelo 2006, 238).
UACDS	The **Uniform Ambulatory Care Data Set (UACDS)**, also by the NCVHS of the DHHS, is a uniform data set of elements for ambulatory care (Giannangelo 2006, 238) that capture a minimum amount of data on patients and outpatient services provided (LaTour and Eichenwald Maki 2006, 150).
DEEDS	The **Data Elements for Emergency Department Systems (DEEDS)** is a data collection set designed for hospital-based emergency departments that the Centers for Disease Control and Prevention (CDC) helped develop (Giannangelo 2006, 241). DEEDS was designed to collect uniform information on emergency departments' services at a hospital (LaTour and Eichenwald Maki 2006, 154).
EMDS	The **Essential Medical Data Set (EMDS)** is a data set that is similar to DEEDS but was developed by the National Information Infrastructure Health Information Network (Giannangelo 2006, 244).
OASIS	The **Outcomes and Assessment Information Set (OASIS)** is a data set developed for home care patients primarily by the Centers for Medicare and Medicaid Services (CMS) and research by the Robert Wood Johnson Foundation (Giannangelo 2006, 240). OASIS helps to trend and analyze the outcomes of home care patients through utilizing a standardized data capture tool used for patients who receive home health services that are covered by Medicare and Medicaid (Giannangelo 2006, 241).
MDS-LTC	The **Minimum Data Set for Long Term Care (MDS-LTC)** is a long-term care data set developed by the National Committee on Vital and Health Statistics of DHHS. The MDS-LTC captures demographic and clinical information on patients receiving nursing home care (LaTour and Eichenwald Maki 2006, 153).
HEDIS	**HEDIS (Health Plan Employer Data and Information Set)** is overseen by the National Committee for Quality Assurance (NCQA). HEDIS is a "standardized set of performance measures designed to allow purchasers and consumers to compare the performance of managed-care plans" (Abdelhak et al. 2007, 14).
ORYX (not an acronym)	Developed and maintained by the Joint Commission (JC). This is a "performance improvement initiative of the Joint Commission used to examine a healthcare organization's internal performance over time and to compare the organization's performance with that of others" (McWay 2008, 462). ORYX uses core measures developed by the JC that are defined and are used across the healthcare continuum so that facilities can compare, analyze, trend, and determine effectiveness in treatment with facilities similar to their own.

and the meaning of their values (such as a laboratory result or other diagnostic test). In addition, a particular facility may have in a patient's health record a current copy of Joint Commission's "Do Not Use" abbreviations list by their facility's medical staff. These examples of data can be universally used in a patient's record but may slightly vary by facility. However, the foundation here is the same everywhere; data must be defined for the user and "with a clear definition and a range of acceptable values" (Johns 2007, 39).

Standardized Data

Attempts have been made for years to standardize data, even with paper-based records. Forms committees have attempted to use standardized forms and templates to help facilitate uniformity across a facility and even across multifaceted organizations. As the electronic health record is developed across the country and around the world, there must exist data elements and data sets that are standard and unified allowing for an electronic platform for data to be exchanged and transmitted. It is imperative that electronic languages are in a version universally acceptable across all networks. It is for this reason that so many agencies are working hard toward this effort.

Duplication of Data

Duplication of any patient data can cause many problems that will be time-consuming and labor-intensive to correct. Data can be duplicated easily and in many ways within the health record. This can become a health information practitioner's nightmare—to rid the database of duplicate data. Any type of patient information in the health record could be duplicated; however, it is found that the medical record number is the most common data to be duplicated in the computer system. The **master patient index (MPI)** contains much information that is easily duplicated by others inadvertently. This occurs when a staff member admits a patient and is not thorough to check for all possible previous admissions. This could happen because of misspelled names, transposed admission and/or discharge dates, incorrect birthdates, incorrect social security numbers, incorrect mother's maiden name, and a host of other incorrect personal identifying information that was not completely searched by the admission person. Therefore, the admission person proceeds to assign the patient a new medical record number for the current admission rather than taking time to identify the previous one. Thus, a duplicate medical record number is created, causing the patient to have two medical record numbers within the MPI database. The MPI would need to be corrected or cleaned up to correct the duplicate.

Cleaning an MPI is not an easy or rapid process. "Cleaning an MPI" is the process of systematically going through each potential problem. This could mean that one problem would be a patient having two record numbers so both health records would have to be reviewed manually page by page to determine if in fact these records are for the same person. The pages must be sorted to the correct patient and to the correct visit dates, then the records can be merged and the original medical record used. The duplicated number can then be deleted (or reused, depending on the facility's policy). If the records are for two different persons, the MPI needs to reflect the differences so others using the system will avoid assigning data to the wrong person. A new record number then needs to be issued to one of the patients to separate the records; this is a time-consuming task. If a facility has hundreds or thousands of duplicates (which can be possible, if an MPI has not been cleaned in years), this can be a task that can take months or even up to one year to complete depending on the number of staff assigned to work on this process. If an MPI is manual and is not "cleaned up" before transitioning to an automated or computerized system, any problems will be transferred to the automated system. Once automated, MPIs need to be maintained and cleaned on a routine basis to prevent problems.

There can also be duplication of data within a patient's health record. Usually these types of mistakes are due to human error. For example a floor nurse on 3rd shift receives a transcribed operative report and places it into the patient's record. At 7 a.m., the health information technician, as part of her regular duties, places another copy of the report into the same chart. The patient is discharged and the chart is released to the HIM department for coding and abstracting for billing purposes. This was a duplication of data error. The coding staff finds the error, removes it, and shreds it.

The Importance of Data Entry

Data Elements

Data is defined as the "collection of elements on a given subject." It is the "raw facts, characters, or symbols" that are communicated manually or electronically (Abdelhak et al. 2007, 711). The data element is synonymous as it, too, is used to "describe a single fact or measurement" (Johns, 159). Data elements are important because these are the building blocks that create the entity that becomes the record. Without the individual data elements, the record is incomplete.

Data elements may sound simple because they typically are one piece of information within a unit, such as gender, age, last name, ethnicity, date of birth (DOB), maiden name, and so on. However, each element is critical to development of the overall record. Data elements within a patient's health record are so vital to the healthcare practitioners that uniform definitions are provided as data are collected. Whether the data elements are paper-based or electronic, the data provides information to healthcare providers during care, as well as to researchers about diseases and treatments, which may ultimately shape future care.

Data Timeliness

The timeliness of data entry is of utmost importance and represents data quality. Healthcare data must reflect the exact time and date at which it was performed during the episode of care. Inaccurate accounting of the treatment may reflect poor quality of care as well as poor documentation of care. Users of the patient's health record depend on accurate and timely data. It is a necessity that all records be timed and dated appropriately during the entire episode of care.

The signatures and/or initials of the healthcare practitioners who oversee each event during a patient's stay are of equal importance. The authentication (signatures and/or initials) of each event during a patient's stay, such as verbal and written orders, verifies that the practitioner has overseen the treatment and/or plans for treatment and that these plans have been carried out. The timeliness of authentication is just as important as the patient's treatment because it represents proof of care, not to mention satisfying medicolegal requirements and billing and claims reimbursement after the patient's discharge.

Data Accuracy

The patient's health record must be accurate and complete. **Data accuracy** "means that data are correct" or "data should represent what was intended or defined by the original source of the data" (Johns 2007, 37). There are a multitude of problem areas that can prevent a health record from being an accurate record; however, quantitative and qualitative analyses are two methods used to help prevent inaccurate data from occurring so frequently within a health record.

Quantitative analysis is used by health information management technicians as a method to detect whether elements of the patient's health record are missing. This may mean that a report could be missing entirely or a section of a report is missing, such as a few hours of progress notes. Reports are either present or absent in a quantitative review (Abdelhak et al. 2007, 124).

A **qualitative analysis** is a detailed review of a patient's health record for the quality of the documentation contained therein. The reviewer usually asks an internal question while reviewing a record: "Would this record hold up in a court of law if it were subpoenaed today?"

Because both qualitative and quantitative reviews are typically done retrospectively, it is difficult to make changes when problems are found. However, reviewers can take advantage of these instances of identifying problems as teaching points for the medical staff and other practitioners who document within patient records, so that future documentation can improve.

Inaccurate data are useless, expensive, and many times harmful to patients. Data forms much of the body of knowledge used by medical professionals, epidemiologists, policy-makers, and public health officials in decision making. Decisions made affect patient lives, policies on healthcare reform, and other major issues regarding health. Resources are allocated at local, state, and national levels based on data collected and entrusted to be accurate. Accurate data are needed to evaluate patient outcomes and quality of life, and to determine satisfaction issues and implement procedures for improvement.

Missing Data

The patient's health record must be complete. Not only is this a state health and Joint Commission standard but also a standard in the bylaws of facilities across the nation. Incomplete health records (missing documents or missing data, or even missing entries or signatures) would not serve any purpose. Any item or element that is not in the patient's health record that should be there is considered missing and qualifies as incomplete data and thus makes the record incomplete.

The HIM profession has been monitoring incomplete patient records since the beginning of record keeping because it is a sound practice of good documentation. Not only is this legally sound, but the primary reason is for the quality of the continuity of patient care. Without accurate and complete data in the health record, practitioners cannot accurately treat the patient. It is in the best interest of the patient and the facility as well as all practitioners to ensure that all data are contained in the health record. This is again why HIM technicians perform a detailed review of health records, with a quantitative and qualitative review to ensure that records are comprehensive. Reviews help ensure that the facility meets legal and regulatory requirements and that the documentation within the records will reinforce this if ever questioned. This documentation also is needed for billing and claims reimbursement issues. If there are data missing, there is good reason that the claim can be rejected or denied by the third-party payer due to this lack of data.

It is true that the HIM technicians are trained to determine quantitative reviews and various levels of qualitative reviews within a health record. If during a qualitative review of a record there appears to be documentation that does not reflect sound practice or the notes appear to have skipped time or "something doesn't look right," the HIM technician is trained to have the record reviewed by a physician advisor (PA). The **physician advisor** volunteers his or her time as part of a hospital committee to review health records for various reasons. The PA can be used for medical record reviews, utilization reviews, quality reviews, surgical case and tissue reviews, other pathological reviews, and a host of blood and laboratory reviews for various medical staff and hospital committees. Several physicians often volunteer as PAs on an annual basis and usually are from diverse backgrounds such as pathology, surgery, medicine, and other disciplines so that reviews can be a true peer review. An example of a true peer review would be a cardiologist reviewing a health record that was documented by another cardiologist and not a physician from any other discipline. **Peer review** is at its best whenever a discipline can review within its own discipline. However, this is not always the case due to the number of PAs who volunteer, especially with smaller facilities or rural facilities that do not have the luxury of a large number of PAs as reviewers each year. These qualitative, quantitative, and peer reviews are more easily done with the electronic health record as data is more readily accessible to reviewers with the need to know basis as defined by HIPAA. Reviews done with the electronic record are assured the data is complete since the record is captured and stored within the system. The review process has greatly benefited from the health record process conversion from a paper-based record to the electronic health record.

Obvious Data Error

Another type of inaccuracy found within patient health records is the obvious data error. Spelling errors are the most common obvious errors and often occur in paper-based health records. As more facilities including hospitals, clinics, and physician offices become computerized, fewer spelling errors will be seen. Many computer systems have built-in regular spell-check and medical spell-check programs helping to reduce errors, and will be discussed further in the next section. Most medical dictionaries are accompanied by a CD that can be downloaded onto the user's PC. This will then only leave errors made by carelessness, such as transposition of numbers when typing a string of numbers. For example:

Original Patient's Medical Record #:	000-47-1039
Transposed Patient's Medical Record #:	000-47-1309

If the admission clerk was hurriedly typing in the medical record number for this patient, it is easy to see how the last three numbers were easily transposed. It is also easy to see how this type of error can be overlooked because the same numbers are there but out of order. Computers can easily find these types of mistakes where humans can easily overlook them.

Wrong Data Codes

Wrong data codes should never occur in any facility. All data codes should be up-to-date. The codes that are used by the HIM department coding staff, such as the ICD coding system, are updated twice annually (October and April) by the **Centers for Medicare and Medicaid Services (CMS)**. Likewise, the CPT coding system is updated annually in January by the American Medical Association (AMA). Because updates for these coding systems are known by the coders, billers, and the computer programmers who update the facility's claims billing computer and chargemaster with the new programs and edits, there should be no reason for using outdated codes. Everyone in the facility, from the administrator to the clerk, is notified of the update schedule because the system usually is scheduled for maintenance at this time for the installation of the updates.

In addition to coding updates, other codes used, such as codes from the state health department, are changed periodically. Whenever codes from various agencies change or there are updates to rules regarding data collection, these are circulated to the facility's administrator for distribution among facility staff as needed. Agencies also post the latest requirements of data rules and collection on their Web sites for those who may not receive the mailings. It is also the responsibility of those technicians who perform data collection to know what agencies send out data changes and when, if they are annual changes, and where to look for updates from each agency that sends out codes.

Data codes must be current or they will not be useful. Outdated information will not be reimbursed; these codes are rejected and payment is denied. This is a waste of time and money. Health information technicians must be proactive and stay on top of data codes to be aware of all changes and when they occur.

Check Your Understanding 3.2

1. The common data set that is overseen by the government agency that oversees the Medicare and Medicaid services is: _____.
   - A. UHDDS
   - B. HEDIS
   - C. OASIS
   - D. ORYX

2. A missing signature from an entry in a health record would be an example of
   _____.
   - A. Retrospective analysis
   - B. Timeliness error
   - C. Qualitative analysis
   - D. Quantitative analysis

3. Who should know of an ICD code change of the healthcare practitioners who are reviewing this record during the patient stay?
   - A. Physician
   - B. Nurse
   - C. In-house coder
   - D. Social worker

Blank Fields

It is imperative to repeat that the patient's health record must be completed. Whether data are entered into fields located as entries on a page in a paper-based record or as entries on a screen in an electronic health record, all data must be entered to be considered complete. If data do not apply, a field usually has several options for the user to choose (such as Not Applicable) so there are no blank fields in the health record. Using the choice of Not Applicable means the user has read the option, there is not a choice that applies from the choices given, and the field was not skipped or left intentionally blank. Other choices when data are not applicable include Not Specified, Not Given, or Not Known.

Multiple Patients, Same Name

Many issues can arise with data accuracy, such as many patients having the same last name or the same first name, raising the possibility that duplicate medical record numbers could be assigned to more than one patient. As an admissions technician processes a patient for admission to the emergency department or the hospital, all concerns about the patient must be questioned to make sure that two different patients with the same or similar name have a different health record number. The technician must be able to question the patient or acquire sufficient data during the admission process to determine that only one patient is given a single unique health record number.

Indexing Errors

For paper-based health records, the MPI was at the mercy of humans for accuracy within the index system. As computers were introduced into healthcare, the MPI was computerized to eliminate many of the indexing errors from handwritten card files. However, errors may still appear due to spelling or a lack of attention to detail when entering data such as patient names into the system.

Errors caused by lack of attention to detail or carelessness result in poor-quality data. The old adage of "garbage in—garbage out" can never be stressed enough. If bad or inaccurate data goes into the system, it is not worth one's time of performing the data entry. This attitude should be the basis for all data entry and data efforts.

HIM professionals are trained to use computer systems to input, manipulate, and collect data, so attention must be paid to the details of the data. Errors made with any index or within the MPI are not acceptable at any level. Error reports are helpful in determining at a surface level if there are errors made at some deeper levels. However, even error reports do not always catch every error. Computer edits also are helpful to the user in identifying some of the errors but again, not every error is caught. It only takes one error for an entire report or collection of data to be considered "unclean". HIM professionals must take ownership individually and pride in efforts to ensure that the quality of work shows in the data entry and data accuracy of the entire data process.

The Importance of Accurate and High-Quality Data—Summary

The significance of data accuracy and data quality cannot be stressed enough. Data must be accurate and precise to reflect what the patient has stated in his or her own words. This type of data is called **subjective data**. An example would be the patient's explanation of his or her chief complaint—how he or she felt on the day of admission in their own words such as "My head is going to burst" or "it hurts really bad." The data in the patient's health record must also be consistent or uniform so that errors are eliminated or greatly reduced. Diagnoses are repeated throughout the health record by practitioners, typically a consistent practice in healthcare.

Earlier in this section, a summary on completeness of the health record was made to review the guidelines that facilities must follow from various regulatory agencies and third-party payers to ensure that health records are complete. (Primarily, completeness of the record is to ensure that patient care is the first priority and so that data elements are not missing and all data are concurrent with regulatory agencies.) Quality data also includes qualitative and quantitative reviews of health records to ensure that the health record is complete with a well-written, peer-reviewed document with no data elements missing. The quality of a well-documented record must be legible, including handwritten orders and notes and signatures, which is a function of the qualitative analysis. Finally, the accessibility of the health record is an issue, primarily for paper-based records in that only one user at a time is able to review the record. For electronic health records, multiple users can view the same health records simultaneously; pending authorization is given for access to these users for permission to view the health record. All of these characteristics that cover data quality in the health record have been published by the American Health Information Management Association (AHIMA) as the **AHIMA Data Quality Model** and are summarized in figure 3.4.

All of these elements have been discussed within the previous section, labeled or not, but have been explained in their simplicity for the beginning health information technician. It is important that the concepts be understood in order for the quality model to function in the HIM and healthcare environment.

Figure 3.4.   AHIMA data quality model

AHIMA Data Quality Model	
Relevancy	Accessibility
Granularity	Timeliness
Consistency	Precision
Accuracy	Currency
Comprehensiveness	

Source: LaTour and Eichenwald Maki 2010, 120–122

Data Integrity: Building It into the Systems

Data integrity must be examined to fully understand accurate and true data. By definition, **data integrity** is the "property that data are true to the source and have not been altered or destroyed in an unauthorized manner or by unauthorized users, the extent to which data are complete, accurate, consistent, and timely" (Abdelhak et al. 2007, 145). Within this section, various threats to data integrity as well as methods that software systems have developed to help keep data safe will be discussed.

Required Fields

To ensure data integrity within the patient's health record, there are many methods that users can build into their paper-based or electronic systems. Because most health records are electronic, they will be the focus of discussion. The data fields within computer screens for capturing data are individual blank fields required to be populated with patient data. A required field is a preset field in which data must be entered before the computer will allow the user to proceed in the program. If these data fields were on paper, the user would interview the patient for data and type the data into the blanks on the paper to complete the data fields. There would be no alerts to let the user know that a data field was skipped or omitted, or if wrong data were entered into a field during entry. With an electronic field, a technician cannot skip ahead in the form, enter other data, and then come back to enter data in this field later. The existence of required fields is one of many reasons why computer-based records are the preferred method for capturing data.

It is determined by the facility which data fields should be set as required, if any. It is good practice to set fields as required for information that is essential for patient care, a facility's needs, or other reporting purposes. A manager must weigh the benefits and disadvantages of required fields to determine what essential information is needed.

Edit Checks

Computerized patient health records have specialized features within the software to minimize errors and aid in data accuracy. **Edit checks** are a standard feature in most health record applications' data entry and data collection software packages. Edit checks are preprogrammed definitions of each data field set up within the software application. So, as data are entered, if any data are different from what has been preprogrammed, an edit message appears on the screen. This edit message is sometimes called a 'flag' because it signals that the user needs to verify the data being entered to ensure that the criteria of the field are met. This serves as a check of the data, hence the term 'edit check,' which basically is a quality verification of data being entered into the system as part of the data collection process.

If the technician has questions, he or she can look at criteria of this data field in greater depth, ask a supervisor to help with this particular data field question, or interview the patient further for more specific data for this field response. Edit checks can be any type of text or number that represents data. For example, 1 = male, 2 = female, and so on, or a drop-down box with several options. Edit checks can also occur when gender does not match for a patient. An example might be similar to the following:

Example Scenario: A 56-year-old Asian male was admitted to the neurology unit with abdominal pains. The workup revealed cholecystitis. The patient was scheduled for a total hysterectomy.

Is there anything unusual about this case? Are men normally scheduled for hysterectomies? This would be an example where an edit check would signal to the technician that something is incorrect.

A message flag would appear on the screen indicating that a hysterectomy is not done for a male patient. The technician would then check the chart for a correct diagnosis and procedure as well as check the patient's gender and verify that the correct patient is in the system.

Drop-Down Menus

With computer-based patient health records, more drop-down menu options are being used with software applications. A drop-down menu is a great option for a technician or health-care practitioner when data needs to be entered. The user simply clicks on the arrow to the right (or left) of a data field and a drop-down menu appears with several choices for selection. Once selected, the data field is automatically populated with the user's selection. A drop-down menu can be used for countless numbers of data fields within the health record. It is used in many documents such as the admission record or the face sheet, the financial record, or the history and physical. Drop-down menus save time because the entire data field item does not have to be typed in the blank.

Help Screens

A help screen built into an application of a computerized health record is comparable to the help function in word processing software. The user can press the designated key on the keyboard to launch the help screen function. The help key can provide tips on functions the system can perform or provide answers regarding "how to" questions about the system. For example, the system can be queried so the user can determine what types of legends are used for the data fields or what the required fields are within the system, especially if the operator's manual is unavailable.

Automatic Save Features

With computerized health records and the easy-to-use features that many software package applications offer, users have the ability to input and save data without the worry of losing valuable information. A built-in automatic save feature will eliminate the need to constantly save data manually every few minutes. An automatic save feature can be set or programmed within the software to save data in the system as often as needed. In Microsoft Word, for example, an automatic Word save function is used and the option to automatically save can be set for a document "from 1 to 120 minutes" (Joos et al. 2006, 124). The automatic save function may save the file, or autorecover files may be saved in various places within different software applications, varying according to the vendor. If a user has ever had a computer crash or has lost power while working in the middle of a document, the value of an automatic save feature is a crucial feature.

Online Reference Linkages

Computerized health records are now advanced enough that software vendors have enabled reference materials to be accessible to the healthcare practitioners through the use of the record software. As a computerized health record is used, a question may arise that may call for some type of reference material. Many software applications have a built-in medical dictionary, drug reference book, table of normal laboratory range values, and other reference aids that healthcare practitioners use daily. In most cases, these built-in reference materials can be accessed quickly and without having to exit the patient's health record screen. A double screen can be used; the computer screen can be minimized on the left (or right) side and the other half of the screen can view the reference book for a quick search of information needed. Online, easy access reference materials save time and enhance the quality of patient care. It is also cost effective because books or reference materials do not need to be purchased separately for each practitioner.

Streamlining Repetitive Data

Data integrity is ensured when data are not compromised. A software application with the ability to streamline data when that data are repetitive is of great benefit to the user. Not all software applications have this feature, but this option is a wonderful bonus that prevents data from being unnecessarily repeated or duplicated. Within a healthcare record, data can easily be repeated accidentally; however, some software applications can detect this and alert the user that duplications have occurred, which allows for the user to rectify the duplicated data immediately. Technology is becoming more effective with each passing day and in this area, streamlining data entry with technology entry to avoid repetitive or duplicate data is a new field and an emerging topic for the future.

User-Friendly Data Fields

The healthcare practitioners who input data into the health record have an enormous duty. As previously discussed, drop-down boxes have proven to be an effective and efficient method for capturing data.

Other types of user-friendly aids within the health record are examples located near a data field to show the user what might be suggested as a possible response for a data field. Many vendors use 'hot spots' throughout their software applications to make the data fields as user friendly as possible. A '**hot spot**' is triggered when the mouse is placed on top of a data field. The mouse changes to another symbol, such as a hand, that for a particular vendor indicates another level of choices from which the user can select. The hot spot is defined at this level and this is where the user can find the explanation for that data field and what data are needed. The exact data fields and which data fields are hot spots depend on each vendor and each software application for the computerized health record software. With this functionality, the facility may set up their software as they wish, so no two applications would be alike.

The Importance of Data Integrity—Summary

Data integrity is as important as the quality of the data: one cannot be more important than the other. Patients, healthcare practitioners, administrators, internal reviewers, external agencies, and all third-party payers (as well as regulatory bodies and accrediting bodies) measure a facility by the data kept. The data must be accurate, timely, consistent, relevant, clear, comprehensive, consistent, and current in its defined state.

Check Your Understanding 3.3

1. What should be done with a data field that has no information that is known or can be entered into this field?

   A. Type in "NA"
   B. Leave it blank
   C. Skip it
   D. Use the return or tab over this field

2. With computerized health records, what is most affected with indexing errors?

   A. MPI
   B. H&P
   C. Discharge summary
   D. Entire health record

3. If every field on the computer screen is a 'required field', what would this affect the most?

   A. Physical resources
   B. Space
   C. Cost
   D. Time

Data Reliability: Uniformity in the System

This section on **data reliability** will focus on the consistency of data. Data should not have any discrepancies within its content. Data must be consistent. There are various methods to ensure that data have reliability, and with technology software applications can aid in this process. This section will focus on data reliability—how various methods of how data can be threatened as well as how technology systems can aid the user in protecting it.

Routine Monitoring of Data

Monitoring of data must be consistent; this is the basis of reliability. The definition of **reliability** is the "repeatability of a measurement" (McWay 2008, 231). In other words, it means that data are checked over and over again, usually by a second person, to determine if the final results are the same as the first results. The data should be monitored regularly, whether daily or on a random basis such as "on every '_nth' number of charts." Monitoring could be at random on whatever the facility determined would provide a good random sample—usually a 10% sample of the total cases is used. This should be a routine process that would be a part of the responsibilities of the data input and collection area because monitoring of the accuracy and monitoring the reliability of data are equally important. During routine monitoring, problems with data can arise to include missing data or lack of quality data. This could be due to the design of the form or screen that collects the data. Usually the vendor or those who design the forms or screens in these systems are not always those who are performing the functions. Those who work with the instrument on a daily basis are the best resource to recommend changes. Other problems that may be encountered while monitoring data consistency could include lack of data because of language barriers in communicating with the patient. Such a barrier could lead to lack of data from the patient's viewpoint, such as the chief complaint and any documentation with follow-up and treatment, including post-discharge instructions.

Data Consistency Checks

Characteristics for data entry should be uniform throughout the patient record to ensure consistency. Health record practitioners must be familiar with the appropriate facility's practices and standards for each record and type of patient visit (that is, inpatient, ambulatory, emergency). Data standards and their quality must be monitored to ensure that consistency in every record is met. For example, one facility may state in their bylaws that records must be completed within 30 days of patient discharge. Another hospital may state in their bylaws that records must be completed within 15 days of patient discharge. The standards can vary by each facility according to their bylaws. Thus, data consistency checks built into software systems aid the healthcare practitioner ensure the documentation is complete for every health record.

The guidelines of data standards as recommended by SDOs as well as regulatory agencies such as Joint Commission and state health departments are the foundations of data documentation. The federal and state rules as well as the facility's own policies and procedures are also guiding principles for healthcare practitioners to follow to help streamline data for consistency. Departments of health information management use procedures such as qualitative and quantitative analysis to aid in checking for data consistency in the records. Quality and utilization (sometimes termed case coordination) departments also review patient records for quality and consistency in documentation. As previously discussed, technology features of computerized software can also help in checking for consistency in the health record data. Built-in software edits verify the data to ensure that data fields match throughout the patient record and that there are no duplicates.

Example: I actually had an abbreviation of "OD OD OD" that I found in a patient record at a specialty hospital. It was written on a progress note some years ago when I was reviewing records. Of course, "overdose" came to my mind first as an abbreviation. I also knew that 'OD' stands for 'oculus dexter' and it also can stand for 'Doctor of Optometry' (Stedman's 2008, 1099). However, to verify the accuracy of these abbreviations in this patient record, I had to query the physician on what these three abbreviations stood for as he was the author of this progress note. You can imagine my surprise when he told me that he wrote this to mean "*one drop* in the *right eye once daily.*"

Abbreviations are extremely easy to use and can be wonderful. However, data must have definitions and be uniform or the type of problem in the above example could be harmful or lethal to patients. If some practitioner had assumed that OD stood for overdose rather than one drop, this would have changed the meaning of the physician's intent. Abbreviations have their place and can be very useful in healthcare, but, they (along with all data) must be defined and all healthcare staff must know the data definitions in order for abbreviations to be consistently used and for the patient to receive the best care possible.

Tracking of Errors and Problems

Technology with computer-based health records has effectively aided healthcare professionals in tracking data errors and other problems of data documentation. Computer software applications continue to improve with the ability to determine data errors made during routine data edits. The analysis of data during system checks can help track errors across systems and networks by comparing the data. This ensures the data are consistent and reliable. Data should agree within the same system and if shared with other systems, the data must agree across networks. If data show inconsistency, the problems must be tracked until the source is found and corrected. Data mining can be the source of tracking data from larger databases and analyzing it downward to the data elements to its primary source. Tracking of errors is not always easy and results are never immediate, but the outcomes are worth the quality time and effort spent during the process.

Trends of Problems Monitored

Data must be monitored on as-needed basis depending on the type of data collected. Data are collected daily, weekly, monthly, and annually. Data types vary tremendously and may include research, billing and claims reimbursement, regulatory agencies, accrediting bodies, quality and utilization studies, administrative duties, risk management functions, statistical reporting, and many other internal and external functions. The types of data collected also vary depending on what agency needs it and for what purpose. Some of the data trends monitored as potential problems include the quality improvement organizations (QIOs) top diagnoses and problem prone areas. As the Centers for Medicare and Medicaid Services (CMS) indicate these areas to the QIOs for review, the top diagnoses listings are collected to review for potential problems. Past scope of services trends identified include heart failure, pneumonia, myocardial infarction, and surgical care improvement. In the same manner, the Joint Commission uses similar core measures as CMS with the addition of pregnancy measures, inpatient psychiatric, children's asthma care, and hospital outpatient department measures (Joint Commission 2009). Trends help to identify areas such as treatment issues or infection rates. Identified trends help to further evaluate and manage such issues for improved overall care and outcomes.

Preventive Maintenance

Data reliability to ensure consistent and accurate data depends on the technological accuracy of the database system used in the storage warehouse and the data retrieval capability as well as the confidentiality, privacy, and security safeguards in place for the data. It is crucial that data are preserved and accurate to the users who are authorized access; in addition, the data must be up-to-date, defined to the users, accessible at all times, consistent, and comprehensive. Users should be trained and know who to contact in the event any problem occurs. An effective preventive maintenance program should have the following:

Policies and Procedures

Policies and procedures should be in place to serve several purposes. They provide protocol to employees to carry out their duties, ensure that problems are resolved properly when encountered, and help to maintain compliance among all. Policies and procedures should be reviewed at least annually, or sooner if changes occur in any processes during the year. These are the step-by-step instructions for the 'how-to' and 'when' in maintaining the system. Policies should include maintenance of the hardware, software, and all peripherals as to the last updates of each and the next scheduled update. Some systems use an electronic reminder system similar to a tickler file to know when it is time for updates. Other systems are notified by vendors with the updates for their software. Policies and procedures must be kept up-to-date on each so that every person knows the maintenance schedule to aid in preventing problems in the system. Policies and procedures also aid in training of new personnel when hired into the facility so that all the information needed about the system is in one place and current.

Maintenance Schedule

It is essential for the facility to develop and follow a maintenance schedule for preventive maintenance and backup of all data retrieval, warehousing, and storage. The facility must follow the policies and procedures that have been developed on the preventive maintenance schedule. The maintenance schedule ensures that data flow processing as well as data retention and all operations are backed up onto other media sources such as optical disks or DVDs for smaller systems or stored in separate systems across the country.

Timely Data Submission and Reporting

If data are collected, they should cover a particular period of time, such as one month or one year. The purpose of collecting data is to have the most accurate and up-to-date information available for the users and those who receive it in reporting, such as internal and external agencies. Collected data usually have a deadline, by which time information must be submitted or reported to the requesting or mandated agency or end user. Data can only be reliable if submitted and reported on a timely basis.

Data Analysis: Assessment of Information

This section of data analysis will focus on the evaluation of data. The quality of data is determined from an assessment of its content. According to McWay, "data quality refers to more than just the 'correctness' of data, inherent in the concept of quality data is that data must be comprehensive, current, relevant, accurate, complete, legible, timely, and appropriate" (McWay 2008, 152). Health information management (HIM) technicians review data in various methods. As previously discussed, qualitative and quantitative analyses are two methods of data analysis used by HIM technicians. There are many other tools of data analysis and assessment to be covered.

Data Analysis Assessment Tools

The instruments used to collect, measure, and display data are extremely vital to the data analysis and outcomes process. Data analysis tools used include charts and graphs, which are effective at evaluating information over time to identify any trends within the data. As information is plotted on a graph, it is easy to see a pattern or trend appear. The trend or a pattern then may indicate a problem area or need for a focused review. Although many problems are found by tracking data over time, charts are also used to denote events or occurrences by frequencies. An example of this is shown in figure 3.5.

Figure 3.5 is an example showing events such as files for data mapping being tracked over time against the number of full-time employees. Even if this example is not fully understandable to its audience, the graph still makes sense to every reader. It can be understood from this graph that over the period of time from March to July, which was more than one year, the number of files for data mapping increased as the number of FTEs decreased. Of course, whether this was a positive or negative outcome is unclear from this example. It is taken out of context from the article and all the parameters of the problem and the factors involved would need to be known for a determination. However, the example graph makes the point that charts and graphs illustrate events or occurrences over time.

Useful Data Tools

Several types of data graphs and charts are effective means of conveying information to the user. The **flowchart** is a tool that is used to show movement of "people, materials, paperwork within a work setting" (Brassard and Ritter 1994). The flowchart is used as an instrument to help see how the flow of work moves so that redundancies can easily be spotted, as well as duplication of efforts. Another tool that is used to show work over time, especially in large projects, is the **Gantt chart**. This tool is an effective instrument for planning and working with large detailed projects. A large project that has many phases or smaller goals can be placed on a Gantt chart. The time period is also plotted using the Gantt chart so that the smaller tasks or goals are planned on the large scale to see how they fit into the scheme of the project.

Other data tools are effective visual instruments when working with information. The PERT chart is useful when working with large projects that are complex and detailed. The **Project Evaluation and Review Technique (PERT) chart** uses numbers and letters to help evaluate the time needed to perform tasks or events and the activities in order. These charts are done by using numbers for the days or hours on the PERT chart and by using letters for the order of the tasks.

Charts and graphs are the best visual displays to aid in making data easily understandable to others. Labels and other easy identifiers make charts and graphs an effective means to communicate data to users both internally and externally.

Figure 3.5.   File count to number of FTEs

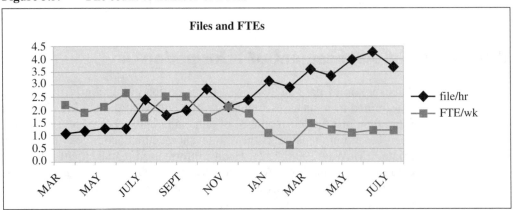

Source: Lambrecht and Wilson 2007

Check Your Understanding 3.4

1. The common graph used for movement of people or flow of work is the

   _____.

   A. Gantt chart
   B. PERT chart
   C. Flowchart
   D. Data Quality Model

2. A graph that is used to denote time and activities for complex projects would be the

   _____.

   A. Gantt chart
   B. PERT chart
   C. Flowchart
   D. Data Quality Model

3. The repeatability of a measure is used for data quality and is called _____.

   A. analysis
   B. reliability
   C. uniformity
   D. clarity

Summary

The quality of data as presented within this chapter depends on the integrity of the data as well as the clarity and currency of the data. The information must be relevant, current, accurate, and appropriate. All of these elements, as discussed in AHIMA's Data Quality Model within this chapter, are of utmost importance when ensuring data quality. SDOs have been created to implement consistency and uniformity in data in the nation and around the world. The timeliness of data submissions in the reporting of information and presenting data to users also is part of the quality process. The quality of data begins with data collection and continues until data are submitted and reported to the end user. Even as data are maintained and stored in the warehouses, networks, and databases, technology must include the quality characteristics discussed in this chapter. Without quality data, there exists no information, only useless data.

References

Abdelhak, M., S. Gnostic, M.A. Hanker, and E. Jacobs. 2007. *Health Information: Management of a Strategic Resource*, 3rd ed. St. Louis, MO: Saunders/Elsevier.

Amatayakul, M.K. 2007. *Electronic Health Records: A Practical Guide for Professionals and Organizations*, 3rd ed. Chicago: AHIMA.

Brassard, M. and D. Ritter. 1994. *The Memory Jogger II*. Methuen, MA: Goal/QPC, Inc.

Burton, L.R. 2003. The life cycle of a project: How to plan for performance improvements. *Journal of AHIMA* 74(9):34ff.

Fenton, S., K. Giannangelo, C. Kale, and R. Scichilone. 2007. Data standards, data quality, and interoperability. *Journal of AHIMA* 78(2):extended online edition.

Giannangelo, K., ed. 2006. *Healthcare Code Sets, Clinical Terminologies, and Classification Systems*. Chicago: AHIMA.

Johns, M.L., ed. 2007. *Health Information Management Technology: An Applied Approach,* 2nd ed. Chicago: AHIMA.

Joint Commission. 2009. Performance Measurement Initiatives. http://www.jointcommission.org/PerformanceMeasurement/PerformanceMeasurement/default.htm.

Joos, I., N.I. Whitman, M.J. Smith, and R. Nelson. 2006. *Introduction to Computers for Healthcare Professionals,* 4th ed. Sudbury, MA: Jones and Bartlett, Publishers.

Lambrecht, J., and P.S. Wilson. 2007 (October). Use of six sigma in data mapping. *Proceedings of the American Health Information Management Association's 79th National Convention and Exhibit.*

LaTour, K.M. and S. Eichenwald Maki, eds. 2006. *Health Information Management: Concepts, Principles, and Practice,* 2nd ed. Chicago: AHIMA.

LaTour, K.M. and S. Eichenwald Maki, eds. 2010. *Health Information Management: Concepts, Principles, and Practice,* 3rd ed. Chicago: AHIMA.

McCoy, M.J., B.J. Bomentre, and K. Crous. 2006. Speaking of EHRS: Parsing EHR systems and the start of IT projects. *Journal of AHIMA* 77(4):24–28.

McWay, D.C. 2008. *Today's Health Information Management: An Integrated Approach.* Clifton Park, NY: Thomson/Delmar Learning.

Nationwide Health Information Network. 2008. Nationwide Health Information Network (NHIN): Background & Scope. http://healthit.hhs.gov/portal/server.pt?open=512&objID=1142&parentname=CommunityPage&parentid=25&mode=2&in_hi_userid=10741&cached=true.

Stedman's, ed. 2008. *Stedman's Medical Dictionary for the Health Professions and Nursing: Illustrated,* 6th ed. Philadelphia, PA: Lippincott, Williams, & Wilkins.

Chapter 4
Databases

Objectives

- Assist in the development of a database.
- Develop and manage the data dictionary.
- Develop queries to retrieve data contained in the database.
- Read and understand an entity-relationship diagram.
- Identify the primary key contained in an entity.
- Differentiate between a data repository and a data warehouse.
- Expound on the ways that data mining can be useful.
- Complete simple normalization of data.
- Differentiate between the various types of data.

Key Terms

Clinical data repository (CDR)
Computer-aided software engineering (CASE) software
Data definition
Data definition language (DDL)
Data flow diagram (DFD)
Data manipulation language (DML)
Data mining
Data modeling

Data repository
Data warehouse
Database
Database management system (DBMS)
Entity-relationship diagram
Foreign key
Hierarchical database model
Java
Natural language queries

Network database model
Normalization
Object-oriented database
Online analytical processing (OLAP)
Query by example
Primary key
Relational database model
Structured query language (SQL)

Healthcare facilities collect and store a tremendous amount of administrative, financial, and clinical data. A database can assist the facility in data sharing and workflow, and clinical and managerial decision making. A **database** is defined as "a collection of data carefully organized to be of value to the user" (Austin and Boxerman 2003, 127). In other words, a database is a tool used to collect, retrieve, report, and analyze data. A database cannot function without a **database management system (DBMS)** to manipulate and control the data stored within the database.

There are many advantages to a database. Databases allow data to be stored in one place and accessed by many different systems. This reduces the redundancy of data and improves data consistency. The decrease in redundancy leads to improved data quality, which in turn saves time by reducing the duplication of data entry. The improved consistency of data improves data quality and ultimately patient care (Austin and Boxerman 2003, 132). The use of a database allows for the standardization of data forms, names of data elements, and documentation, which makes moving from various screens and various information systems easier for the users. A database requires a database administrator to keep the database operational and working at peak performance (Hebda et al. 2005). A database allows the database administrator to implement security measures to control access to the data (Kroenke 2008). These security measures may include requiring a username and password for each user, control measures of what data the user has access to, and what the user can do with the data. Another advantage of a database is that the data are independent of software applications and therefore data can be shared (Austin and Boxerman 2003, 132).

Data Definitions

Data Elements

The healthcare facility must develop a database that meets its needs. These needs are identified by researching the needs of the users and the external stakeholders such as the Joint Commission. The core data elements stored in the data are often controlled by data sets such as those described in chapter 3. The facility can add other data elements to meet the needs of the organization, such as accreditation and other needs. The data elements may be related to administration, such as patient name and medical record number; or they may be financial in nature, such as the charge for the hospital room or the laboratory test performed; or clinical in nature, such as history of present illness or follow-up plan.

Structure of Table

Within a database exists a file made up of a number of tables containing all of the data related to a facility. Within these tables are the hierarchical levels previously described as fields and records of data in chapter 2. The table contains all data related to a particular subject or concept such as a patient and each of these tables contains records pertaining to each individual patient. Within each record are individual fields. Examples of fields are patient last name, social security number, or date of birth. Database managers are able to display the information about the data onscreen when a user has a request for particular data. The **query** is a search for data that meet specific criteria the user requests within subsets of the database (White 2008, 121). The queries sort and filter the data with the database manager software to display all records that meet the criteria for user review. If the results of the query are too great, the criteria for the search can be narrowed to provide further filtering for a more desirable result.

Within the database, the tables organize the information of all records into rows and columns. With the enormous amount of information stored in a database, how can a query within a single record locate information? Each record is set up with a primary key as it is entered into the database. One of the fields will be the unique identifier that identifies each record. This unique identifier is called the primary key. A **primary key** is a unique patient identifier used in a healthcare database (Abdelhak et al. 2007, 276). When the database software was created, the developer chose one field to be the primary key. Historically, this was sometimes a patient's social security number; however, because of privacy issues, this is not recommended now. Many facilities use a patient's health record number or another uniquely assigned number from the facility for this purpose. The primary key is used in the relational database model discussed later in the chapter. The value contained in the primary key field cannot be duplicated; thus, two patients cannot have the same medical record number. Sometimes the primary key of one table is included in another table. When this happens, the second key is called a **foreign key**.

The standard language for a relational data model is structured query language (SQL) (Austin and Boxerman 2003, 139). This language is used to manage the database and to retrieve data. For details, see chapter 6.

Types of Fields

The data collected in each field can take a number of formats based on the needs of the field.

- Alphabetic fields accept only alphabetic characters. Data elements of this field type include patient name.

- Numeric fields accept only numbers that can be calculated. This would include charges, but would not include zip codes and the medical record number.

- Alphanumeric fields accept alphabetic characters, numbers, or a combination of the two. Alphanumeric fields include street address, zip codes, and phone numbers.

- Time/date fields contain only a date or dates.

- Auto-numbering fields create a unique number that will never be assigned again. This could be the medical record number.

The type of data collected in each field is identified in the data dictionary, which is described later in this chapter.

When developing the data elements that go into a database, the fields should be normalized. **Normalization** is breaking the data elements into the level of detail desired by the facility. For example, last name and first name should be in separate fields as should city, state, and zip code. This allows the user to search or otherwise manipulate any of the data elements. Conversely, if the city and state were stored in the same field, the user would not be able to run reports or query the database based on state; because the name of the city varies widely in length, the computer does not know where the city ends and where the state begins. For example, the city of Opp, Alabama is much shorter than San Luis Obispo, California. The latter also has three words in the name so the computer cannot be made to look for a space or a number of characters. By breaking the city and state into different fields, searches by city or state can be done with ease.

Normalized Data	Unnormalized Data
Last name	Last name, first name
First name	Middle initial
Middle initial	Address
Address	City, state, zip
City	
State	
Zip	

Once all of the necessary individual data elements are determined, a common **data definition** should be developed for each of the data elements because not everyone defines terms in the same way. For example, time of admission could be the time that the patient walked into the healthcare facility, the time that the patient's admission was entered into the registration system, or the time that the patient reaches the assigned patient room.

Check Your Understanding 4.1

1. The best choice for field type used for the medical record number is:

   A. alphanumeric
   B. numeric
   C. auto-numbering
   D. alphabetic

2. The term used to describe breaking data elements into the level of detail needed to retrieve the data is:

   A. normalization
   B. data definitions
   C. primary key
   D. database management system

3. In a database, which term describes how data about an individual patient are stored?

   A. Field
   B. Table
   C. Row
   D. File

4. The term used to describe a key from one table that is located in another table is:

   A. primary key
   B. foreign key
   C. normalization
   D. data definitions

5. What type of field is used to enter numbers that cannot be calculated?

   A. Alphanumeric
   B. Numeric
   C. Auto-numbering
   D. Alphabetic

Database Management System

The **DBMS** controls and manipulates the database to meet the needs of the user. It controls the ability to create, read, write, and delete data stored in the database. Examples of a DBMS are Oracle, Sybase, and Microsoft Access (Oppel 2004). Oppel identifies six functions for a DBMS. These are:

- Moving data to and from the physical data files as needed.

- Managing concurrent data access by multiple users, including provisions to prevent simultaneous updates from conflicting with one another.

- Managing transactions so that each transaction's database changes are an all-or-nothing unit of work. In other words, if the transaction succeeds, all database changes made by it are recorded in the database.

- Support for a query language, which is a system of commands that a database user employs to retrieve data from the database.

- Provisions for backing up the database and recovering from failures.

- Security mechanisms to prevent unauthorized data access and modification (Oppel 2004).

There are three parts to the DBMS:

- Data definition language (DDL)
- Data manipulation language (DML)
- Data dictionary

The **data definition language** (DDL) translates how data are stored in the computer from the physical view to one that is understandable by the user. This user view is called the logical view. The DDL creates the tables utilized in a relational data. Another task of the DDL is to define relationships between data (Austin and Boxerman 2003, 137). In addition, the DDL controls the security of the database.

The **data manipulation language** (DML) accesses, makes changes to, and retrieves data from the database. These capabilities can easily be performed in a database without the user being an experienced computer programmer. To retrieve data, a query is generated. The term 'query' is used to describe selecting records that meet specific criteria. Queries may also perform calculations on the data, such as calculating the average length of stay. Queries can also screen data for inclusion or exclusion. Three user methods to access data contained in the database are (Austin and Boxerman 2003, 138):

- Natural language queries
- Query by example (QBE)
- Structured query language

Natural Language Queries

Natural language queries allow the user to use common English words to tell the database which data are needed (Austin and Boxerman 2003, 138). For example, the user may enter a query by typing "list all of the patients whose principal procedure is 47.01." This command would generate a list of patients who had the principal procedure of laparoscopic appendectomy. Another example may be, "How many patients were discharged on August 1, 2009?" Although natural language queries are easy for the user to learn and use, the concept is still in its infancy and therefore is not robust enough to be widely used. To process the query, the system searches key words in the question in order to fulfill the request. Some systems may allow the use of voice recognition, thus eliminating the need to type in the request.

Query by Example

Query by example (QBE) is a query method commonly used by microcomputers (Austin and Boxerman 2003, 138). The user only has to point and click to choose tables and fields contained in the database. The system then allows the user to choose whether the entries that meet those criteria should be included or excluded from the query. For example, the user may choose the patient table and discharge date as the field. The user can then tell the system to include patients discharged May 1 through May 31, 2009. Only the patients with a discharge date within that range would be included in the results of the query. Boolean search capabilities such as "and," "or," and "not" may be used to narrow down the data to specifically what the user needs. For example, the query could be to retrieve patients who had a principal diagnosis of cholecystitis and a principal procedure of laparoscopic cholecystectomy. Truncation such as the wildcard may be used to look for variations in spelling or characters (Englebardt and Nelson 2002). For example, the user could search for patients whose admission date is greater than, or before, a specific date. The wildcard would be used to indicate that the query should identify data that meet the partial information provided. For example, a query of 250.* would retrieve all diabetes codes such as 250.00, 250.02, 250.10 and so on. Other query tools include the greater than and less than options.

Structured Query Language

Structured query language, better known as SQL, is used to query data. SQL uses simple commands such as "select" to control the query. SQL is discussed in more detail in chapter 6.

Data Dictionary

The data dictionary describes the data used by the system. It also controls the quality of data. This control is accomplished by standardizing data collection (AHIMA e-HIM Work Group on EHR Data Content 2006). The data dictionary is used to improve data consistency because fields are known by the same title from system to system. For example, the data element that describes the number assigned to each patient visit is identified by a number of names such as encounter number, billing number, and patient number. The data dictionary would require this field to be called encounter number or some other title consistently throughout all systems.

There should be two types of data dictionaries. One is a DBMS that defines the data, catalogs attributes of the data element, and defines relationships between the data. According to LaTour and Eichenwald Maki (2006), a DBMS data dictionary should have at least the following information:

- Table name

- All attribute or field names

- A description of each attribute

- The data type of the attribute (text, number, data, and so on)

- The format of each attribute, such as DD-MM-YYYY

- The size of each attribute such as 11 characters in a social security number (including dashes)

- An appropriate range of values, such as integers 1000000–999999 for the health record number

- Whether the attribute is required

- Relationships among attributes

The data dictionary may also control if a mask is used and if so, what form it takes. For example, if a patient's home telephone number is entered as 5555555555, numbers could appear as (555) 555-5555. Another example of where a mask could be used is social security number. The social security number of 123456789 could be entered and it appears in the system as 123-45-6789.

Austin and Boxerman's (2003) view of the data dictionary adds several other pieces of information to the information collected on each data elements. These added attributes are:

- Person in the organization with the right to make changes to the data elements

- The date that the data element was last changed

- Programs and reports that use the data elements

The second type of data dictionary is an organization-wide data dictionary. The purpose of this data dictionary is to encourage data quality. Members within the organization meet to identify the definitions of each data element and their formats (LaTour and Eichenwald Maki 2006). Table 4.1 shows an abbreviated sample of a data dictionary.

Table 4.1.   Abbreviated data dictionary

Field Name	Last Name	First Name	Medical Record Number	Date of Birth	Gender
Data type	Text	Text	Text	Alphanumeric	Alphanumeric
Format	A–Z, ', -	A–Z	0–9	MM-DD-YYYY	M, F, U
Field size	25	25	10	8	1
Range			0000000001-0009999999		
Required	Yes	Yes	Yes	Yes	Yes

Check Your Understanding 4.2

1. What is the term used to describe a search that uses commands such as "and" and "not"?

   A. Boolean search
   B. Natural language queries
   C. SQL
   D. Data dictionary

2. What component of the DBMS controls security?

   A. Data manipulation language
   B. Data definition language
   C. Data dictionary
   D. All of these control security

3. The term used to describe how a data element is displayed is:

   A. Queries
   B. DBMS
   C. Mask
   D. Wildcard

4. The type of query that uses wildcards and Boolean searches is:

   A. Query by example
   B. SQL
   C. Natural language queries
   D. All of these queries use them

5. The title of a data element is recorded in the:

   A. Data manipulation language
   B. Data definition language
   C. Data dictionary
   D. Natural language query

Data Modeling

Data modeling is the design of the database needed for the organization. The model should be based on the organization's strategic plan and should identify the data elements to be collected and the relationship between the data elements. The data model is a pictorial representation of what the database should represent to the users. This pictorial representation contains all of the entities appropriate for the facility. It also shows the technical database structure to be used in the database.

There are three levels of data models—conceptual data model, logical data model, and physical data model (Johns 2002). The conceptual data model is not tied to a particular database model, but rather defines the requirements for the database to be developed. This conceptual data model is the basis for the logical and physical data models.

According to Johns (2002, 146), the logical data model "is the view of the data by a specific group of users or by a specific processing application." For example, the nursing department would look at the data differently than the HIM department and the HIM department would look at it differently than the marketing department. The tools used vary by the type of database involved, but may include the entity-relationship diagram. Data modeling generally includes the entity-relationship diagram or the semantic object model. The **entity-relationship diagram** is a common type of data modeling that focuses on relationships between entities. An entity is a person, location, thing, or concept that is to be tracked in the database. In healthcare, entities would include items such as patient, physician, or laboratory test. Each entity has attributes, which are facts or data about the entity. Some examples of attributes of the entity patient include:

- Medical record number (primary key)
- Last name
- First name
- Middle initial
- Street address
- City
- State
- Zip
- Home phone
- Cell phone
- Work phone
- Date of birth
- Social security number

Each entity would have a unique identifier. A patient's unique identifier could be the medical record number or social security number. In an entity-relationship diagram, entities are linked together to show relationships between the two. There are several types of relationships, such as one-to-one, one-to-many, and many-to-many. For example, a patient may have many physicians, a patient may have many laboratory tests, and a physician may have many patients. Examples of these relationships are shown in Figures 4.1 and 4.2.

Figure 4.1. **One-to-one relationship**

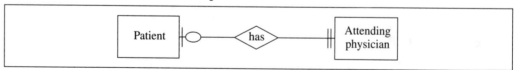

Figure 4.2. **One-to-many relationship**

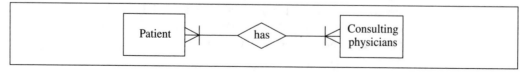

The physical data model shows how the data are physically stored within the database. The users are not involved with this level of the database due to the technical complexity of the physical data model. With the current sophisticated databases, the emphasis on the physical data model has diminished (Johns 2002).

Data modeling tools are used to create the data model. **Computer-aided software engineering (CASE) software** is designed to create many of the diagrams and other tools used in the data model. CASE software can develop tools such as the entity-relationship diagrams described above as well as **data flow diagrams** (DFDs). A DFD is a diagram of how data flows within the database. The DFD is a good way to show management and other nontechnical users the system design. It is also a way to introduce the overall design of the system without getting bogged down in the details. These details can be shown on other diagrams. Unfortunately, developing and updating a DFD is a timely process and may be difficult to design if the user does not have the necessary level of detail or if the data flow is constantly changing.

Another tool is the semantic object model. This model is similar to the entity-relationship diagrams in that there are entities, attributes, and identifiers. The difference is that the semantic object model objects also document what the objects can do (McWay 2008).

Check Your Understanding 4.3

1. The software used to generate data flow diagrams and other data modeling tools is called:

   A. CASE
   B. entity-relationship diagram
   C. database management system
   D. logical data model

2. The data model that defines the requirement of the database is:

   A. conceptual data model
   B. logical data model
   C. physical data model
   D. all three models define the requirements

3. In a database the concept of patient is an example of a(n):

   A. entity
   B. relationship
   C. data flow diagram
   D. CASE software

4. The entity-relationship diagram is used in which type of data model?

   A. Conceptual data model
   B. Logical data model
   C. Physical data model
   D. All three models

5. An attribute:

   A. is an assumption about an entity
   B. is defined by the data dictionary
   C. is a fact about an entity
   D. is a type of data model

Common Database Models

A database model is the logical constructs used to represent how data are stored and the relationships between the data. Four database models can be used (Johns 2002):

- Relational
- Hierarchical
- Network
- Object-oriented

Relational

The most common database model is the **relational database model** (Amatayakul 2007, 211). It is "one of the older models developed by E.F. Codd in the early 1970s on the premise that all data are stored in tables with relationships among the tables" (Abdelhak et al. 2007, 276).

In the table, the data are stored in rows and columns much like a spreadsheet. An example of the relational database model is Microsoft Access. Each row in the table is called a record and each column or field is a single piece of data. A relational database must have two or more tables to be a database; otherwise, it would be a flat file.

In relational models, a certain field can be designated as a primary key. As previously discussed, this means that a search for certain criteria of this field will speed up the process. Furthermore, in a relational model two tables can be matched by using the search criteria so searching can be done across tables. "Because rows in a table have no inherent order, they are simply added to as they grow" (Amatayakul 2007, 211).

The relational database has a number of advantages. First, it is flexible because the file is not tied to a specific application, like a .docx file is tied to Microsoft Word 2007. The database can be used by many different applications. The relational database allows the database administrator to control access to certain tables in order to provide security for the data contained in that database. Also, because data are entered only one time, data consistency and quality are improved. This one-time data entry not only improves the data but the efficiency of the healthcare organization. Finally, because data are stored in a single location, the user will have the most current data available (Johns 2002). Please see Table 4.2 for an example of the table in the relational database.

Hierarchical

Another database model is the **hierarchical model.** This model, like the name implies, structures the data in a hierarchy very similar to an organization chart. Similar to a tree structure, the trunk of the tree would be the starting point or the initial query by the user, and as the search narrows or goes forward, each branch of the tree becomes smaller, progressing outward toward the leaves of the tree, which is the endpoint of the search. Each piece of data in the database is called a node. A hierarchical data model stores data in a tree structure. Pointers indicate where in this tree structure the data are stored. A parent-child relationship is created by the relationships developed by the pointer. The relationship can be described as one to many. This means that a parent can have many children but a child can have only one parent (Austin and Boxerman 2003, 134).

Table 4.2.   Example of table in a relational database

Medical Record Number	Last Name	First Name	DOB	Admitting Date	Discharge Date
123456	Smith	Harry	10/10/1963	4/17/2008	4/21/2008
234567	Jones	Patricia	11/8/1956	5/14/2008	5/27/2008
345678	Adams	Georgia	1/31/1920	4/23/2008	4/25/2008
134534	Warren	Barbara	3/12/2003	5/1/2008	5/4/2008

As mentioned before, in the hierarchical data model, access to data starts at the top of the hierarchy and moves downward. For example in figure 4.3, the hierarchy moves from patient, to laboratory test, and then to name of test. An example of parents and nodes is given in figure 4.3. In that example, the node patient is parent to three child nodes. These three nodes are: laboratory test, attending physician, and radiology examination. The node laboratory test has four child nodes. Then at the next level, laboratory test becomes a parent to four children: name of test, date of test, time of test, and test results.

The hierarchical database model is not always user friendly because it may require developers of the system to program through the records and system to connect records. The platform is an older model and is not compatible with the current EHR systems (Amatayakul 2007, 210). Two other disadvantages of the hierarchical database model is that many-to-many relationships are difficult to depict and it is challenging to use the data for more than one purpose (Abdelhak, 2007, 277).

Network

The **network database model**, illustrated in figure 4.4, uses pointers to connect data. The nodes are called owners and members rather than parent and child nodes as in the hierarchical model. A node in the network data model can have more than one parent, unlike in the hierarchical data model (Austin and Boxerman 2003).

Object-Oriented

The **object-oriented database** is a database model that handles text, images, audio, video, and other objects. In the model these images and other nontext items are stored as objects with hierarchy and a navigational style of programming. (Oppel 2004, 15) defines an object as "a logical grouping of related data and program logic that represents a real world thing" such as a patient, physician, or test. Each data element is called a variable.

Figure 4.3.   Example of a hierarchical data model

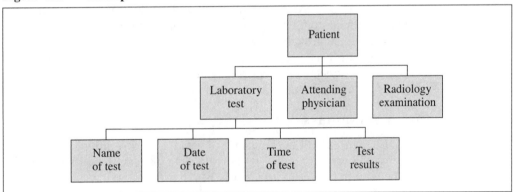

Figure 4.4.   Example of a network data model

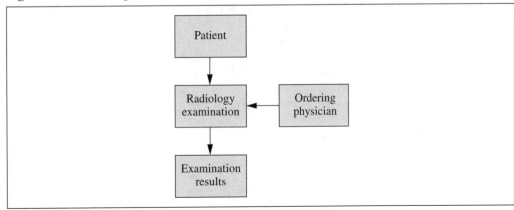

The object-oriented database uses programming tools such as Java. **Java** is a programming language that was designed to be used on the Internet. It uses applets, which are programs that reside on HTML Web pages (Oppel 2004). When the users access the Web page, a window appears, asking the user to install the Java applet.

Two concepts related to the object-oriented model are encapsulation and inheritance. Encapsulation is defining the characteristics of an object. For example, a laboratory test would have a name, test result, time, and date. In the object-orientated database an object can inherit properties from another object. This characteristic is called inheritance (Oppel 2004). An example of this is attending physician and consultant. Both have name, address, specialty, phone number, and other data elements in common.

Data Warehouses and Data Repository

Data in healthcare facilities are collected in many different systems, both clinical and administrative. The data from these systems are frequently centralized into a single database. Two options for this single database are the data warehouse and the data repository. The **data repository** is a database that stores patient-specific data from many different systems. A **data warehouse** also stores data from many different systems and includes historical and current information. The data warehouse is designed to quickly analyze data.

Data Repository

A data repository is a database that is developed in an open format, thus allowing the facility to use it for multiple systems. This open format allows the facility to access data stored in various systems from one source (Amatayakul 2007). The data repository is updated by the various systems in real time, thus providing users with access to the most current information available. This real-time access to data is called online/real-time transaction processing. A data repository may utilize a relational database model.

The database may store clinical, administrative, and financial information data. Other data repositories store one specific type of data—for example, a data repository that stores clinical information such as that from a laboratory information system or a pharmacy information system. This type of data repository is called a **clinical data repository (CDR)** (Tan 2005). Object-oriented databases may also be used to store video, audio, images, and other types of data. The primary key is used to link the data between the various data repositories.

Data Warehouse

Data warehouses hold an abundance of data from many different source systems. The source systems will vary depending on how the data warehouse will be used. The data warehouse can be used in healthcare to identify best practices in patient care, to identify data that can provide the competitive advantage, and to improve efficiency. The data warehouse is designed for specific types of analysis such as patient care or business. For example, a data warehouse may be designed to look for trends in patient care. This type of data warehouse will require information from all of the clinical information systems, the financial information system, the clinical provider order entry, and other information systems. These systems would be chosen for inclusion in the data warehouse because they provide data on the care provided to the patient, the costs of that care, the tests ordered, and the alerts identified, for example. It does not include systems such as the chart locator and chart deficiency systems used in the HIM department; these systems have no bearing on identifying trends in patient care. The data warehouse is updated periodically, rather than in real time as is the EHR or the data repository. There should be a predetermined policy about the frequency of the updates and how long data should be retained.

Data Mart

A data mart is a subset of the data warehouse designed for a single purpose or specialized use. The data mart performs the same type of analyses as a data warehouse; however, the target area is narrower. There are a number of reasons why a data mart is desired; for example, the costs of managing the data mart are lower than those associated with the data warehouse, and the data in the system can be scaled down to only those data required for the project. The facility may choose to develop the data warehouse before the data mart, or the data mart can be developed first, or both can be developed at the same time. This order of development depends on the needs of the organization. Examples of how a data mart may be used include patient satisfaction and research. Patient satisfaction would not require the patient-specific information that would be stored in the data warehouse, but it would include the types of services, the nursing unit, and other basic information in addition to the patient survey or other patient satisfaction information collected. The data mart can be used in research because it can be used to provide de-identified information and the limited information required to conduct the research, and protect the confidentiality of the patient by providing only the minimum information necessary.

Data Mining

McWay (2002) defines **data mining** as "the process of finding unknown dependencies in large data sets using automated means." Data mining may also be called database exploration or information discovery. Data mining is used to analyze data to identify patterns that would be unnoticed without the analysis. Data mining requires sophisticated software such as decision trees, genetic algorithms, neural networks, predictive models, rule induction, and fuzzy logic. These techniques are described as follows:

- A decision tree is visually diagrammed as a tree-shaped configuration. This configuration allows rules to be defined that are used to make a decision.

- Genetic algorithms determine the best model to be used because they are able to enhance other algorithms.

- Neural networks are used to predict actions and classify data. They are nonlinear predictive models that improve with practice.

- Predictive models identify patterns. Once a pattern is identified, the model is able to calculate the odds that a specific action will occur.

- Rule induction identifies patterns from if/then statements. Statistical significance tests are used on the data.

- Fuzzy logic is the method of data mining used when concepts are imprecise.

Once the data pattern has been identified, the facility must decide how to use the information.

Online Analytical Processing

According to LaTour and Eichenwald Maki (2006, 581), **online analytical processing (OLAP)** is a "computing technique for summarizing, consolidating, viewing, and applying formula to and synthesizing data according to multiple dimensions." The use of OLAP turns the data warehouse into a decision support tool because it can analyze large amounts of data quickly by drilling down into the data. It can help the facility use operational data that it already has and use it to make strategic decisions.

Common Uses/Examples on Healthcare and Health Information Management

Healthcare collects an abundance of data and retains these data for years. Unless the data are turned into information, they have no real value to the organization. HIM professionals work together with database administrators, other information technology staff, and the end users to ensure that the data stored within the data warehouse will meet the needs of the users. The HIM professional is often a liaison between the information technology staff and the end user. The HIM professional can be involved in data mining by defining the data to be collected and stored in the data warehouse. The HIM professional can build data quality into the databases contained in the data warehouse. This can be done by building a data dictionary, populating drop-down boxes, building edits, and by building other data quality measures into the system. Examples of how data mining can be used in healthcare, including HIM, include identifying:

- Best practices in patient care
- Medication adverse effects
- Potential fraud and abuse violations
- Patterns of mortality and morbidity

Having this type of information enables the facility to use new information to improve services, patient care, and other functions. As more data are entered, the facility can continue to run analyses to determine if other patterns appear.

Check Your Understanding 4.4

1. Which of the following is a technique used in data mining?

   A. Java
   B. Data repository
   C. Data mart
   D. Fuzzy logic

2. The database model that uses a table as the basis for the design is:

   A. relational
   B. network
   C. hierarchical
   D. object-oriented

3. The concept of parent/child is used in which database model?

   A. Relational
   B. Network
   C. Hierarchical
   D. Object-oriented

4. Which term is a true statement about the data warehouse?

   A. The data warehouse is updated in real-time.
   B. The data warehouse stores a subset of data from the clinical data repository.
   C. The data warehouse is used for a single purpose.
   D. The data warehouse is updated periodically.

5. A programming language designed to be used over the Internet that is used in an object-oriented database model is called:

   A. CASE software
   B. applet
   C. Java
   D. object query language

References

Abdelhak, M., S. Grostick, M.A. Hanken, and E. Jacobs. 2007. *Health Information: Management of a Strategic Resource*. St. Louis, MO: Saunders Elsevier.

AHIMA e-HIM Work Group on EHR Data Content. 2006. Guidelines for Developing a Data Dictionary. *Journal of AHIMA* 77(2): 64A-D.

Amatayakul, M.K. 2007. *Electronic Health Records: A Practical Guide for Professionals and Organizations,* 3rd ed. Chicago: AHIMA.

Austin, C.J. and S.B. Boxerman. 2003. *Information Systems for Healthcare Management.* Chicago: Health Administration Press.

Burke, L. and B. Weill. 2009. *Information Technology for the Health Professions.* Upper Saddle River, NJ: Pearson Prentice Hall.

Duffy, P.G. 1997. Data dictionaries: An overview. *Journal of AHIMA* 68(2):30–34.

Englebardt, S.P. and R. Nelson. 2002. *Health Care Informatics: An Interdisciplinary Approach.* St. Louis, MO: Mosby.

Farishta, M. 2001. More than a DATABASE: Mining your data for decision making success. *Journal of AHIMA* 72(10):28–32.

Hebda, T., P. Czar, and C. Mascara. 2005. *Handbook of Informatics for Nurses and Health Care Professionals.* Upper Saddle River, NJ: Pearson Prentice Hall.

Johns, M.L. ed. *Health Information Management Technology: An Applied Approach.* Chicago: AHIMA.

Johns, M.L. 2002. *Information Management for Health Care Professions,* 2nd ed. Clinton Park, NY: Delmar Learning.

Kroenke, D.M. 2008. *Experiencing MIS.* Upper Saddle River, NJ: Pearson Prentice Hall.

LaTour, K.M. and S. Eichenwald Maki, eds. 2006. *Health Information Management: Concepts, Principles, and Practice.* Chicago: AHIMA.

McWay, D. 2008. *Today's Health Information Management: An Integrated Approach.* Clifton Park, NY: Delmar Learning.

Mon, D.T. 2003. Relational database management: What you need to know. *Journal of AHIMA* 74(10):40–45.

Oppel, A. 2004. *Databases DeMYSTiFieD: A Self-Teaching Guide.* Emeryville, CA: McGraw-Hill Osborne.

Tan, J.K. H. 2001. *Health Management Information Systems: Methods and Practical Applications.* Gaithersburg, MD: Aspen Publications.

Chapter 5
System Selection and Implementation

Objectives

- Assist in the system selection process.
- Assist in the system implementation.
- Participate in the implementation team.
- Develop training materials.
- Assist in the development review of the request for proposal.
- Assist in the system analysis process.
- Conduct training classes for users.

Key Terms

Alpha site
Application service provider (ASP)
Best of breed
Best of fit
Beta site
Chief information officer
Computer-assisted instruction
Data conversion
Escrow
Feasibility study
Force majeure
Functional requirements
Gantt chart
Go-live
Graphical user interface (GUI)
Information systems project steering committee

Information systems strategic planning
Interface
Interface engine
Middleware
Payment milestone
Project
Project definition
Project Evaluation and Review Technique (PERT) chart
Project management
Project manager
Project team
Prototype
Reengineering
Report design
Request for information (RFI)
Request for proposal (RFP)

Scope creep
Screen design
Setting configuration
Site preparation
Site visits
Source code
System analysis
System development life cycle (SDLC)
System evaluation
System implementation
System selection
Test environment
Testing
Train the trainer
User preparation
User task force
Weighted system

Introduction

System selection and **system implementation** is the process of deciding on an information system (IS), preparing it, and training facility staff for use of the system in the healthcare facility. The system selection and implementation process begins with the idea that the facility should consider obtaining a particular system such as the electronic health record (EHR), for example. The process continues until the system is in use and has been evaluated as to whether or not it meets the established objectives.

The complexity of the system selection and implementation process varies widely, from implementing Microsoft Office or other standard software products to the very complex implementation of an EHR system. The length of time required thus varies from a few days or weeks to months or even several years. The number of people involved will also vary based on who is impacted by the system and the complexity of the system to be implemented.

Systems selected should support the facility's business objectives. The systems should be identified and prioritized during the **information systems strategic planning** process, as more systems are usually identified than the facility's resources can handle. Strategic information system planning is defined as "the process of identifying and assigning priorities to the application of information technology that will assist an organization in executing its business plans and achieving its strategic goals and objectives" (Austin and Boxerman 2003, 259). For example, if a facility's business objective is to meet a goal of improved quality of care, then the facility should look for information systems that would support this goal, such as the EHR or clinical provider order entry (CPOE). The EHR would improve the quality of care because of the immediate access to patient information as well as the use of alerts and other features. The CPOE would improve care because the orders would be immediately available to the ancillary department, and the healthcare provider would be able to take advantage of reminders and alerts regarding contraindications, the need for laboratory tests to monitor blood levels, and so on.

Steps included in the system selection process are:

- Planning
- Organization of the project
- System analysis
- Request for proposal
- Evaluation of systems
- Selection of a system
- Contract negotiation

Steps included in the implementation process are:

- Site/space preparation
- Installation of hardware/software/networks
- Programming modifications to software
- User configurations and settings
- Interface development
- Report design
- Screen design
- Testing
- Training

- Go-live

- Evaluation

Some of the system selection and implementation steps are linear, but others can be performed concurrently. For example, the contract has to be signed before the software can be installed, but the organization can design screens and reports at the same time. It is imperative to remember that throughout implementation and planning, the plan itself is a working document and will continuously change and evolve. Flexibility is necessary. Each of the system selection and implementation steps will be covered in this chapter.

Planning

Planning is critical to the system selection and implementation process. Planning for an information system is a complex process and includes many steps such as:

- Conducting a feasibility study

- Setting the budget

- Setting the goals and objectives

- Identifying the project manager

- Identifying the project team

- Determining who will build and maintain the system

- Choosing between integrated and interfaced systems

- Obtaining buy-in from management and users

- Training

Planning a major system implementation requires a lot of work by a lot of people. A lack of planning can and will cause problems with the system, which can cause the system to fail or delay the implementation date, thus costing the facility money. An example of poor planning is ordering hardware without evaluating the space. Insufficient space can lead to inability to install the hardware due to insufficient electrical wiring, inadequate space, or other problems with the physical plant.

Conducting a Feasibility Study

A **feasibility study** determines if a proposed information system is an appropriate option to meet the objectives of the organization (Englebardt and Nelson 2002). The study examines the costs, the benefits, and any expected problems and determines whether or not to proceed with the proposed system. The benefits should be both tangible and intangible. Tangible benefits are easy to quantify (Austin and Boxerman 2003), such as elimination of duplicate tests. Intangible benefits, while critical, are not easy to quantify. An example of an intangible benefit would be to improve quality of care. If the benefits do outweigh the costs, then the project should be considered.

Setting the Budget

Developing the budget for a system implementation is important since cost is a key determining factor in deciding whether or not to implement. The budget should be comprehensive and as accurate as possible because it is used in the decision-making process. The budget should include system selection and implementation expenses as well as the cost of maintaining the system for a specified period of time, such as 2 to 5 years. Additionally, the budget should include items such as cost of software, upgrading infrastructure, hardware, training, renovations to the physical plant, maintenance of the system, project management, and travel expenses for site visits.

Goals and Objectives

Goals and objectives for the system must be established as part of the planning process. The goals and objectives identify what the facility wants to accomplish with the implementation of the proposed system and how these goals will be achieved. These system goals should be based on the facility's business goals (Austin and Boxerman 2003). As with any goals, they should be measurable yet realistic and attainable. It never hurts to add on some cushion time for any unforeseen issues. Examples of goals are: to reduce the number of staff by five, to reduce the discharge not final billed (DNFB) report to $500,000, and to reduce the number of duplicate tests by 75 percent. Goals will be determined by the type of system and the needs of the facility. Once established, goals should be used to identify which information system best meets the desired outcomes.

Once the system is implemented, it should be evaluated regularly thereafter as to whether the system met and will continue to meet or exceed the stated goals and objectives. For example, the post-implementation evaluation will identify whether the duplicate tests were reduced by 75 percent or whether staffing was reduced by five.

Identifying the Project Manager and Project Team

The project manager and project teams are an important part of project management. **Project management** is "a formal set of principles and procedures that help control the activities associated with implementing a usually large undertaking to achieve a specific goal, such as an information system project" (Amtayakul 2007, 467). Project Leadership including the project manager and the **project team** members should be identified before the project begins. The **project manager** leads the project, and therefore must have an understanding of the system being implemented, knowledge of project management, leadership skills, and conflict management skills (Amatayakul 2007). A sample project manager job description is presented in figure 5.1. The project manager is responsible for ensuring that the project plan stays within the designated timeline, issues are resolved, desired outcomes are met, and customer satisfaction is achieved. A project team is a collection of multi-disciplinary individuals (that is, billing, clinician, administration, IT) assigned to work on a project. Their role is important because they are responsible for ensuring that the system implementation plan is carried out according to the project manager's specifications. Their backgrounds will vary according to the needs of the project (Amatayakul 2007). For example, implementation of an EHR will require information system staff, health information management, physicians, nursing, and other clinical users of the system. The project team will be discussed in detail later in the chapter.

Determining Who Will Build and Maintain the System

One of the critical decisions to be made during the planning process is whether a facility should build the system itself, purchase it from a vendor, or use an **application service provider (ASP)** (Austin and Boxerman 2003).

An ASP is a third-party service company that delivers, manages, and remotely hosts (off-site, usually at the host location) standardized applications software via a network through an outsourcing contract based on fixed, monthly usage or transaction-based pricing (Amatayakul 2007).

With an ASP, a user simply logs into the system and accesses it exactly as if the data center were located in-house, although the data center may be located at a great distance from the facility. An ASP is similar to paying rent and can significantly reduce the capital expenditures up front, and monthly expenditures are a preapproved flat-fee structure so expenses are always known. This method is favored by facilities that do not have staff with the necessary skills to develop and maintain a system. A disadvantage to the ASP format is that the user may not have as much control over the system. For example, the scheduling of maintenance and upgrades is up to the host, and the client has no say in the matter. Another disadvantage is that since an organization is "renting" the system, it is not investing in its

Figure 5.1.   Project manager job description

Position: EHR Project Manager

Reports to: Chief Science Officer

Key Functions and Responsibilities

Integrated Healthcare Information

1. Using an evidence-based approach, facilitate culture of having integrated healthcare information by screening clinical systems for appropriate fit, integration potential, and timing of projects based on EHR architecture. This will be done in partnership with the chief information officer and person(s) championing the specific clinical system.

Electronic Health Record System

2. Direct selection and implementation of EHR components to include:
   a. Enterprisewide master person index
   b. Clinical data repository
   c. Document imaging to include medical (for example, PACS) and administrative images
   d. Physician order-entry and electronic signature capabilities
   e. Patient care documentation
   f. Clinical decision support tools to include:
      (1) Clinical alerts and reminders
      (2) Care management protocols
   g. Other information systems and emerging technology as necessary and feasible
3. Lead break-through project team to deliver the following:
   a. Longitudinal record of patient care across the organization's continuum of care sites
   b. Clinician utilization of EHR that facilitates and enhances patient care delivery processes at the point of care and remotely as appropriate
   c. Patient interaction with clinicians, access to their personal health record of care at the organization, and quality education
   d. Tools that facilitate cost-effective care management and respond to a growing number of managed care contracts
   e. Capacity to perform large patient database searches and studies without impacting the performance of the EHR in day-to-day activities
   f. Support for the organization's training and research programs

Business Process Redesign and Information Protection

4. Coordinate reengineering of work flows and patient care documentation with clinical users to leverage and maximize organizational and personal productivity to improve patient care delivery processes.
5. Ensure that systems selected are compliant with all applicable laws, regulations, and standards, and that their storage, retention, authentication, accuracy, and transmission integrity support admissibility.
6. Develop processes for determining who has access to specific health information; how users will be educated, trained, and kept continually aware of patient privacy and security requirements to provide data confidentiality, integrity, and availability; and ensure that ongoing auditing of access is performed and supported by appropriate sanctions and disciplinary processes.

Budgetary/Operational Responsibility

7. Develop and account for operating and capital budgets for above processes.
8. Determine appropriate staffing and resource requirements for the EHR project.
9. Establish appropriate metrics and monitor benefits realization.

Skills/Experience Required:

- Knowledge of health information management and technology, clinical user needs, and healthcare work flow
- Extensive and progressive healthcare management experience
- Experience with the selection and implementation of healthcare information systems
- Ability to enroll and build strong relationships with all levels of management, physicians, and staff
- Ability to lead a project team through uncharted territory, shift paradigms, take risks, and bring ideas from concept to reality
- Relentless focus on outcomes

Adapted from Job Description for Director, Integrated Healthcare Information, Central DuPage Health System, Ann Ogorzalek, RHIA own structure and therefore would have to make a large investment should it ever decide to bring the system in-house.

The second option would be for the facility to build the system. If a facility decides to build a system, it would be designed to meet the specific needs of that facility. The system would have the look and feel that is desired as well as the desired functionality. There are, however, disadvantages such as:

- It could take longer to develop.

- The planning must be more detailed than if purchasing a system.

- If the facility loses the staff that developed the system, it may be difficult to upgrade the system to meet the needs of the facility over time.

The final option mentioned here would be to purchase a predeveloped software system from a vendor. As with the other options, there are advantages and disadvantages to this option. A system purchased from a vendor may not be exactly what the facility wants, but it would be faster to implement, and the facility would benefit from extensive research and development conducted by the vendor. The design of the system would be less detailed, but the facility would have the use of the vendor's customer support system to assist with upgrades and problems that arise.

When working with a vendor, the healthcare facility may have the opportunity to be an alpha site. An **alpha site** is the first healthcare facility to implement the information system. The facility generally receives a discount for the system in exchange for participation in the development of the system. Because the system is still being developed, the facility may face problems with the implementation that would not be encountered with a more mature version of the same system. It also takes more time than a typical implementation. The facility may also be asked to be a **beta site**. Beta sites are the next few healthcare facilities who subsequently implement the system. Many of the problems with the system are resolved with the alpha site but these beta sites are likely to encounter numerous problems as well.

Choosing Between Integrated and Interfaced Systems

If the decision is made to purchase an information system from a vendor, the next decision is whether the product should be integrated or interfaced.

Integrated Systems

Integrated systems are designed to work together. A good example of an integrated system is Microsoft Office. The user can share information among Microsoft Word, Microsoft Excel, and other products within the Office suite. Many healthcare vendors use this model to interface systems used by healthcare facilities. This type of system is much easier to manage than an interfaced system because of the lack of interfaces. Integrated systems collect, store, and retrieve information from the same database and, further, technologies allow that they support each other. The user is quickly able to move between systems because they have the same look and feel, which can also make it easier to use (Austin and Boxerman 2003). The decision to purchase software from a single vendor is frequently called **best of fit** (Amtayakul 2007).

Interfaced Systems

In an interfaced system, the products are not designed to work together, but rather are linked through an interface. An **interface** takes data from one system and plugs that data into another system. In other words, an interface acts as a bridge between two systems/databases to translate data into each system's respective language. Interfaces will be discussed in detail later in the chapter. An interface has to know what data to retrieve, where the data are located in the first database, whether any data manipulation has to be performed, what that manipulation is, and where the data are to be entered into the second database. If the interface is not working, the systems will not be able to share information until the problems with the interface are resolved (Austin and Boxerman 2003).

Although an interfaced system takes more effort to manage, many facilities choose this method because the facility's users can choose the various products that they want instead of choosing a single vendor's product, which may have a wonderful encoder but an inadequate laboratory information system, for example. Choosing the systems based on functionality rather than by vendor and interfacing them is frequently the option selected. Choosing the best product for your organization regardless of vendor is called choosing the **best of breed** (Amatayakul 2007).

Obtaining Buy-in from Management and Users

It is critical that the facility's upper management support the project from the very beginning of the process. If management shows support for the system, the employees will follow suit and support it. However, if management displays discontent or lack of support, the employees will be most likely to resist the change. Support can be shown by attending meetings, talking about the system's benefits to the organization, its employees, and its customers, and generally demonstrating that the system is valued. Communication is critical here. Remember to keep staff and all those to be affected by the system updated to the decisions, the changes, and all expectations. The more the personnel are informed, the less likely for resistance to occur because they will know what to expect.

The Importance of Planning

The importance of planning becomes evident when the most common reasons for project failures are examined. According to Young (2000) these reasons are:

- Lack of clear vision

- Inadequate resources

- Lack of planning

- Use of inappropriate resources

- Lack of experienced staff to complete assigned tasks

- Unrealistic expectations

Other reasons for project failure include lack of training, poor communication, and an inadequate system.

If a facility spends more time and energy on the front end of a system implementation project, it will be better positioned to succeed. Adequate planning is demonstrated, in part, when the facility has from the outset of the project the necessary staff, money, and other resources, as well as an understanding of what is needed and what the desired outcomes are expected to be.

Organization of Project

Once the decision is made to implement a system, the project's formal organizational structure must be put in place. A **project** is a plan and course of action that will address a specific objective, made up of a series of activities and tasks with a defined start and stop date. The plan has a targeted objective and deliverable to be accomplished. The project will need specific resources assigned to it in order to be completed (Abdelhak et al. 2007).

Project Team

Most, if not all, information system projects require a team of individuals to successfully implement the system. The number of individuals needed and the make-up of this team vary from project to project depending on the needs of the implementation (Austin and Boxerman 2003). For example, if the facility is implementing a chart deficiency system for use only in the health information management (HIM) department, the team should include the appropriate people in HIM and information systems. The team would not need to include physicians, nurses, risk managers, or laboratory staff. If the facility is implementing an order entry system, the team would need representatives from the physician staff, as well as from the HIM, nursing, laboratory, and pharmacy departments to ensure that the system is properly planned and developed.

An HIM professional will frequently sit on the committee because the system may impact the HIM department indirectly, and having an HIM professional involved in the process can help ensure that the department's needs are addressed. Additionally, the HIM professional can serve as a consultant and source of information for compliance, legal, and other concerns. For example, the HIM professional can assist with retention, privacy, security, and documentation issues, among many other considerations of the system, which may ultimately affect the HIM department.

The major participants in the project management team are the **information systems project steering committee**, the project manager, the **user task force**, the project team, the vendor, and, possibly, one or more consultants. These roles are described here:

- The **information systems project steering committee** is responsible for every information system acquisition project in the facility (Wager et al. 2005). Each project team will report back to the steering committee. The steering committee's role is to ensure that the strategic information system plan is being efficiently and effectively implemented and that the project stays on target (LaTour and Eichenwald Maki 2006). This committee is frequently led by the **chief information officer** (CIO). The CIO is generally at the vice president level and is responsible for all information resource management functions at the facility. The information system, HIM, and other information management departments frequently report to the CIO. The CIO must be a visionary and have strong management skills. While the CIO is not a technical role, the individual must understand enough about information technology to ensure the proper management of the systems (Glandon et al. 2008). Other team members may be administrators, managers, project managers, and other leaders in the facility.

- The project team works with the project manager to implement and manage the project. This team will meet periodically, based on project needs, to discuss progress of the project and any issues that arise. The project team generally meets less frequently in the early stages of the project; the frequency increases as the implementation date gets closer. The team may even meet daily right before go-live. This team should be multidisciplinary. The makeup of the team will be determined by the type of system being implemented and its complexity. The team should include information system staff, clinicians, HIM personnel, and others as appropriate. It is important to include a representative from facility management if possible, to show support for the system.

- The **project manager** is responsible for coordinating the individual project, monitoring the budget, managing the resources, conducting negotiations, and keeping the project on schedule. These roles require the project manager to have both technical and analytical skills as well as people skills. The project manager should be skilled in conflict resolution, communication, and project management. Leadership skills are also important because the project manager must be able to develop a consensus and manage meetings for the project team.

- The **user task force** is a group of users, who will ultimately be using the system, that test the system and perform other project-related tasks for which the committee receives feedback. These users are generally on loan from various departments to assist in the project. Some members of the user task force may be deployed as needed for **testing** (performing an examination or evaluation) and other tasks, whereas others are pulled out of their department for the duration of the project. This reassignment may last a year or more depending on the project (Kreider and Haselton 1997).

- The vendor representative is the expert on the system and so will be an extremely valuable team member. This individual will be the liaison between the facility and the leadership at the vendor's company. The vendor representative knows the product and can be a valuable resource with regard to how best to implement and use the system. Additionally, he or she can give the project team information on what has (and has not) worked for other facilities. This information can help the facility recognize and use best practices, and help it avoid costly mistakes. If not scheduled to be on site during a meeting, the vendor representative may need to meet via telephone conference due to their expertise (Kreider and Haselton 1997).

- If the facility decides to hire a consultant, the consultant will be a valuable member of the team as well. The consultant hired should not have ties to a particular vendor's product, but rather be objective to help the facility obtain the product that best meets its needs. The consultant should have experience in system selection and implementation.

Project Identification

Before any decisions are made, the facility must define what the accomplished project is. The **project definition** is defined during the project planning process to tell the facility exactly what it is trying to do with the system being implemented and the expected outcomes (Kreider and Haselton 2003). The facility must identify:

- The purpose of the system

- How the system links to the facility's business strategy

- The goals for and scope of the project

The scope of the project determines exactly what work is—and is not—to be included in the project based on resources available. Identifying the project's scope is important to prevent scope creep. **Scope creep** happens when items not included in the original scope are added after the project has begun. The additions to the project will increase the time needed for the project and the money and resources required to accomplish it (Englebardt and Nelson 2002).

Once the facility knows what it plans to do, the project team can begin dividing the project into specific activities or tasks. The team may start out with a basic skeleton of a project plan and continue to add substance to it as they go along. This plan should describe each task to be completed, how it will be completed, who is responsible for its completion, when a task should begin, and when the task should be finished. The basic components of the plan are:

- Feasibility study: This study defines the objectives and need for the project and justifies the plan.

- Resources: The resource plan identifies the resources needed in order to meet the objectives of the plan. This includes money, time, staff, space, and other resources.

- Design: In the design stage, the project team identifies the specific details required to implement the plan. For every task identified, the plan must provide a start and end date and a person responsible. If the project requires programming, the team must establish the standards that will be used in writing the program.

- Hardware and software procurement: This stage includes ensuring that the facility has all of the hardware and software needed and that any missing components arrive in a timely manner. Hardware delivery may take 6 weeks, for example, so ordering needs to be done early in the process.

- Transition: The transition phase prepares the facility for the conversion from the old system to the new. This stage includes not only the actual conversion of data, but preparing staff for the change.

- Implementation: The implementation stage includes the steps to be taken to prepare for the implementation and the actual conversion to the new system.

- Postimplementation: The postimplementation stage begins immediately after implementation is complete. The team must evaluate itself to prepare for the new project. It should also include an evaluation process to determine if the objectives of the project were met and how the process could have been improved (Kreider and Haselton 1997).

The level of organization for the project depends on the level of complexity of the system being implemented. If it is a small department system, it may only require two to three people to implement. Large systems that impact the entire facility can take hundreds of people. In large projects, there are frequently subcommittees that are responsible for small areas of the project. The subcommittees meet and work on their segment of the project. The chair of the subcommittee then reports back to the full project committee.

Project Tools

There are a number of tools that can be used to control the project. These tools include Gantt charts and PERT charts, project plans, trouble tickets, and status reports.

- The project plan provides details for how to accomplish the project. It directs and guides the team on activities, time, costs, and sequencing of activities. It also provides a narrative description of the project. The project plan could include project tools such as the Gantt chart and the PERT chart (Abdelhak et al. 2007).

- The **Gantt chart** (see figure 5.2) is a project management tool that records specific tasks, their start and end dates, the person responsible for the tasks, and any connections between tasks. The Gantt chart can easily show which tasks are behind schedule, which are on target, and which are ahead of schedule (Abdelhak et al. 2007).

- A Project Evaluation and Review Technique **(PERT)** chart (see figure 5.3) is a management tool that evaluates the tasks, dependencies on other activities, activity sequence, and the time required to complete the task. Because the PERT chart shows interdependencies between tasks, it will help determine whether the implementation date is slipping due to delinquent tasks (Abdelhak et al. 2007). This slippage is shown by review of the critical path. Because the critical path shows the longest amount of time to complete the project, if key tasks along the critical path are delayed, the critical path itself lengthens, thus lengthening the duration of the project.

- Status reports are periodic updates on where the project is, what has been accomplished, and what problems have been encountered. Solutions for the problems should be identified in the report. Status reports are typically directed to the information systems project steering committee to keep that group informed on the project's progress. The status report is generally written by the project manager, but could be written by a designee.

- The trouble ticket is a tool used during the implementation phase to document and track problems encountered. The project manager keeps track of all trouble tickets turned in, assigns someone to be responsible for the resolution of the problems, and monitors the tickets for closure. Some of the issues recorded may be minor, whereas others may be major. Either way, all of the problems recorded by the trouble tickets should be resolved prior to implementation of the system.

Figure 5.2 shows an example of a Gantt chart, and figure 5.3 shows an example of a PERT chart.

Additionally, software such as Microsoft Project can be used to help manage a project. Project management software can create the Gantt and PERT charts as well as other types of tools for the project team to review. It can also track how much of each task is complete (0 to 100 percent), who has been given the responsibility for each task, the beginning and ending dates, the sequencing of tasks, and more.

Figure 5.2.   Sample Gantt chart

		Task Name	Duratio	Start	Finish
1		Identify project manager	1 day	Fri 8/8/08	Fri 8/8/08
2		Identify project team	1 wk	Mon 8/11/08	Fri 8/15/08
3		Conduct systems analysis	6 mons	Mon 8/18/08	Fri 1/30/09
4		Write RFP	6 wks	Mon 2/2/09	Fri 3/13/09
5		Distribute RFPs to vendors	2 days	Mon 3/16/09	Tue 3/17/09
6		Meet with vendors	1 day	Mon 4/6/09	Mon 4/6/09
7		Receive RFP submissions	1 mon	Tue 4/7/09	Mon 5/4/09
8		Review RFPs	1 mon	Tue 5/5/09	Mon 6/1/09
9		Site visits	1 mon	Tue 6/2/09	Mon 6/29/09
10		Check references	1 wk	Tue 6/30/09	Mon 7/6/09
11		Make decision on system	1 wk	Tue 7/7/09	Mon 7/13/09
12		Sign contract	1 wk	Tue 7/14/09	Mon 7/20/09
13		Order hardware for users and data center	1 wk	Tue 7/21/09	Mon 7/27/09
14		Site preparation (add outlet, shift existing computers)	3 days	Tue 7/21/09	Thu 7/23/09
15		Install hardware in computer room and units	######	Mon 9/7/09	Thu 9/24/09
16		Update network to accommodate increased traffic	######	Mon 9/7/09	Thu 9/24/09
17		Install software on file server	1 day	Fri 9/25/09	Fri 9/25/09
18		Configure settings in system	1 mon	Mon 9/28/09	Fri 10/23/09
19		Write routine reports	3 mons	Mon 9/28/09	Fri 12/18/09
20		Develop new screens	3 mons	Mon 9/28/09	Fri 12/18/09
21		Develop training plan	2 mons	Mon 9/7/09	Fri 10/30/09
22		Identify data conversion needs	5 days	Mon 9/29/08	Fri 10/3/08
23		Write interfaces	2 mons	Mon 9/28/09	Fri 11/20/09
24		Write program required for data conversion	1 mon	Mon 10/6/08	Fri 10/31/08
25		Write user manual, training materials and policies and procedures	6 mons	Mon 10/26/09	Fri 4/9/10
26		Test software	2 mons	Tue 12/1/09	Mon 1/25/10
27		Correct errors identified in testing	1 mon	Tue 1/26/10	Mon 2/22/10
28		Train the trainers	2 wks	Mon 4/12/10	Fri 4/23/10
29		Conduct training	2 mons	Mon 4/26/10	Fri 6/18/10
30		Go-live	3 days	Mon 6/21/10	Wed 6/23/10
31		Acceptance testing	2 mons	Thu 6/24/10	Wed 8/18/10
32		Evaluation of implementation	2 wks	Thu 8/19/10	Wed 9/1/10

Project: chapter 5 gantt Date: Fri 1/29/10	Task		Project Summary		
	Split		External Tasks		
	Progress		External Milestone		
	Milestone		Deadline		
	Summary				

Figure 5.3. Sample PERT chart

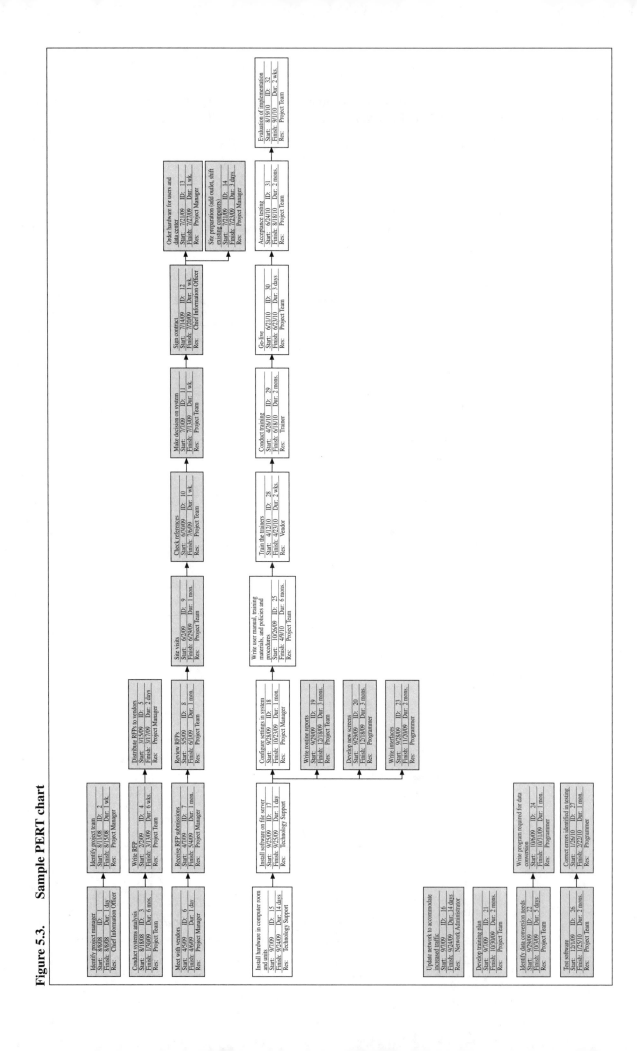

Check Your Understanding 5.1

1. True or False: The information systems project steering committee is responsible for the day-to-day implementation of new systems.

2. The process that outlines the cost, benefits, and disadvantages of the proposed systems is the:

   A. feasibility study
   B. project plan
   C. trouble ticket
   D. status reports

3. The PERT chart shows if there is slippage in the implementation date. This slippage is shown by:

   A. dependencies
   B. Gantt chart
   C. project plan
   D. critical path

4. The coding supervisor performs a monthly audit of coding quality. Is this a project?

   A. Yes
   B. No

5. Differentiate between integrated and interfaced.

   A. Integrated systems are designed to work together, and interfaced systems must be linked.
   B. Interfaced systems are designed to work together, and integrated systems must be linked.
   C. Integrated systems are designed to be embedded in your hospital information system, and interfaced systems are part of your hospital information system.
   D. Interfaced systems are designed to be embedded in your hospital information system, and integrated systems are part of your hospital information system.

System Analysis

System Development Life Cycle

Abdelhak (2007, 306) defines the **system development life cycle (SDLC)** as the "process used to identify, investigate, design, select, and implement information systems." Generally the SDLC (illustrated in figure 5.4) has five steps:

- Initiation

- Analysis

- Design

- Implementation

- Maintenance/evaluation (LaTour and Eichenwald Maki 2006)

Benefits of the SDLC

The SDLC is an important part of the system selection process because it helps you understand your organization and its needs. The SDLC is a structured process that can be useful by identifying users' needs and alternatives, selecting the information system, system

Figure 5.4.   System development life cycle (SDLC) diagram

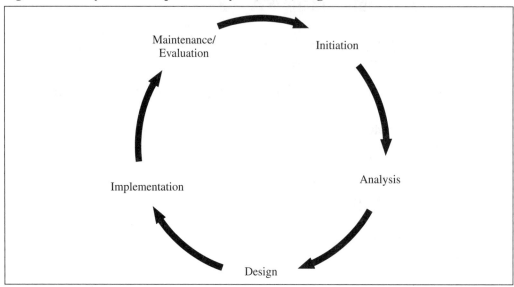

implementation, and other steps in managing information systems. SDLC requires the involvement of people throughout the organization including those who use the system (Johns 2006). The use of people throughout the organization who are impacted by the organization ensures that the needs of all of the users and the organization are met.

SDLC Process

The SDLC is an ongoing process as demonstrated by the circular nature of Figure 5.4. There are a number of models used to describe the SDLC. Each of the four stages in the model used in this book is described below.

Initiation

Initiation is where the facility decides to acquire a specific information system (Abdelhak et al. 2007). This decision may come about because of an information system strategic plan, the obsolescence of an existing system, or some other reason. In analysis, the facility determines what users need from the proposed system. This stage reviews the current processes of the facility, the proposed processes, and the desired **functional requirements.** Functional requirements describe "what, not how, nor to what degree of accuracy, nor to what format" (Mikulski 1993). The design phase determines how the system will be selected or developed. It includes the specific design of a system to be developed by the facility or how the facility will identify the system for purchase. The implementation phase begins with the signing of the contract and ends when the system is operational. Some of the steps in this stage are installation of hardware or software, training, testing, and change management. The final stage is maintenance/evaluation of where the system is used, updated, and evaluated. The facility needs to know if the system meets the goals established for it and to conduct the day-to-day operations to keep the system up and running. This is a cyclical process; once the system no longer meets the needs of the users, the process begins again (LaTour and Eichenwald Maki 2006).

Systems Analysis

Systems analysis is "the process of collecting, organizing, and evaluating data about IS requirements and the environment in which the system will operate" (Austin and Boxerman 2003). Systems analysis is generally the first step in the SDLC after the decision to implement the system has been made. It helps determine the needs for data, storage, reporting, and functionality. To identify the needs of the facility, the team would look at the existing systems and the needs of the users, and identify and evaluate alternatives. During systems analysis, users are asked questions such as:

- What do you like about the current system?
- What problems do you have with the current system?
- What changes do you foresee that will impact this system?
- What information do you need from the system?

Answering these questions helps the project team understand the current system and how it meets or does not meet the needs of the users. A system will be used by the facility for a long time and therefore must be adequate both at the time of go-live and in the foreseeable future.

To identify the needs of the facility for the foreseeable future, the team needs to understand the environment in which the system will operate. No one can see into the future with certainty, but internal and external environmental scanning can identify some issues that must be addressed. Internal scanning is identifying changes within the facility that will impact the information system. External scanning is identifying changes outside of the facility that will impact the information system. For example, if a facility was developing a new system that contained protected health information in 2002, it would have to ensure that the system would meet the strict Health Insurance Portability and Accountability Act (HIPAA) privacy rule that was implemented in April 2003. The facility may be aware of other pending legislation, trends, or other issues that may impact the system under consideration. Understanding the environment helps ensure that the system will work today and for the expected future.

Questionnaires, interviews, observations, flowcharts, and other data collection tools may be used to obtain the data needed to answer these questions (Austin and Boxerman 2003). The team should collect data from all levels and types of users. The needs of the clerical staff will be very different from the needs of management staff. Many managers think they know the needs of their staff, but many of these managers know what the policy states, not what is actually happening. The information gathered should include all aspects of the system such as data elements, reports, privacy, security, and overall functionality.

Questionnaires allow for a large number of users to provide input about the needs of the system (Austin and Boxerman 2003). This is especially true if closed-ended questions are used so that the responses can be tabulated quickly and easily. Closed-ended questions can be answered with yes or no, Likert type scales, and other limited choice responses. Likert type scales are great for obtaining the users' beliefs regarding a statement. An example of a Likert scale begins with a statement such as: "On a scale of 1 to 5 with 1 being strongly agree and 5 being strongly disagree, rate the following statement." An example of a belief could be "The new EHR will improve the efficiency of the facility." An example of a typical closed-ended question could be, "Do you generate reports as a part of your job?" Obviously, the response to this question is limited to yes or no. Computerized tools such as Survey Monkey and even machine-readable Scantron forms make the aggregation and analysis of the responses quicker. The downside of questionnaires is that the correct questions may not be asked, so there may be gaps in the data collected. The use of open-ended questions may help fill some of these gaps, but they slow down the aggregation of data and data analysis (Austin and Boxerman 2003). Open-ended questions allow the participants to expand on their response; however, the team must collect, read, and analyze each statement individually. An example of an open-ended question is: "How does the current information system help you in your job?"

Interviews are powerful tools for obtaining information. There are three types of interviews: structured, unstructured, and semi-structured. In the structured interview, everyone is asked the same questions. This improves analysis of the findings, but does not encourage the interviewee to talk openly about pertinent issues, thus taking the risk that important data will be overlooked. In the unstructured interview, the interviewer does not have a list of questions but rather gets the interviewee talking about their job, their data needs, and other issues related to the information system. The semi-structured interview is a combination of the structured and unstructured formats. There are questions that interviewees are asked, but they are also encouraged to discuss in detail their job, data needs, and other issues related to their information system needs. The unstructured and semi-structured formats make it harder to identify trends and to analyze data, but major issues that could have been overlooked otherwise may be identified.

Typically, two members of the team are needed to conduct interviews because one person interacts with the interviewee and the other person takes notes (Abdelhak et al. 2007). Because of the increased staffing needs, the amount of time required to collect and analyze the data, and the need to meet with users individually, interviews are very time-consuming, which makes them costly. This means that the planning team may interview fewer individuals than those who may respond to a questionnaire.

Observation is watching an action being performed. It is useful in determining what employees are actually doing. This is important because frequently supervisors or others may tell the interviewers what they think is happening but in reality something very different is occurring. The use of observation is a way to validate what the interviewee has been told. If using observations, each observation session should be short—maybe 30 to 40 minutes—because the observer becomes bored and misses details (Abdelhak et al. 2007). Also, observation sessions should be scheduled throughout the day because different tasks may be performed at different times.

Flowcharts may be used to "provide a concise, logical, and standardized mechanism for depicting and analyzing current information flows" (Austin and Boxerman 2003) (see figure 5.5). The flowchart frequently uses geographic symbols to demonstrate the steps performed (McWay 2008). Problems and inconsistencies may be identified through the development and analysis of the flowchart. The process on the flowchart would depend on the type of system being developed but could represent the flow of the medical record in the HIM department, the flow of a physician query, or the steps in denial management. The flowchart would identify critical points in the process as well as problem areas. This

Figure 5.5.   Sample flowchart

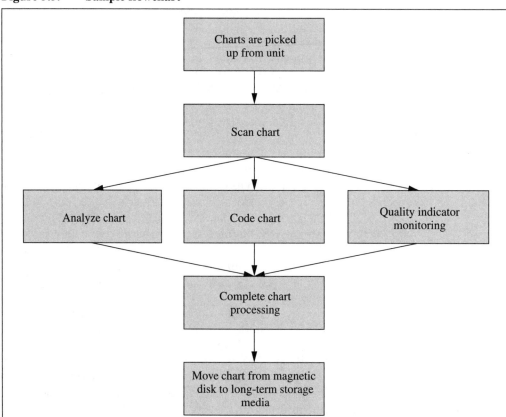

information can be used to improve new processes implemented along with the new information system.

Many facilities use a combination of questionnaires, interviews, observations, and other data collection tools to obtain the best information. The use of multiple tools also allows the team to involve more users and at the same time obtain detailed, validated information. The large number of participants helps to foster buy-in from the users. Buy-in refers to the acceptance of the system and recognizing its value to the user and to the facility. Users who buy-in to the system are supportive and less likely to resist using the system into their job role.

System analysis is a "process of studying organizational operations and determining information systems requirements for a given application" (Glandon et al. 2008, 75). It is frequently ignored or given only minimal attention during the system implementation process. This is a mistake. System analysis is critical because it forces the facility to evaluate itself and to look at how it does business. This understanding will help select the system that will best meet the needs of the facility.

Design

In the design phase, the standards upon which the system will be evaluated and selected are identified (Abdelhak et al. 2007). This includes functionality, purchase vs. develop vs. ASP, and other attributes desired in the IS. This will be further described in the system selection section of this chapter.

Implementation

This stage of the SDLC addresses the steps required to implement the IS. This includes a comprehensive plan for the implementation process. (LaTour and Eichenwald Maki 2007). This will be discussed in the implementation section of this chapter.

Maintenance and Evaluation

The maintenance and evaluation stage addresses the day-to-day operations of the IS after implementation. The system should be evaluated on an ongoing basis in order to ensure that the IS continues to meet the needs of the organization (LaTour and Eichenwald Maki 2007). This is discussed further in the implementation section of this chapter.

System Selection

Most facilities today decide to purchase a system from an IS vendor. The vendor has invested millions of dollars in research and development and has a support system to assist the facility in the implementation of the IS being purchased. The facility must identify what they demand from an IS. This information is used to determine which system best meets the needs of the organization.

Request for Information

The **request for information (RFI)** is a formal document requesting information on information systems. The RFI asks the information system vendor for basic information about the product and how their information system would meet the requirements outlined in the RFI (Abdelhak et al. 2007). The RFI can be used to select minor information systems, or the information gathered in the RFI can be used to determine who will receive the more rigorous **request for proposal (RFP),** which "details all required system functionality, including functional, technical, training, and implementation requirements" (Abdelhak et al. 2007, 343).

Request for Proposal

The RFP is a much more detailed document than the RFI and is critical to the selection process. The purpose of the RFP is to give the vendor all the information needed to propose an information system that meets the needs of the facility. The RFP describes what system is needed, how many people will be using the system, and how the system will be used. Common components of the RFP are:

- Letter of introduction
- Information for potential vendors, including:
  — Information about bidders' conference
  — Description of facility
  — Patient (or other) volume statistics
- Description of the proposed system, including:
  — Technology requirements
  — Functional requirements
  — Required format of response
- Instructions for RFP
- Request for sample documentation
- Request for sample contract
- Vendor profile
- System testing requirements
- Sample résumés of implementation staff
- System selection criteria
- Training requirements
- References

Appendix B shows a detailed template for an RFP (AHIMA 2007).

Letter of Introduction

The letter of introduction is a cover letter that is sent to the vendor along with the RFP. The letter introduces the vendor to the RFP, and identifies who the vendor should contact at the facility. It may also provide some information that did not make it into the RFP. The information on the bidders' conference gives the date, time, location, and other information.

The bidders' conference is a meeting for vendors to come to the healthcare facility to ask questions about the RFP, the facility, and more. This meeting enables all of the potential vendors to hear the same information and to get all of their questions answered so that they can completely respond to the RFP.

Information for Potential Vendors

The description of the facility section provides the vendor with enough information about the facility to enable the vendor to properly respond to the RFP. This information includes the size of facility, number of employees, number of employees who would use the system, and number of locations that would use the system (Austin and Boxerman 2003). This section also should describe the facility's existing systems so the vendor can respond as to how they can work with the existing system.

It should also include patient (or other) volume statistics that would be related to the system (see table 5.1). The statistics may include number of discharges, number of surgeries, number of emergency department visits, and the number of outpatient visits—whatever is needed for the proposed system (Abdelhak et al. 2007).

Description of the Proposed System

In the proposed system section, the vendor describes the system that it is proposing to meet the needs of the facility. The vendor should describe the infrastructure required, licensing, the capabilities of system, the benefits that would be realized, and more.

Table 5.1.   Sample of requested volume

Imaging System Statistics Facility Findings	Number
Average number of discharges per day	45
Average number of emergency department visits per day	60
Average number of outpatient surgeries per day	25
Average number of outpatient visits per day	125
Average number of pages—inpatient discharge	100
Average number of pages per emergency department visit	12
Average number of pages per outpatient surgery record	40
Average number of pages for each outpatient visit	2
Average number of release of information requests per day	21
Average number of pages copied for release of information/day	475
Number of forms utilized in medical record	325
Number of forms already having barcodes	200
Percentage of medical record to be entered into the imaging system via COLD technology	40%
Projected number of change in workload over the next 5 years	10%

The functional requirements identify the desired functions of the IS, which makes this a significant part of the RFP. This document is developed during the system analysis process and outlines all of the functions expected of the system. The functions should include all aspects of the information, including but not limited to, individual data elements, data entry methods, reporting, management of the system, functionality, and technical issues. Technical issues can include topics such as the type of database used and the ability to work with a certain operating system or interface with existing products.

Each functional requirement is listed. The vendor indicates whether the function is available, is available with customization, will be available in the future, or is not available (Hebda et al. 2005). The facility will take this same list of functional requirements and use it to evaluate the RFP. There are at least two ways to classify each functional requirement. The first is that each functional requirement should be designated at least as mandatory or desirable (Austin and Boxerman 2003). Some RFPs use three categories: mandatory, desirable, and luxury. Each functional requirement is categorized into one of the designations. A numeric rating system can be used as well; in other words, "scoring" each function based on its importance. For example, each function is rated on a scale of 1 to 5, 1 = unimportant, 5 = highly important. The functional requirements with the available, not available, and other categories are part of the RFP, but the version with the evaluation ratings is not. The functional requirements are used in the system evaluation to determine if a vendor has all of the functionality, and also to determine if the missing functionality is important. For example, if there is a functional requirement to combine duplicate medical record numbers, and it is missing from one of the products under review, the rating would help the reviewer determine whether this is a serious gap.

Other RFP Requirements

The required format of response tells the vendor what the facility requires regarding the RFP. For instance, the facility might require a specified number of paper copies and an electronic copy in Microsoft Word or Portable Document Format (PDF). The facility may also limit the number of pages, or the look of the document. The facility may even provide an electronic template for the vendor to complete. The instructions for RFP may include rules regarding whom the vendor can talk to at the facility, the deadline for submission, and a statement that the vendor assumes responsibilities for the expenses to complete the RFP as well as the expenses for any on-site demonstrations, along with expenses for RFP preparation.

The request for sample documentation and request for sample contract is simply that—a request for a copy of the documents. The vendor profile is a description of the vendor and is designed to ensure that the company is financially sound and capable of meeting the needs of the facility for years to come (Abdelhak et al. 2007). The RFP asks for information on the number of installations of similar systems the vendor has performed, financial viability of vendor, and the number of years the product has been available.

System testing requirements would outline the expectations the facility has regarding testing. The RFP would provide the types of testing to be performed and the role of the vendor in that testing.

Many facilities request sample résumés from the vendor's staff, which provide details of the experience and qualifications of the staff who could be assigned as consultants to that particular project. These sample résumés are used to ensure the vendor has experienced staff members who can support the facility throughout an implementation. It is not a guarantee that any of the individuals represented would be assigned to the project, but rather a sample of the experience that the vendor's employees have.

The system selection criteria are used to select the system. This would include major steps such as findings of the demonstration, findings of site visits, review of the RFP, costs, expected benefits, and reliability of vendor's products. It would not include rankings of importance and other details that the project team will utilize to make the final decisions.

Finally, the RFP should request the training requirements for the system, including the number of people trained by the vendor, cost of training, the estimated time it should take to train each user, types of training required, and other recommendations regarding the training process.

Check Your Understanding 5.2

1. Which stage of the SDLC includes a comprehensive plan?

   A. Analysis
   B. Design
   C. Implementation
   D. Maintenance/evaluation

2. I am collecting data as part of the system analysis function. If I want to get the most system users involved as possible, which would be the BEST method of data collection?

   A. Observation
   B. Questionnaires
   C. Interviews
   D. Flowchart

3. I have asked a vendor for detailed written information on their product. This would be:

   A. RFI
   B. RFP
   C. flowchart
   D. vendor profile

4. I am calling six hospitals that use XYZ's EHR. This is an example of:

   A. reference check
   B. site visit
   C. demonstration
   D. RFP review

5. What problems do you encounter with the existing hospital information system? Is this an open or closed question?

   A. Open
   B. Closed

Evaluation of Proposed Systems

The evaluation process used to select a system should be established during the planning process. The process should include multiple components including:

- On-site demonstrations
- Site visits
- Review of RFP
- Reference checks

On-Site Demonstrations

In an on-site demonstration, the vendor brings its product to the healthcare facility, either as a demonstration version or a full version of the product. Project team members and other users gather to view the product and to ask questions of the sales team. The idea is to have as many people as possible watch the demonstration to see what the product can and cannot do. All attendees should come to the demonstration with situations they encounter in their daily tasks and ask how the system would handle it. The on-site demonstration allows for multiple user involvement and is an important method to learn about the product. This may be the only chance for some team members or other users to see the system before implementation; not everyone can go to site visits to see the system in a live environment (Abdelhak et al. 2007).

Site Visits

Site visits are a great way to view the products in a live environment. A site visit usually consists of a small group of team members (usually key players) visiting a facility, preferably similar in size and characteristics, which has the product implemented, to observe the system in use. During the visit, the team asks questions of the site visit facility's staff involved in the system. The salesperson for the product will attend the site visit as well to answer questions and ensure that the project team obtains the information needed to make a decision. It is recommended that the project team ask the vendor's staff to step outside the room for a few minutes. The philosophy behind this is that the facility staff may be more open about problems with the system if the vendor is not in the room. Seeing the system operating in a real environment is quite different from a demonstration environment and thus gives the project team a much more realistic view of the system and how it works.

Reviewing RFP Responses

The vendor spends a lot of time responding to an RFP, so the RFP should only be sent to the vendors who are seriously being considered (Abdelhak et al. 2007). It is also very expensive (Wager et al. 2005). The number of RFPs submitted is typically limited to three to five vendors. The healthcare facility also spends hours reviewing the RFP responses because for major information systems purchases, the responses could fill a 3- or 4-inch binder. A spreadsheet is frequently developed to assist in the analysis of the RFPs, and this enables the decision makers to compare key information between products more easily when making their decision.

Some of the information that could be included in the spreadsheet includes:

- Cost
- Compatibility with existing system
- Level to which the system meets functional requirements
- Reaction to site visits

A sample comparison is shown in table 5.2.

Table 5.2.   Sample of comparisons between vendors responding to RFP

Comparison of Vendor Systems			
System Capabilities	**System A**	**System B**	**System C**
Works with existing hospital information system	Yes	Yes	Yes
One-time costs	$654,000	$498,500	$576,000
Ongoing costs (3 years)	$65,000	$89,000	$79,000
Hardware needed	File server, PCs throughout facility, barcode scanners, and printers	File server, PCs throughout facility, barcode scanners, and printers	File server, PCs throughout facility, barcode scanners, and printers
Works with existing database	Yes	Yes	Yes
Number of years vendor in existence	31	12	6
Number of installations	123	26	2
RFP shows financial viability	Yes	Yes	Yes

Reference Checks

The facility should contact several facilities where the product under consideration is in use. These reference checks are a great way to learn if other facilities are satisfied with the product without the expense and time it takes to go on site visits. The vendor will provide a list of references, and the evaluating facility should try to obtain a complete list of client sites from the vendor or independently identify client facilities that are not on the reference list (Amtayakul 2007). Best practices recommend that the evaluating project team contact facilities from the vendor's reference list, as well as facilities that are clients of the vendor but are not included on the reference list. The reference list may only contain customers who are satisfied with the product and leave off the unsatisfied ones. Facilities not on the list may be identified through the corporate offices, networking, or cold calls. Notes from these reference checks should be collected and used as part of the decision-making process.

Making the Decision

It is the responsibility of the project team to review the responses to the RFP and other evaluation tools to determine which system will best meet the needs of the facility. To prevent arguments over which system to choose, there should be a quantifiable means of evaluating the systems. One way is to assign points to the RFP review, site visits, observations, and other evaluation methods. If a point system is used during the evaluation process, then the system with the highest number of points should theoretically be the best system and therefore the one that is chosen. However, this is not always the case, because a vendor may have the overall highest score but have low scores in key functions; not only should the total points be used, but each individual task should also be considered. A **weighted system** is one method of a point system that can be used (see table 5.3) (Abdelhak et al. 2007). With the weighted system each function would be listed along with a score showing how important the functionality is. The project team would give each function a score and the score would be multiplied by the weight. The weighted scores would then be totaled. There should also be a tiebreaking process, just in case. Examples of tiebreakers could be cost, site visit findings, or other evaluation criteria. As an example of the importance of a complete evaluation system, one corporate entity had all of their HIM directors critique an information system and vote on

Table 5.3.   Sample weighted scores for system selection

Weighted Scores for System Selection					
Functionality	**Weight**	**Vendor A Score**	**Vendor B Score**	**Vendor A Weighted Score**	**Vendor B Weighted Score**
System is user friendly	3	4	6	12	18
EHR can easily access knowledge-based resources on the Internet	3	10	6	30	18
EHR allows patient to view PHR information	2	4	6	8	12
EHR allows patient to enter PHR information	1	2	5	2	5
Total				52	53

the one they wanted. There was a tie and none of the directors would change their vote. The project was cancelled because of the inability to select a system.

In the weighted score example, system B has the highest score and does beat system A in every criteria except one. The one function where it is lower is "EHR can easily access knowledge-based resources on the Internet," where its score is substantially lower than that of System B. The weight of this function is higher than the other functions so decision makers would have to determine what is more important, a higher score or the ability for providers to access knowledge-based materials quickly and easily.

Contract Negotiation

Once the decision on which system to purchase has been made, the contract negotiation process begins. Some hospitals start negotiations with more than one vendor. Based on the initial meetings, the facility chooses one vendor to continue on with negotiations. Typically, a contact team, not the project team, negotiates the contract. The negotiating team should include at least the CIO and an attorney; however, with a minor implementation, the HIM director may work with a member of administration. A minor system might be a chart location system that is used only by the HIM department and is quickly and easily implemented and has a simple contract. A major implementation would involve multiple areas of the healthcare facility, a significant period of time to implement, and a complex contract. The goal of the contract negotiations is a win-win situation. Obviously, the healthcare facility wants a good product at a reasonable cost that is implemented in a reasonable time period. The facility should not try to secure the product under such strict requirements that the relationship with the vendor is negatively impacted from the beginning. With many of these installations, the facility will be working with the vendor for 10 years or longer; therefore, it is in the facility's best interest to create a good working relationship. The facility should not accept the sample contract provided by the vendor because this contract is written in favor of the vendor. The negotiation team is responsible for working with the vendor to develop a contract that works for both parties.

Some of the clauses covered by the contract include:

- Delivery dates
- Licensee grant
- Warranties and guarantees

- Responsibilities of each party

- The state whose laws govern the contract

- Cost

- Milestones for payment

- Force majeure

- Software in escrow

- Version of software

- Penalties

- Cancellation of contract

- Acceptance testing

- Maintenance and updates

- Training

- Documentation (Austin and Boxerman 2003)

A licensee grant is the section of the contract that controls what the healthcare organization can do with the software. It controls the locations that can use it, who can use it, and how it can be used (AHIMA 2006).

Delivery dates are the dates that the software and hardware will be delivered to the healthcare facility. The inclusion of these dates in the contract is important because nothing can be done until the software is available and installed at the facility. Warranties and guarantees are affirmations the vendor makes that if broken, they can be held accountable. Samples of warranties are:

- Vendor has the legal right to sell software.

- If it is found that the vendor does not have the right to sell the software, then the vendor is legally responsible.

- Information systems will be available 99.9 percent of the time.

- Information systems will perform query within 3 seconds.

- Response time for technical support.

Contract law varies by state; therefore, the contract must specify which state's laws cover the terms of the contract. The vendor generally asks for the laws of their state and the hospital asks for their state, so negotiation is required.

It is important to detail the responsibility of each party in the contract (see table 5.4). This helps ensure that no problems will arise later over whom is responsible for what. This information will be used in the negotiation of the price. Obviously, the more participatory a vendor is during implementation, the more the vendor should be paid.

The cost of the system is one of the last clauses negotiated. The amount of money paid to the vendor will be based on the responsibilities of the vendor, the number of users specified in the contract, and other clauses. The facility should require a fixed price so they know exactly what the cost of the system will be. Healthcare facilities should never pay the entire negotiated amount or a large percentage of the cost up front. The contract should establish **payment milestone**s (see table 5.5) (Mikulski 1993). A payment milestone is an action that once occurring triggers payment to the vendor. This payment is a specified percent of the total cost of the system. This must be negotiated and spelled out in the control. Typical milestones include delivery of software, go-live, and acceptance

Table 5.4.   Sample allocation of responsibility list

Task	Responsible Party
Train the trainer	Vendor
Train end users	Facility
Develop interfaces	Facility and vendor
Design screens	Facility
Testing	Facility and vendor

Table 5.5.   Sample milestones for payment

Milestones for Payment	
Milestone	**Percent of Vendor's Payment**
Signing of contract	20 percent
Delivery of software	10 percent
Commencement of testing	10 percent
Go-live	30 percent
Completion of acceptance testing	30 percent

testing. A significant percentage of the payment should be held until acceptance testing is complete. Failure to do so could result in the vendor moving to the next installation and not responding in a timely manner to any outstanding issues. If there is a significant amount of money involved, the vendor is more likely to be responsive to the needs of the facility.

Force majeure is a legal term that refers to an "act of God" (Merriam-Webster 2009). This contract clause is designed so that the parties of the contract cannot be held accountable to a deadline if there was an "act of God" that prevented compliance. For example, say there was a hospital in New Orleans implementing a computer system and the vendor was responsible for a task due in the middle of Hurricane Katrina. In this case, the vendor would not be held accountable for any penalties as specified in the contract.

Healthcare facilities have the need to protect themselves in the event the vendor goes bankrupt. One way of doing this is to place a clause in the contract that requires the vendor to place the source code in escrow (Dolan 2006). **Source code** is the programming code that was used to develop the system. **Escrow** is a situation in which a third party holds a copy of the software in case the vendor goes bankrupt (AHIMA 2006). This means that if the vendor goes out of business, the healthcare facility can obtain access to the code behind the software so they can maintain the system themselves or hire someone else to do so. Both parties prefer to use escrow rather than obtaining access up front. The vendor prefers this method as well because it does not want its trade secrets to be widely available.

Cancellation of the contract becomes important if for some reason the product or vendor does not meet the needs of the facility. This clause allows the vendor or healthcare facility to void the contract with appropriate notice. There should also be a period of time in which the contract is in force unless cancelled earlier by either party. This clause may require a 30- or 60-day notice to the other party in the event of a cancellation (Austin and Boxerman 2003).

The version of software that will be delivered to the facility should be specified in the contract. The vendor will know when the next version is scheduled for release. Depending on the time frame of implementation, the facility may receive the current version or the new version. The contract may also state that the facility will install the current version but will receive the upgrade to the new system as part of the contract or at a reduced cost (Austin and Boxerman 2003).

The contract should specify penalties for both the vendor and the facility for failure to meet the dates specified in the contract. Penalties vary widely and can be monetary or in the form of free training, free software modules, or other forms. The penalties should be serious enough to keep the parties on target, but not so punitive they would seriously risk the financial stability of the facilities. One facility had negotiated such a tight time frame with major penalties that the information systems department essentially did not do anything other than implement the new system and keep the current systems operational for an entire year. If departments needed assistance with the information system, they were told to hire someone to do it for them. Placing this amount of pressure on the vendor or the project team is not the purpose behind the penalties in the contract. The purpose is to keep everyone on task and on target.

Acceptance testing is a critical part of the information system implementation because it establishes whether the terms of the contract have been met regarding performance and functionality. The contract must spell out what outcomes are acceptable. These outcomes will be used to determine when the acceptance testing is complete and the vendor can receive payment (Austin and Boxerman 2003).

Information systems are constantly changing. Maintenance must be an ongoing responsibility for both the vendor and the facility. The contract should spell out the responsibilities of both parties. The contract should also specify if upgrades to the information system are included in the contract and the costs for those upgrades. These upgrades will assist the facility in remaining compliant with accreditation, regulations, and other mandates. The system updates also repairs any problems found in the system and keeps the system operational (Austin and Boxerman 2003).

Training responsibilities of the vendor, including issues such as the number of people to be trained, where they will be trained, the cost of the training, and the length of the training, should be spelled out in the contract (Austin and Boxerman 2003).

The contract should include the type of documentation provided by the vendor to the facility. This documentation generally includes technical manuals for technical support as well as user manuals (Austin and Boxerman 2003).

System Design

As discussed earlier in the chapter, a decision will be made during the planning phase in which a facility will purchase a system, use an ASP, or design a system. The requirements identified in the system analysis phase are used to create specifications for the system. The specifications will be used for programming the system in-house or for evaluating vendor systems. If the facility is designing its own system, the facility could create a formal system design or use a prototype. Creating a **prototype** is a way to quickly design and develop a system (Abdelhak et al. 2007). With prototyping, programmers quickly develop a system, show it to the users, obtain feedback, make revisions to the program, and continue until the system is developed. Although this is an option for system design, most system designs are much more formal and detailed.

The design should include system objectives, output specifications, input specifications, database design, and expected costs of the system. The objectives are the goals the facility wants to achieve with the implementation of the system. The output specification would be reports and screens to be produced in detail. Input specifications identify the data needed to accomplish the goals and produce the outputs. The design should specify what data are collected, from where the data will originate, and in what format the data should be stored. The design should specify the size of the database and amount of activity expected. Once the specifications are developed, administration must approve them before proceeding with the project (Abdelhak 2007).

Check Your Understanding 5.3

1. Our new system is operated on a computer that is physically located at a remote location for our facility. We pay a monthly fee to the company that owns the computer and in return they manage our system for us. This is:

   A. vendor product
   B. ASP
   C. facility developed product
   D. site visits

2. The vendor will be paid 20 percent of the negotiated amount of the contract at the time of the contract signing. This is an example of:

   A. warranty
   B. force majeure
   C. escrow
   D. payment milestone

3. Evaluate this statement: A hospital should be tough in contract negotiating and insist on obtaining the software code.

   A. This is a true statement.
   B. This statement is true only if there is staff to make changes.
   C. This statement is not true. The hospital does not need or want access to the code.
   D. The hospital would be best served by escrow.

4. True or False: In a point-based evaluation system, the information system selected should always have the highest score.

5. True or False: System design must be more detailed for evaluation of software for purchase than for an in-house developed product.

System Implementation

There are many tasks involved in system implementation. Some of these steps can be completed concurrently, whereas others must have one or more of the previous steps completed before proceeding. If any of these tasks are omitted or given little attention, the project will fail. The plan should implement the information system in such a way as to have the least impact on the facility. For example, the new system can be implemented at midnight when the activity in the hospital is low.

Hardware/Software

Because it may take a long time to receive hardware (that is, computers, monitors, and servers), staff needs to plan accordingly and place the order early. The most critical piece of hardware is the file server or other computer storage component that will house the application software. System implementation may be delayed if the file server or other hardware is not available according to the project plan.

The application software will be provided to the healthcare facility by the computer vendor based on the date specified in the contract. The version of the software provided will also be controlled by the contract. If the vendor is late in sending the software for installation, the implementation of the system will be delayed.

Site Preparation

Site preparation is making any needed changes to the physical location where the computer, workstations, printers, or other hardware will be installed (Abdelhak et al. 2007). Site preparation needs vary widely, from construction of a new building, to renovations of an old one, to use of existing structures and upgrades to the infrastructure. Modifications needed may require the installation of special air conditioning and/or floors designed to run cables under it, added security measures, or more electrical outlets to name a few. However, site preparation may be as simple as moving existing hardware around to make room for the new. The nursing units, the HIM department, and other locations may need to be renovated to add space for computer terminals, barcode printers, network printers, and other hardware, but the data center must be completed first because the nursing units and other departments will not use the system until go-live. In addition to the physical plant, the facility network may need to be updated to accommodate the extra traffic resulting from the new system.

Failure to properly prepare the site and infrastructure will result in delays in the installation of hardware and software, which will in turn delay the entire implementation plan of the system. One facility learned this lesson when they attempted to plug in the hardware and did not have an available electrical outlet.

User Preparation

User preparation is providing the users with enough information about the system being implemented so that they are prepared both psychologically and through training to use the system. It is important for system users to be notified and updated throughout the system selection and implementation process. The users need to know that the system is being implemented and should have an accurate understanding of what to expect from the system and what is expected of them. Many people have doubts about their job security or fear computers when new systems are installed; therefore, these fears must be addressed. Management must be open and honest with the users regarding expectations, downsizing, changes in job descriptions, and other concerns. The information must be accurate; otherwise, users will lose trust in the manager's word. Sometimes a new system is promoted so intently that users expect more from the system than it can provide. These unrealistic expectations lead to disappointment and, in turn, a lack of support from the users. There should be as many users involved in the system as possible to obtain their support. Their involvement can be through the system analysis function, being part of the implementation team, assisting in testing, and other ways. Even those users not involved in the selection and implementation need to have realistic expectations. Their expectations can be managed through training, articles in the facility newsletter, updates at department meetings, and other formal and informal means of communication (Abdelhak et al. 2007).

Installing Hardware/Software

Once the hardware arrives, it will need to be set up and installed in the data center. Computers will also need to be installed in the nursing units, training rooms, and all locations decided upon according to the project plan. The printers, network, scanners, and all of the other hardware will also need to be installed according to the project plan.

The software will then need to be loaded onto the file server, mainframe, or other computer in the data center. Some applications require software to be used on the individual user computers. If this is the case, the software has to be loaded on to each individual computer to be used in development and testing. The software on the user computers will have to be installed on all authorized computers prior to implementation. Any failures in the site preparation will be identified in this stage.

Setting Configuration

Most computer software purchased by hospitals or other healthcare facilities provides the facility with at least some flexibility in the implementation of the system. This flexibility is allowed through setting configuration. **Setting configuration** is the entry of the desired behaviors of the system into tables or setting fields. For example, if the computer system will keep track of the patient type, the hospital gets to determine if patients will be classified as inpatient, outpatient, emergency department, testing, outpatient surgery, or another patient type. The facility may even be able to determine that an "I" means inpatient.

The project team sets up the specifications by filling in tables and other fields with the desired setup. They will also be able to update tables that provide their reimbursement rates, tax identification number, national provider identifier, or other appropriate values. Other settings may include time frame before bills drop, data/format of claims submitted to fiscal intermediary, and what fields are required. The settings will ensure that the system works according to the needs of the healthcare facility.

It can take minutes or months to get all the specifications and tables updated, depending on the complexity of the specifications and the system. For example, each user's information must be entered into the system, including their username, initial password, location, type of access, and permissions as to what they can perform within the system. For example, Mary Smith may have access to the laboratory results, but she can only view these results—not delete or modify them. Determining who has access to what and what they can do with it, especially if the system's security controls screens and individual data elements, is a time-consuming task.

Programming and Customization

There may or may not be programming required depending on the type of system, complexity of the system, and whether the facility is purchasing a system or programming one themselves. If the system interfaces with other systems to share information such as demographic or other information, the interfaces will have to be programmed. If the facility is converting data from another computer system, programming will have to be done to perform **data conversion**. Data conversion is the process where data is copied from the existing system, manipulated into the format required by the new system, and entered into the new system.

The facility may want to have some changes made to the software to better meet the needs of the facility. This customization of the system can be completed by either the facility or the vendor. Although customization may better prepare the system to meet the needs of the facility, there are reasons why the facility should not customize the software beyond what is already built into the system by the vendor. Some of these reasons are:

- If the facility makes changes to the software and then has trouble with the system, the vendor can blame the modifications. The vendor may then refuse to work on the system.

- The vendor may not give the facility a service agreement.

- Every time that the facility receives a software update from the computer vendor, the information system staff will have to check the modifications to see if they are affected by the new update. Because the facility may receive several updates a year, this can be an onerous task (Rollins 2006).

Screen Design

The information system may allow the facility to make changes to the computer screen so that it works the best for the facility. **Screen design** is developing screens of an information system to meet the needs of the user and to promote job efficiency. To accomplish this goal, team members involved in this process must be aware of the needs of the users and the work they perform. Reasons why the facility may want to change the computer screen include:

- No single screen contains the data needed to make data entry or viewing efficient.

- The vendor's screens do not have data elements in a logical order for the workflow of the users.

- The existing screens are too cluttered for the users' preference.

The screen design may include designing computer views for various types of users. This flexibility would allow nurses to see new orders, care plans, or other information first; the cardiologist and neurologist would have first access to cardiac and neurologic tests, respectively.

When designing screens, the fields should be in a logical flow to facilitate data entry. The flow of data entry should be from left to right and top to bottom. Screen design is very different from form design. Screens have about one-third of the view that a paper form has (Rhodes 1997). Screens, like paper, should have a title and/or a control number to manage the screen. Screens should be simple to use and have a standardized terminology across screens to facilitate data entry, training, and data quality. For example, the data element medical record number should be called that on all screens—not medical record number on one and patient identifier on another. Screens should also have the same look and feel so that the user can easily move from screen to screen. Instructions can be posted on the screen where necessary to assist users. Color, blinking, and reverse video can be used to draw the user's attention to important data such as allergies. Special features such as color should be used sparingly so the user's attention is drawn to the information displayed. The color of the screen and text should be pleasing to the eye and comfortable for users to view for long periods of time.

A **graphical user interface** (GUI) is a method of screen display that uses icons, menus, and other tools to assist in the use of the system (Hebda et al. 2005). These icons are shown on a toolbar. Icons provide shortcuts to functionality within the system, along with buttons and menus, allowing the user to command the software to perform specific tasks and providing shortcuts to functionality within the system (Williams 2006). The most common and recognized GUI interface is the Windows GUI.

Report Design

Report design is the process of creating and formatting a report. This design includes the content of the report, the order of the data on the report, and any desired formatting specifications. The system may come with standard reports, but most likely will not have all those needed by the facility. In addition, the reports provided will probably not be presented the way users want them to look. Because of this, the facility will need to design new reports and/or alter existing "canned" reports to make sure that users have all of the information routinely needed. This does not mean that the implementation team has to write every report the facility will ever need now. The report design discussed here is for the standard reports that users will need daily, weekly, monthly, quarterly, semiannually, or annually. Ad hoc reports, which are one-time reports, can be created as needed. Many information systems have a report writer built into them. Many allow data to be exported into various reporting systems such as Crystal Reports, Cognos, and Microsoft Access.

Typical characteristics of reports are report title, the date and time that the report was run, the time period that the data covers, the page number where appropriate, appropriate column headings, and data. These reports may be in a multitude of formats, some of which can be changed or manipulated and others that cannot. For example, a report may be generated in Microsoft Excel format, which would allow the user to sort data, run calculations, group, and perform other data manipulations. Other reports may be in Adobe Acrobat format, which is generally used for the display of data only. A sample report is shown in figure 5.6.

Interfaces

According to AHIMA (2010, 155), an **interface** is "the zone between different computer systems across which users want to pass information (for example, a computer program written to exchange information between systems or the graphic display of an application program designed to make the program easier to use)." Interfaces link two or more systems together, enabling them to share data such as demographics. In other words, an interface acts as a bridge between systems transporting and translating data into each system's respective programmed language. Interfaces can be one-way or two-way. One-way interfaces send data from one system to another without any data returning. In a two-way or bidirectional interface, data is exchanged between systems regularly.

Writing interfaces is a difficult and time-consuming process because a program has to be written and maintained for sending and receiving data. Representatives from both computer vendors must be involved in the process. If one system has the insurance type Medicare stored as MED and the other system has it stored as MCR, this information must be converted. This conversion can be performed by an **interface engine.** An interface engine allows "two applications to exchange information without having to build a customized interface for each application" (Abdelhak et al. 2007, 280). The interface engine has to convert the data so that it can be accepted by the system receiving the information. The interface must know where the insurance type is stored in the originating system, retrieve the data, convert the data, and then plug the converted data into the correct field in the new system. As a tool, the interface engine has made interfaces easier to work with, but there is still a lot of work to do. An interface engine is a type of middleware. **Middleware** is software and hardware that connects applications (Abdelhak et al. 2007). The interface engine does not eliminate the work necessary to transmit data between systems, but, rather, reduces it. If the interface engine goes down, no data can be transmitted, which can cause issues especially with patient care and the need for current information. Figure 5.7 illustrates interface engine connectivity.

Figure 5.6.　　Sample report

		Macon General Hospital				
		Admission Register				
		March 31, 20XX				
Encounter Number	**MR Number**	**Patient Name**	**Admit Date**	**Admit Time**	**Attending MD**	**Bed**
123456812	1123568	Benson, Mary	3/31/08	19:22	Scott, A	264
123456800	0568745	Johnson, Claude	3/31/08	13:26	Wilson, J	547
123456789	1234567	Smith, Amanda	3/31/08	01:23	Scott, A	246
123456806	0984562	Thomas, Frank	3/31/08	17:47	Jones, X	534

Number of admissions　　4

Figure 5.7.　　Example of interface engine connectivity

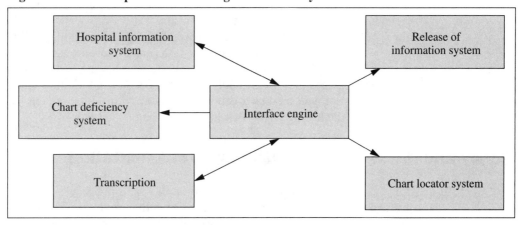

Conversion

With most new information systems, a facility is converting from one system to another—even if the first system is paper. The facility cannot ignore the historical data but, rather, must bring some (if not all of it) to the new system. In a paper system, the historical data must be captured through abstracting, scanning, or other data entry methods. In an information system implementation, conversion is transferring data from one computer system to another while simultaneously making any necessary changes in format or content. A conversion is more difficult than it sounds because systems frequently store data very differently or the facility may be making changes to how it wants data to be collected. During conversion planning, the implementation team has to determine how much data is being converted and what data fields will need to be converted from one format to another. The amount of data transferred is a decision that must be made by the facility. The decision will be influenced by the type of system, laws and regulations, whether or not the old system will remain operational, and other issues. Sometimes facilities decide to transfer data from a specified time period only into the new system. For example, they may decide to convert only the last 2 years. Other conversions require all data be transferred. The facility may also choose to enter data for all time periods, but only selected data elements rather than all data collected.

Planning is critical to ensure the quality of data in the new system. Once the conversion planning is finished, a program needs to be written that will make the necessary changes. A formal testing plan is required to determine how the implementation team will test the conversion to work out any problems before go-live.

Reengineering Processes

Reengineering, also known as business process reengineering, is reevaluating the way the facility does business in order to improve efficiency. Reengineering is a task that is frequently overlooked in the efforts to implement the IS. Every task and every preconceived notion must be challenged. The question "why" should be asked over and over. There are no exemptions from being subjected to evaluation and change—everything is subject to change. This is challenging to employees who are comfortable with the status quo. Some of the tasks performed by the employees have been performed for years. The reason behind the task may be outdated, but the task continues because the employee is afraid to stop. At one facility, an employee received a report generated by the information system department every day. The report was filed away and never reviewed. When asked how the report was utilized, the employee stated that it was never reviewed. The employee balked at the idea of stopping the report—just in case it was ever needed. The implementation of a new information system is a perfect time to critique the tasks performed to try and improve efficiency, costs, and effectiveness (Abdelhak et al. 636).

The employees may feel threatened and afraid because of the changes impacting their job, but reengineering is a necessary part of the information system process. The facility cannot implement a computer system and expect the work processes to remain the same. The facility will need to change procedures, update the policy and procedure manual, change workflow, eliminate unnecessary tasks, and add new tasks. Failure to do so can decrease efficiency rather than maximize on the benefits the system affords. The information system changes the way a facility conducts business and impacts the manual processes and workflow as well as their overall interaction with the computer. The documentation tested during the testing phase should contain the revised processes.

Policy and Procedure Development/Documentation

After the reengineering is completed, the policy and procedure manual must be updated to reflect the new way of doing business (Abdelhak et al. 2007). Policies and procedures should blend together the manual processes and decision-making processes. Management and maintenance of the system itself must also be clearly outlined. Examples of system policies are backups, downtime policies for routine maintenance, upgrades, testing of upgrades, and disaster planning.

The policies and procedures need to address how the system will be used by the various users throughout the facility such as coders, admission clerks, and other staff. In addition, the healthcare facility must create training manuals and user guides for reference. These materials will be available to the users as resources on how to use the system, how to incorporate it into their job, and how to identify how their job has changed.

Check Your Understanding 5.4

1. An interface engine is an example of:

   A. system analysis tool
   B. functional requirements
   C. setting configuration
   D. middleware

2. The type of testing where both the old system and the new system are operating at the same time is:

   A. interface testing
   B. application testing
   C. parallel testing
   D. conversion testing

3. The form used to report problems with the new system is frequently called:

   A. trouble ticket
   B. request for proposal
   C. functional requirements
   D. testing plan

4. The implementation stage that looks at the way the business does business is called:

   A. testing
   B. reengineering
   C. conversion
   D. system analysis

5. True or False: A graphical user interface is the process of creating and formatting reports.

Training

Training is crucial to the success of the implementation process. There needs to be a well-designed training plan that addresses the timing and methods used to train the users (Englebardt and Nelson 2002). The plan must be properly executed or negative repercussions can occur. Users may be concerned they are reverting back to being a novice employee after being an expert in their position. They may also be concerned about whether or not they will be able to keep their job if they are unable to learn the new computer system. Individuals who are most concerned with the new computer systems are those who are not comfortable with computers at all. Communicating with employees and keeping them informed of changes, impact, and expectations of their position will help prepare them for training.

Each person learns differently. Learning ability is impacted by their age, maturity level, and experience, so their preferred learning style may change over time. Because of these factors, instructors should use a variety of methods that will reach all learning styles. Typical learning styles are:

- Sensory: Is the learner auditory (prefers to listen), visual (prefers to read), or kinesthetic (prefers to practice)?

- Personality: Various personality traits shape our orientation to the world.

- Information processing: People differ in how they receive and process information.

- Instructional and environmental preference: Sound, light, structure, and learning relationships affect perceptions. (LaTour and Eichenwald Maki 2007, 717)

Instructors and trainers should have a basic understanding of adult learning principles and practice them in the development of training and its implementation. Some key adult learning principles are:

- Adults like being responsible for their own decisions: They resent not having control, so the instructor should let the learners have a say in the program. This can take the form of helping to set the agenda, deciding which of two or three activities to do, and so on (Bryant and Reimer 2007).

- Adults are experienced: Adult learners come to the training session with a lot of experience and knowledge upon which they can draw. Not all adults have the same knowledge and experience. The instructor and students can learn from each other. The varied backgrounds and knowledge can make for an interesting discussion and an improved learning experience (Bryant and Reimer 2007).

- Adults need to know why: Instructors should get into a habit of telling the adults why they need to do or learn what they are being taught. They need to know why something is important just as much as they need to know how to do something (Bryant and Reimer 2007).

- Adults need to see relevance: Adults do not want to waste their time. They want to learn what they need to know for the immediate future. The instructor will need to tie the material in the class to what the individuals in the course will be doing. In other words, do not teach nurses how to do something with the computer system that only the HIM department will be doing in the future. The nurses need to know what they will be doing. If an adult learner does not see relevance to themselves, they will not be motivated to learn (Bryant and Reimer 2007).

- The adult needs to be ready to learn: Training sessions may be mandatory and the learners may show up physically to the session, but they cannot be made to learn. The instructor must engage the learner and encourage the desire to learn (LaTour and Eichenwald Maki 2006).

- The learner has to be motivated to learn: Some healthcare facilities have motivated learners by making them take a competency test at the end of the training session. This test makes the learner use skills they learned in class. The motivation comes in because the healthcare facility usually ties the future of their job to successfully completing this test. These tests are generally very easy, but there are people who cannot pass them. These users are usually given a second or third chance before they are terminated. The threat of termination is not the best motivation because motivation to learn should come from within; however, the facility must know that the users are competent to use the systems (Bryant and Reimer 2007).

Planning for Training

There should be someone on the project team who is responsible for planning the complete training process. This trainer has a wide range of responsibilities including developing objectives, developing the training plan, and implementing the training.

The trainer would attend implementation team meetings in order to keep up with the status of the project. The trainer needs to know when training will be needed, the type of training needed, and also be a superuser (or expert) on the new system. With this knowledge, the trainer will be prepared to develop the training program necessary to teach others to use the system. The trainer is responsible for sharing and providing the necessary knowledge needed to prepare other trainers to teach as well.

The trainer will also work with the training staff from the vendor. The vendor's staff knows the product well and will be able to offer the team suggestions on different teaching methods directly related to the system. The vendor should provide the trainers with resources that can be customized for the facility.

Keep in mind, that as the trainer, he or she will be working with both management and end users during the training planning and training implementation stages. These interactions make the trainer an excellent liaison between the two groups. The trainer will be able to communicate expectations of administration to users as well as communicate the fears and concerns of the users back to administration.

Contents of the Plan

The project team should create a training schedule that allows everyone who needs training to participate (Englebardt and Nelson 2002). The schedule should include sessions for all work shifts. This may mean training sessions are conducted for the day, evening, night, and weekend shifts. The training plan should contain learning objectives providing both trainer and trainees with information about what will be accomplished throughout the training sessions. The training plan should also outline the agenda, which describes the functions of the computer system that will be covered, how they will be covered, and how much time will be spent on each topic (Englebardt and Nelson 2002). The "how it will be covered" section includes teaching tools such as PowerPoint, hands-on training, demonstrations, and computer-assisted instruction to be used during training.

The training plan should also address the content that will be covered. These may include topics such as rollout schedule, policies and procedures, confidentiality, and security. When planning content, trainers need to determine the level of computer literacy each trainee possesses before determining what training is needed. For example, have they ever used a mouse? Do they need to learn Windows? The trainer will need to determine how many students will attend each session so that the number of trainers and training sessions can be determined. The planners will also have to determine the resources that will be needed such as a training room, computers, Internet access, training database, data projector, and handouts.

Another decision to be made is how the training will be divided into sessions, because not all users need the same training. Two examples for the division of sessions are by department (such as nursing) or by function (such as order entry). In other words, the planner needs to decide whether the session will teach all nurses together or will the session teach people how to look up test results and have everyone who needs to know how to do this included in the same session. The division of the training will impact the number of teachers, the schedule, and the training materials.

Selecting the Training Location

Not every trainer is fortunate enough to have a dedicated training facility. Trainers may be forced to reserve computer classrooms throughout the facility. If so, the rooms need to be reserved early. Whether there is a dedicated room or not, the trainer should make sure the room is physically comfortable. This means that the room is at a comfortable temperature, has appropriate lighting, and the workstations are ergonomically sound. Cellular phones and beepers should be turned off in order to prevent distractions.

Scheduling the Training

Scheduling can be a very tricky task because trainers have to conduct different training classes required by patient care providers, administrative office staff, and other groups of users. Many healthcare facilities are open 24 hours, 7 days a week, thus employees work a variety of shifts. Because of this, training must be offered on all shifts including weekends. Issues to consider are as follows:

- If there is more than one class required, the team must make sure that they are offered in a logical format. Breaking modules down into separate classes is wise because otherwise the students become confused. For example, the trainers would need to teach an introduction to computers class before the trainers teach Windows, and the trainer would need to teach Windows before they can teach people to use a Windows-based application.

- This is further complicated by the fact that the trainers need to schedule the classes as close as possible to go-live while starting training early enough to get everyone trained in time. Completing training too early is also problematic because the users can forget what they learned before the system is implemented, thus making the transition difficult for the user and the facility.

- Length of a session matters. Short sessions tend to work better because most healthcare professionals are used to being on their feet while working. They are unaccustomed to sitting down and may become frustrated by inactivity (Abdelhak et al. 2007).

- The training sessions should not be scheduled during holidays because many people take time off, which causes scheduling problems with getting everyone trained.

- Physicians should be scheduled for one-on-one training sessions. The reason for this is that physicians do not like to appear less than competent in front of peers. Some physicians do not know how to use the computers and do not want others to know about their lack of knowledge. Physician training is scheduled at the convenience of the physician, which is basically any time. It could be early in the morning, at lunch, late in afternoon, the evening, or on weekends in order to avoid interfering with physicians' schedules.

Resources Needed

Each user should be provided a handout at the training session to take back to their work area. Training materials are excellent resources to be utilized by users to look up how to do some task that may have been forgotten. Several days, weeks, or even months may pass between the initial training session and the implementation of the computer system. During that time, it is likely for users to forget much of the material learned. To help users retain the knowledge acquired in training, the facility may also want to make the system available (in test mode) to users for practice throughout this interim period.

Content suggestions to the development of educational materials provided to the students are as follows:

- The objectives should be clearly outlined.

- The agenda for the course should be sent to the scheduled attendees ahead of time. The agenda is subject to change, but acts as a guide to help keep trainers on track.

Train the Trainer

"**Train the trainer**" is a phrase used to describe a group of one or a few people sent to the vendor to be trained on how to use the new system and then go back to the facility to train more trainers (Wager et al. 2005). These people are generally called "superusers." Superusers return to the healthcare facility and train other trainers who will in turn help conduct training sessions (Englebardt and Nelson 2002).

The trainer is the one person whom the user associates with knowledge of the system and its uses, so the trainer is very likely to receive calls from former students about it. This visibility will make the trainer a key player in the hours and days following go-live. It will likely be the trainer that users turn to with questions and fears.

Conducting the Training

Now that all of the work planning the training is finished, it is time to conduct the class. Instructors should be prepared to enter the classroom to make sure it is ready for training. Trainers should use a variety of instructional methods during the session as this has been found to improve learning. Students should be provided with handouts, policies and procedures, and other materials that they can keep (Hebda et al. 2005).

Evaluating the Training

Trainers must be evaluated on their delivery, impact, and knowledge of the application to make sure objectives of the training are being met.

LaTour and Eichenwald Maki (2007) identified four outcomes of training that should be critiqued. These are:

- Reaction: What is the reaction of the trainees immediately after the program? Are they excited about what they learned?

- Learning: What have the trainees actually learned? Can they now use a new software program?

- Behavior: Have supervisors noticed a change in employee behavior? Has morale improved?

- Results: How does the actual level of performance compare with the established objectives? Can the employees assign codes more accurately? (LaTour and Eichenwald Maki 2007, 731)

A valuable method for obtaining feedback is to have each trainee complete a written evaluation at the completion of the session, answering questions about the overall training and the ability of the trainer. These evaluations can help to identify what is and is not working. Findings may identify needed improvements such as in the handouts, poor instructors, or not enough time for hands-on activities. Findings from the trainee evaluations should be shared with the instructors anonymously so that any needed modifications can be identified, and to just evaluate the overall training plan performance. Evaluation results should be used to improve the quality and method of training where needed. There is always room for improvement.

The overall training program should also be evaluated on an ongoing basis to ensure that goals of training are met. A formal plan for evaluation should be developed prior to the start of the training sessions.

Additional and Ongoing Training

After the training phase and before go-live, the facility eventually won't need the same number of trainers or frequency of class sessions. Training needs should be reassessed to determine frequency and structure of needs. Training may be reorganized to be in conjunction with the facility's human resources department new employee orientation program or it may be separate. Training may be required before the employee is issued a user identification and password.

In a perfect world, the system on which users are trained would remain the same as the one implemented. However, changes to the system will be made and are necessary for technology advances, resolving glitches, and other issues. Therefore, training does not end with go-live of the system. When significant changes are made, training may have to occur to update and prepare users for the changes. Also, existing employees may need additional training to learn advanced capabilities, reinforce what they've already learned, or if they transfer jobs or their job changes over time.

Computer-Assisted Instruction

Computer-assisted instruction (CAI) will not be used by most healthcare facilities, but it is a viable option. CAI is a software program designed to use multimedia and interactive technology to teach a topic. A good example of CAI is the CD that comes with many medical terminology textbooks. Multimedia can use audio, video, simulation, self-quizzes, and other tools to engage the student. Drill and practice CAI reinforce material that the learner already knows, whereas problem-solving addresses issues that the learner may face in his or her discipline (Kreider and Haselton 1997).

The benefit to CAI is that it has been proven to increase learning while decrease learning time (Hebda et al. 2005). Students are able to work at their own pace and on their own schedule. They are able to receive immediate feedback on whether or not they do something right (Kreider and Haselton 1997). CAI also reduces costs, provides standardized training, and is designed to use multiple learning styles. The student is actively engaged in the training (Hebda et al. 2005).

Documenting the Training

Documentation of all training provided is critical. Students should sign into each training session to provide proof of attendance for both employee's and employer's benefit. If a competency test is given, documentation of the results also should be maintained. Copies of all training materials and objectives for the training also should be retained.

Testing Plan

All components of the information system will need testing before the go-live. The purpose of testing the computer system is to ensure that everything is functioning properly (Austin and Boxerman 2007). Testing helps the implementation team identify any bugs (problems) with the system. This is a cyclical process so the team will test the system, identify problems, fix problems, and test the system again. The test cycle will continue until all problems have been resolved. Testing requires careful and detailed planning to ensure that complete and accurate testing is carried out in a timely manner.

Types of Testing

There are many types of testing that must be performed in preparation for a system implementation. The types of testing include:

- Interface Testing: Ensures that the interfaces function properly. The facility must test to confirm that data from the feeder system are transferred into the new system in the correct field and in the right format. Data to be transferred varies by system but commonly include the patient's name, medical record number, date of birth, and other demographic information. Other types of data that may be transferred include laboratory tests, radiology results, or any other data that are collected.

- Hardware Testing: Ensures that all hardware, including computers, printers, and scanners, work together as they should. Examples of testing to be performed include the ability to scan documents, print a report, or scan barcode. Some computers may have limitations placed on their abilities for privacy, security, or other reasons. For example, the facility may choose not to print laboratory results on the nursing units to protect confidentiality, thus forcing users to look up the most current results available.

- Application Testing: Ensures that every function of the new computer system works. Application testing also ensures that the system meets the functional requirements and other required specifications in the RFP or contract. Application testing should also ensure that every conceivable situation that the computer will be used to address can be handled. The team must also test the reports to ensure that the data and statistics contained therein are correct.

- Documentation Testing: During the implementation process a number of documents, including user guides, policies and procedures, and training materials, are created. These documents should be followed during the testing process to ensure that the instructions in the documents are accurate. In testing the documentation, the tester follows and tests the information system documentation that will be provided to the users. Errors in the documentation will be identified and corrected so that the user will have the proper instructions.

- Conversion Testing: Ensures that the team is able to transfer data from the old system to the new system. Conversion testing will confirm that the data conversion is performed correctly. Testing usually begins with a small amount of real data that have been copied. After the initial test has been run, the team would fix any problems, rerun the test, and then continue to add larger and larger amounts of data. This testing will continue until the team is sure that the problems have been resolved prior to the actual data conversion.

- Training Testing: The team should train a group to see how well the training materials, agenda, format of training, time allotted for training, and other attributes work. Changes are made to the training process as needed before real training begins.

- Volume Testing: Most of the testing performed on the application is done with a handful of people sitting at a computer system trying to identify problems. The system may work fine with a small group of people, but most systems are used by large groups of people simultaneously. To test the system in as real an environment as possible, volume testing should be performed. Volume testing gets as many people to use the system at one time as possible. Volume testing confirms that the computer system and the network can handle the large volume of users and data. The user task force as well as other users throughout the facility can be brought in for volume testing. The project team will need to recruit as many users as possible to use the system at the same time (Abdelhak et al. 2007).

- Parallel Testing: Unlike most other testing, parallel testing occurs when the new system is operational. This is not a required test, but can be a valuable one. Parallel testing is when the facility runs the old and the new system simultaneously and compares the reports and data from the two systems to validate both performance and synchronization. For example, the facility could compare the number of admissions for a specific date, the number of tests ordered, or the number of times that a test was ordered. Because of the extra resources needed to operate both systems, this test is frequently omitted. The benefit to parallel testing is that if the new system does not work as expected and the facility has to shut the system down, then the existing system is current, thus not impacting the operations of the facility.

- Acceptance Testing: Like parallel testing, acceptance testing occurs after go-live. It is a time to verify that the system is working as expected in a live environment. It gives the healthcare facility time to confirm that the new system meets response time, functional requirements, and other standards guaranteed in the contract (Amatayakul 2007).

Test Plan

The testing plan must cover areas such as what is to be tested, who will be involved in the testing, dates of testing, documentation of testing results, and types of testing. The testing must continue until all problems are fixed. The testing must include the documentation created for use with the system as well.

The testing plan should create a realistic testing environment. For example, the settings in the test system should be the ones that the facility will utilize during operation. The testing plan will identify a "laundry list" of functions that must be tested before the system is implemented. One way to test the functions is scenario or use-case testing, during which users bring real-life situations to be addressed by the system. These scenarios should be documented in the plan. The use of scenarios allows the user to think through how a situation will be handled by actually using the system. Scenario testing thoroughly tests the system because it addresses entries into the system, tasks, and output from the system (Amatayakul 2007).

Testing Documentation

Many healthcare facilities use what is frequently called a trouble ticket to report problems encountered during the testing phase. The trouble ticket is simply a form that is used to give specific information on problems encountered. The information provided may include: screen where problem occurred, function being performed, error message received, data entered, report with incorrect data, or other problems encountered. The information provided must be as detailed as possible so that the problem can be replicated by the project manager or designee. The trouble ticket is logged into some type of tracking system when received, assigned a tracking number, and assigned to the appropriate person to solve. Once the problem has been resolved, the resolution is recorded, and the system testing begins again. The team cannot just test the part that was broken because the change that was made to fix the problem may have broken something else.

Conversion

Once the system is ready for use and the facility is ready for the system, the data conversion plan must be implemented to move the existing data into the new system in the appropriate format (Wager, Lee, and Glaser, 2005). If data conversion is successful, the facility is then ready to start using the new computer system. Facilities frequently capture the information available in the system at midnight so that they can determine what data are in the old system and what data are in the new system. A specific time period of transition is useful in case the facility has to go back to the old system because the new system did not work.

Go-Live

Go-live is the official time and date that the facility begins using the new system. The go-live is generally scheduled for a time when the facility is the least busy. For example, a hospital will generally go-live during the night shift because there is less activity at that time.

Go-Live Models

There are four philosophies with regard to go-live: parallel, phased, pilot, and big bang (Young 2000).

Parallel Approach

Although parallel start-up works well, it is labor intensive and therefore expensive. Because the old system is in place and current, this approach provides a safety net and has the least amount of risk involved.

Phased Approach

Another method is the phased approach. In this method, the implementation starts with one module of the system, and then gradually other modules of the system are added. A module is a subset of an information system such as pharmacy orders in a clinical provider order entry system. All units, departments, and other entities utilize the system, but they only use it for one module at a time. For example, a hospital could start using their order entry system by ordering medications only. After the medication ordering is successful, then laboratory will be added and so on. With an optical disk system, hospitals frequently start scanning emergency department records, then outpatient surgery, and then other record types until they work their way up to inpatient records. The advantage of this method is that staff is not overwhelmed by trying to do everything at once and the impact on the staff is lessened. The disadvantage is that it seems to take forever to finish the start-up process.

Pilot Method

The next philosophy is the pilot method in which only one nursing unit, department, or other entity starts using the new system at a time. Once consistently successful, the next group is implemented. For example, the 3W nursing unit starts ordering everything using the new system, but nobody else uses the system. The next unit scheduled would be unit 3E. Again, this method is designed to limit the impact on the facility.

Big Bang Method

The last method, the big bang method which is also called the cutover method, is the most risky. With this method, the facility stops using the old system and starts using the new system. It is the riskiest because the facility no longer has the old system as a backup and the new system is being used all over the hospital, so there are a lot of scared people trying to use a computer system they are not comfortable with.

Planning for Go-Live

Whichever method is chosen, planning is critical because system implementation cannot interfere with patient care. There are some steps that should be taken no matter which plan is selected.

Initial Support

First of all there needs to be a member of the implementation team in every unit or department when the system goes live. These team members should be highly visible. They could all wear the same t-shirts or buttons or some other means of identifying them as a member of the implementation team. Team members are needed to answer questions and generally ensure that the system start-up runs as smoothly as possible. Keep in mind that users will be scared and will want to see someone who can help them. Trainers play an important role not only in the training but during go-live, which means they are a key part of the implementation presence throughout the facility.

Ongoing Support

Initially someone must be available 24 hours a day, 7 days a week to assist users. The length of time that this intensive support is needed will depend on how major a system it is and how well the implementation is going. Generally this intensive support is needed no longer than a week (Englebardt and Nelson 2002). There should be a special help desk users can call for help when needed. The amount of coverage needed will eventually be reduced to the use of beepers and the regular help desk support. The implementation team must be prepared to go back to the old system if the new one does not work.

System Evaluation

After the system is implemented and functioning properly, the implementation team will need to evaluate how well the system implementation went. "The purpose of **system evaluation** is to determine whether the system functions in the way intended" (Abdelhak et al. 337). The team needs to learn what did and did not work and determine how they can improve the next implementation. The team will also want to know if the facility met the goals that were established for the project and if the project came in on budget. This evaluation allows the team to learn from mistakes and from the experience. After a predetermined time period, the team will need to determine if the facility has realized all expected benefits (Johns 2007). Some examples include goals such as, did the number of staff get reduced, or did the facility save the money that was expected, or did it reduce the turnaround time on obtaining test results?

Post-Implementation

Post-implementation, or maintenance, is the final step of the implementation process. In this stage, the system is operational and the goal is to provide ongoing maintenance and improve the system where needed (Hebda et al. 2005). In the immediate post-implementation period, problems may be found that were not revealed during the system testing and will need to be resolved. Changes may need to be made to correct the problems and more testing will need to be done. Even after the system is working well, there will be periodic updates to ensure the system is current. There will also be routine maintenance and upgrades such as backing up data, increasing storage capacity, and upgrading hardware and software. As discussed earlier, major computer systems have what is called a test system or a **test environment** (Hebda et al. 2005). This is an exact duplicate of the system in use, excluding data. In this test environment, changes can be made to the system and tested to see what happens.

Because it is in the test and not the production environment, the software changes can be tested without worrying about problems resulting from the changes. This will enable support staff to solve problems before the update is moved to the live. Once the system is working appropriately in the test environment, it can be implemented into the live one.

Check Your Understanding 5.5

1. True or False: The active learner prefers to learn by case studies rather than writing papers.

2. The go-live model where the old system is stopped and the new system used is:

   A. phased
   B. pilot
   C. cutover
   D. parallel

3. Which of the following is an adult learning principle?

   A. Adults need to see relevance
   B. Adults like to be told what to do
   C. Adults learn well even if not motivated
   D. Adults have the same knowledge and experience

4. True or False: System training should be broken into short sessions for healthcare professionals.

5. The implementation stage where the team determines what they could have done better is:

   A. training
   B. post-implementation
   C. evaluation
   D. system analysis

References

Abdelhak, M., S. Grostick, M.A. Hanken, and E. Jacobs. 2007. *Health Information: Management of a Strategic Resource.* St. Louis, MO: Saunders Elsevier.

Amatayakul, M.K. 2007. *Electronic Health Records: A Practical Guide for Professionals and Organizations.* Chicago: AHIMA.

American Health Information Management Association. 2006. Wordpower: A glossary of software licensing terms. *Journal of AHIMA* 77(4):42, 44.

American Health Information Management Association. 2007. RFI/RFP template. *Journal of AHIMA* 78(6): web extra. http://library.ahima.org/xpedio/groups/public/documents/ahima/bok1_034278. hcsp?dDocName=bok1_034278.

American Health Information Management Association. 2010. *Pocket Glossary of Health Information Management and Technology*, 2nd ed. Chicago: AHIMA.

Austin, C.J. and S.B. Boxerman. 2003. *Information Systems for Healthcare Management.* Chicago: AUPHA Press Health Administration Press.

Bryant, G. and J. Reimer. 2006. E-learning for HIM, theory and practice: A new world order or reinforcement of existing (e-) learning theory. *Proceedings of the American Health Information Management Association's 79th National Convention and Exhibit.*

Dolan, T.G. 2006. Contracting for ASP services: When signing for the benefits, remember to manage the risks. *Journal of AHIMA* 77(5):48–50.

Englebardt, S.P. and R. Nelson. 2002. *Healthcare Informatics: An Interdisciplinary Approach.* St. Louis, MO: Moseby.

Glandon, G.L., D.H. Smaltz, and D.J. Slovensky. 2008. *Austin and Boxerman's Information Systems for Healthcare Management.* Chicago: Health Administration Press/AUPHA.

Hebda, T, P. Czar, and C. Mascara. 2005. *Handbook of Informatics for Nurses & Health Care Professionals.* Upper Saddle River: Pearson Prentice Hall.

Johns, M.L., ed. 2006. *Health Information Management Technology: An Applied Approach.* Chicago: AHIMA.

Kreider, N.A. and B.J. Haselton. 1997. *The Systems Challenge.* Chicago: American Hospital Association.

LaTour, K.M. and S. Eichenwald Maki, eds. 2006. *Health Information Management: Concepts, Principles, and Practice.* Chicago: AHIMA.

McWay, D.C. 2008. *Today's Health Information Management: An Integrated Approach.* Clifton Park, NY: Thompson Delmar Learning.

Merriam-Webster. 2009. Force majeure. http://www.merriam-webster.com/dictionary/force+majeure.

Mikulski, F.A. 1993. Managing Your Vendors. Englewood Cliffs, NJ: Prentice-Hall, Inc.

Rhodes, H. 1997 (March). Practice brief: Developing information capture tools.

Rollins, G. 2006. The perils of customization. *Journal of AHIMA* 77(6):24–28.

Wager, K.A., F.W. Lee, and J.P. Glaser. 2005. *Managing Health Care Information Systems.* San Francisco: Jossey-Bass.

Williams, A. Design for better data: How software and users interact onscreen matters to data quality. *Journal of AHIMA* 77(2):56–60.

Young, K.M. 2000. *Informatics for Healthcare Professionals.* Philadelphia, PA: F.A. Davis.

Chapter 6
Data Storage and Retrieval

Objectives

- Assist in the planning for an EDMS.
- Differentiate between an EDMS and an EHR.
- Develop policies and procedures to manage HIM in an EDMS environment.
- Design reports.
- Manage the day-to-day activities of a document imaging system.
- Prepare forms for document imaging.
- Determine the best way to index documents.
- Develop data retention schedule.
- Determine storage needs for the facility.
- Design screens.
- Understand the importance of destruction, its methods and techniques.

Key Terms

Ad hoc report
Administrative data
Aggregate data
Annotation
Backscanning
Bar code
Boolean search
Business continuity planning
  (BCP)
Clinical data
Code 39

Computer output to laser disk
  (COLD)
Data manipulation
Data retention
Document imaging
Electronic document
  management system (EDMS)
Enterprise report management
  (ERM)
External data
Hybrid record
Internal data

Jukebox
Patient-specific data
Primary data
Routine reports
Scanner
Scanning workstation
Secondary data
Structured query language (SQL)
Symbology
Target sheet
Workflow technology
WORM technology

Introduction

Patient information traditionally has been stored in paper files in open shelving, mobile shelving, or other storage units in the health information management (HIM) department. With the advent of electronic document management system (EDMS), the electronic health record (EHR), and other clinical information systems, more information is being moved to digital storage media. Rather than managing filing of medical records and loose materials, the HIM professional is now managing the EDMS, jukeboxes, scanners, retention of digital data, hybrid records, and more. These methods of storage create new challenges for the HIM professional.

During this time of transition from the paper record to the EHR, HIM professionals must be prepared to manage both paper and electronic data. This combination of paper and electronic medical record data is called the **hybrid record**. Even when the EHR has been implemented, the EHR must still be prepared to accommodate paper documents received from external sources. Examples of documents that may be received in paper format are records from other facilities, consent forms the patient has to sign, and the personal health record.

Data Sources

To understand data storage and retrieval, it is important to understand the data as well as the sources from which they came. Data are generally broken down in two different ways: primary and secondary data sources. **Primary data** come directly from the source. The medical record is a primary data source because the information comes directly from the patient and the healthcare providers. Data taken from a primary source (such as the medical record) and abstracted into another database or registry are called a **secondary data** source. Examples of secondary data sources are cancer registry, master patient index, and disease index.

Other ways to differentiate between data sources include patient-specific data and aggregate data. **Patient-specific data** identify the individual patient to whom the information describes. Patient-specific data are used in patient care and in databases where the identity of the patient matters. For example, in the tumor registry, the registry staff follows the patient for the patient's lifetime, so it is necessary to be able to identify the particular patient. **Aggregate data** come from multiple patients and are grouped together without the ability to identify the particular patient. Aggregate data are used for research, quality improvement activities, and other statistical analyses.

Types of Data

The content of the medical record, whether paper or electronic, comes from many sources. The two types of data found in the medical record are administrative and clinical. In a paper environment, the information is written on forms and filed in the medical record. In an electronic environment, much of the data in the EHR come from other information systems. These information systems feed administrative data, clinical data, and other types of data into the EHR, the EDMS, and other systems.

Administrative data typically include basic demographic information, insurance information, and other information used to identify the patient and perform billing and other administrative tasks. Much of the administrative data are collected from the patient during preregistration and registration. This information is generally entered into the admission/discharge/transfer system and then is transferred to the EHR.

Clinical data generally is collected by healthcare providers, including physicians, nurses, respiratory therapists, and physical therapists, as they care for the patient. Some of the clinical information found in the medical record includes:

- Medical history

- Observations

- Treatments

- Test results

- Plans

- Discharge instructions

The specific content of the medical record is controlled by state licensure regulations, accreditation standards, and hospital policies and procedures as well as medical staff bylaws. Data sets such as the Uniform Hospital Discharge Data Set (UHDDS), Uniform Ambulatory Care Data Set (UACDS), Data Elements for Emergency Department Systems (DEEDS), and other data also control the individual data elements collected by the healthcare facility.

Internal and External Sources

Data come from internal and external sources. **Internal data** come from within the facility and include the administrative and clinical data previously discussed. **External data** come from outside the facility and can be used to compare the facility with other similar facilities. For example, a teaching hospital can compare their nosocomial infection rate with that of another teaching hospital to determine if there is a statistical difference between the two. When discrepancies are found, the facility can then take the necessary steps to improve performance. Not only is this an important quality improvement tool, but one mandated by Joint Commission's accreditation standards. There are many sources of comparison data such as professional organizations, government agencies, and accreditation agencies. Four major sources of external data are the Centers for Disease Control and Prevention (CDC), National Center for Health Statistics (NCHS), Agency for Healthcare Research and Quality (AHRQ), and Joint Commission. The CDC is a governmental agency whose mission is "to promote health and quality of life by preventing and controlling disease, injury, and disability." On the CDC Web site are many different data sets that can be downloaded and used in benchmarking. These data sets cover cancer, fatal accidents, mortality, and natality (CDC 2009). The NCHS is part of the CDC. Their mission is to collect information on healthcare in the United States that can be used to improve the quality of the citizens' health. From the NCHS Web site, facilities can access data on births, deaths, injuries, and more (NCHS 2008). The AHRQ is a federal agency whose mission is to research the quality of care provided to Americans, the costs associated with that care, the outcomes, and patient safety (AHRQ 2009b). AHRQ maintains a database called Healthcare Cost and Utilization Project (HCUP) that provides data that can be used for benchmarking. HCUP contains data from state hospital associations, private data organizations, and the federal government. The data in the HCUP database include inpatient discharges, emergency care, and ambulatory surgery (AHRQ 2009a). Joint Commission developed performance standards known as ORYX. ORYX collects core measurement data from their accredited hospitals and uses that data to monitor and compare the quality of care provided. For hospitals, Joint Commission is currently collecting data on acute myocardial infarction, heart failure, pneumonia, pregnancy and related conditions, hospital-based inpatient psychiatric services, children's asthma care, surgical care improvement project, and hospital outpatient measures (Joint Commission 2009).

Check Your Understanding 6.1

1. ORYX is sponsored by what organization?

   A. Joint Commission
   B. AHRQ
   C. NCHS
   D. CDC

2. The data in the database contain national data on costs of care. This is an example of:

   A. internal data
   B. external data
   C. aggregate data
   D. patient-specific data

3. This system collects data on the patient's vital signs, medications, test results, and more, collected from patient care activities. This is what type of data?

   A. Administrative
   B. Secondary
   C. Clinical
   D. External

4. Part of the medical record is stored electronically, some is on microfilm, and the rest is still stored on paper. This is called:

   A. primary data
   B. secondary data
   C. hybrid record
   D. clinical data

5. What controls the specific data elements collected?

   A. Data sets
   B. Hybrid record
   C. Aggregate data
   D. Primary data

Electronic Document Management System

The AHIMA e-HIM Work Group on Electronic Document Management as a Component of the EHR defines the **electronic document management system** (EDMS) as "any electronic system that manages documents (not data) to realize significant improvement in business work processes. Like most information systems, EDMSs consist of a number of component technologies that support both analog and digital document management" (AHIMA e-HIM Work Group on Electronic Document Management as a Component of EHR 2003, 64.A). The work group identified six basic functions expected of an EDMS:

1. Automated forms processing

2. Electronic signature, document annotation, and editing

3. Document capture

4. Document indexing, barcoding, character and form recognition, and forms redesign

5. Document retrieval, viewing, and distribution

6. Document management (AHIMA e-HIM Work Group on Electronic Document Management as a Component of EHR 2003, 5)

Automated forms processing technology allows the user to type data directly into the computer, eliminating the need to manually complete a paper form and then scan it into the computer. By entering the data directly into the system, the data are available for manipulation. Electronic signature, document annotation, and editing are critical to the EDMS because physicians and other users can electronically sign the documentation entered into the system—a feature important in both the electronic and paper environment. The user also should be able to add notes to existing documentation and to edit documents when errors are identified. Because the medical record is a legal document, the original documentation must be retained so that the differences between the two documents are shown.

Document capture is much more than scanning paper images into the EDMS. Voice, video, electronic transactions, and other technologies may be used to capture data. One example is optical character recognition (OCR), Amatayakul defines OCR as "a method of encoding text from analog paper into bit-mapped images and translating the images into a form that is computer readable" (Amatayakul 2007, 466). With OCR, a document can be scanned and the content is editable. Document indexing, barcoding, character and form recognition, and forms redesign are ways to link documents to a particular patient, thus allowing for retrieval. These indexing tools allow the user to locate and retrieve a specific patient's medical records, a specific encounter, and even a specific document through the use of indexing by entering search criteria into one or more of the index fields. The user is then able to view the desired document as well as print, fax, or use another method of transmission. The purpose of the EDMS is not to eliminate paper, but rather to manage documents. To manage these documents, the facility needs to use the EDMS not only for document imaging alone. It must also use character recognition along with imaging to manage all documents for the organization and not just the medical record. The EDMS also uses work flow in order to facilitate the business process of the facility. The EDMS also includes multimedia technologies and moving documents from one system to another without printing the document on paper.

Document Imaging vs. EHR

Some people erroneously believe that document imaging is the EHR. LaTour and Eichenwald Maki (2006) describe the EHR as "a comprehensive system of applications that afford access to longitudinal health information about an individual across the continuum of care, assist in documentation, support clinical decision making, and provide for knowledge building" (LaTour and Eichenwald Maki 2006, 218). Based on this definition, document imaging does not qualify as an EHR because it does not assist in documentation and meet other attributes of this description. If employee's expectations are not managed and they believe that the document imaging system is the EHR, they are often disappointed in the system when it is implemented. The employees will soon recognize that the document imaging system will not be able to perform the functionality of the EHR. For example, the document imaging system will not be able to perform searches on the content of the records because the images are "pictures" of the paper documents. The document imaging system also will not assist in clinical decision support.

Document Imaging Overview

Document imaging is the process of scanning a document into the computer and creating a picture of the document. This image can be retrieved by any authorized user from essentially any location. Multiple users can also view the same image at the same time, enhancing communication between care providers. The scanned document cannot be searched, edited, or changed. Although document imaging is not an EHR, it is a valuable tool to healthcare facilities that do not have the space needed to store paper records and that do not want to use microfilm. Many of the healthcare facilities that elect to implement a document imaging system use it as an intermediate step toward the EHR.

Implementation Issues—The Legal Health Record

When implementing a document imaging system, or other system that contains clinical information, the facility must define the legal health record. According to the AHIMA e-HIM Work Group on the Legal Health Record, the legal health record "is the documentation of healthcare services provided to an individual during any aspect of healthcare delivery in any type of healthcare organization" (AHIMA e-HIM Workgroup on the Legal Health Record 2005). When defining what constitutes the legal health record in an EDMS environment, there are a number of characteristics that should be addressed. These are:

- The record is created in the normal course of business.

- The individual responsible for recording the entry authenticates medical record entries.

- The record is protected from alteration and tampering.

- Amendments and corrections are made according to industry standards.

- The organization adopts a policy statement that the scanned record is a legal, archival record (as opposed to the original documentation).

- A scanning quality management program is created and strictly adhered to by the organization.

- A functional system backup and disaster recovery program is implemented. Backup copies of the data are securely stored off-site. The backup and disaster recovery process is certified to ensure that all data can in fact be recovered.

- Direct electronic interfaces from ancillary systems such as radiology, pathology, laboratory, and transcription to the document imaging system will eliminate the need to scan documents and integrate data from department systems.

- A minimum set of data should be required for indexing scanned health information.

- Storage media used and format of the scanned documents must protect information from loss and damage.

- The storage format must be efficient, manageable, and in compliance with laws and regulations.

- System security should be consistent with the HIPAA final security rule and current industry standards.

- Health records that are not considered official business records for the healthcare provider should not be scanned and made a part of the scanned health record.

- Access to the scanned record should be carefully controlled and limited to a need-to-know basis (Rhodes and Dougherty 2003, 56D).

The legal health record may consist of paper and electronic formats. The facility must determine if a scanned record meets the definition of the legal health record for their state so that they know what record is necessary when responding to subpoenas. If the paper medical record is retained when the chart is scanned, the original paper copy is generally the legal health record. If the paper medical record is destroyed, the imaging record would be the legal record. This may not be the case if the paper record is retained. State laws generally view the original medical record as the legal health record when it is available. Some facilities destroy the medical record after scanning; others do not. Those who choose to destroy the original medical record may do so within weeks, months, or years of scanning. The decision whether or not to destroy the record, when to destroy the record, and the definition of the legal record should be made after consulting with the facility's attorney.

Check Your Understanding 6.2

1. When using a document imaging system, what happens to the paper record?

   A. It is destroyed
   B. It is retained
   C. It is the decision of the facility whether to destroy or retain
   D. It must be retained for 1 year before destruction

2. Document imaging is _____.

   A. the same as the EHR
   B. different from the EHR
   C. better than the EHR
   D. the same as the EHR except it does not have knowledge-based resources

3. Document capture is:

   A. scanning
   B. scanning, OCR, forms recognition, and barcodes
   C. scanning, OCR, indexing, and barcodes
   D. scanning and barcodes

4. What technology allows for direct data entry of clinical data into the imaging system?

   A. OCR
   B. Automated forms processing
   C. Indexing
   D. Document annotation

5. The purpose of an EDMS is to:

   A. scan documents
   B. reduce filing space needed
   C. document retrieval
   D. document management

Advantages and Disadvantages

There are many advantages and disadvantages to the document imaging system. Some facilities choose to focus on the advantages and implement the system in their progression toward the EHR; others choose to skip this step and go directly to the EHR. Examples of advantages are space savings, productivity gains, and immediate access to patient information. Disadvantages include increased use of technology, lack of manipulation/reporting, and fear of change.

Advantages

Space Savings

Space savings is a definite advantage of the document imaging system because paper records take up a lot of space. Space in a healthcare facility is a valuable commodity, and facilities are always looking for ways to improve space utilization. To realize the space savings, many facilities destroy the paper medical record after a predetermined period of time. This practice ultimately eliminates the need for the file area, opening the space for other needs. Based on the needs of the facility, the freed-up space may be used to allow expansion of the HIM department or reallocated to other departments. The elimination of the file room may take several years as charts are destroyed, scanned, or microfilmed.

Retrieval of Large Number of Records

The HIM department is constantly pulling large numbers of charts for audits, research, and other purposes. HIM staff must pull the charts for review and later refile them once the review is complete. This process takes up a lot of time and space because the charts have to be stored during the review process and space has to be allocated for the reviewers to work. With a document imaging system, medical records are stored electronically. If a researcher or auditor needs to access large numbers of medical records, these records can be placed in a work queue. The reviewer can view the medical record from any location as long as proper authorization is provided, thus eliminating the need to pull, manage, and refile the medical records.

Productivity Gains

Through the use of document imaging technology and workflow technology, employee productivity is improved because they no longer have to look for records and move charts from one location to another. Document imaging eliminates record retrieval, chart assembly, and many other routine paper-based traditional medical record functions. Other functions, such as coding, analysis, and qualitative analysis can be done electronically. With imaging systems, patient care providers have 24-hour access to patient information without the need for around-the-clock staff. Another productivity gain comes from the elimination of lost records. Hours spent looking for medical records could be better spent on other tasks such as eliminating duplicate medical record numbers, documentation improvement, compliance audits, and privacy audits.

Online Availability of Information

When it comes to emergency patient care, minutes count. The availability of the patient's past medical history can be the difference between life and death. For example, if the patient has an allergy and the physician does not know, the medication could be inappropriately prescribed to the patient, thus resulting in harm to the patient and possibly death. The ability to access critical information in seconds—not minutes or hours—improves the quality of the care to patients and can prevent unnecessary or duplicate testing. Another benefit to the online availability of information is that multiple users view the same record simultaneously, even the same document at the same time. This accessibility improves user satisfaction and ultimately improves patient care through improved communication and accessibility.

System Security and Control

With access controls, audit trails, and other security measures, the security of the medical record is improved over that of the traditional paper record. Admittedly, with the paper record there is only one point of access, but there is no way to know who viewed the medical record and what they looked at. With proper security measures, only authorized individuals will be able to view what they have a need to know and there will be a record of not only the medical record viewed but also the specific documents. See Chapter 12 for details.

Database Retrieval

Document imaging systems allow for searches based on indexed data. For example, a search could retrieve all patients who were discharged from the facility on July 4, 2009, or all of Dr. Smith's patients, or John Brown's medical record. This function is great for research and saves time from having to identify patients and then retrieve their data individually. The searching is limited to the data elements captured during indexing.

Disadvantages

Increased Use of Computer Technology

Although increasing the use of computer technology is a benefit in many ways, for some individuals it is a disadvantage. In order to utilize document imaging, the user must be able to use a computer to retrieve the medical record. Even in the current digital environment, many people do not know the basic functions of a computer. The addition of technology changes the culture of an organization, which leads to fear. The fear of job security, lack of competency, failure, and the overall fear of change overwhelms not only employees, but management as well.

Fear of Change

Many employees are scared of losing their jobs when told that computers are going to be used to replace the paper records. Research has shown that, at least initially, the number of employees needed increases because the HIM department is still managing the paper record in addition to the computerized record. Because of this, management must let the employees know the status of their position. Usually staff will maintain their current job, but that job may change. Instead of filing reports, they may be scanning documents. Keeping employees informed of the changes will keep their fear manageable and may prevent the department from losing good employees. Fear can develop not only in staff, but also within management. Fears such as the risk of not being able to access information because of technology failure, power outages, bad media, or other reasons adds to the responsibility and accountability expected of management.

Lack of Manipulation/Reporting

Because the images are pictures of the medical record document and not entries into the EHR, the user is unable to manipulate the data to show trends or other views. Likewise, the user cannot generate reports related to the images rather than entered data.

Implementation

Healthcare facilities must manage the existing medical records when a document imaging system is implemented. The facility has to decide how many or if these existing records will be scanned into the system. Facilities vary widely on what they decide. Some start with the implementation date of the document imaging system, and only records with a discharge date on or after the implementation date are scanned. Other facilities choose to backscan some or all existing records to provide users electronic access to the old charts. **Backscanning** is the process of scanning past medical records into the system so that there is an existing database of patient information, making the system valuable to the user from the first day of implementation. Although this methodology provides an immediate database of medical records in the system on the first day of the go-live, it also gives the facility a 2-year or longer backlog of information to be scanned, preferably before implementation. Many of these patients may never come back to the facility, so the facility is not realizing the benefit of having online records. The facility would choose how far back to go with the scanning, such as 6 months or 2 years. Facilities that choose to backscan documents participate in research and have high readmission rates to the facility. Other facilities start scanning at the implementation date; however, when a patient is admitted, their old records are scanned into the system so only active patients are scanned into the system. The decision should be based on the needs of the facility, cost, filing space, and other resources. The decision should balance the needs of the user and the resources available. Many facilities only provide access to the document imaging system to the HIM department initially if the decision was made not to backscan. The logic behind this decision is to prevent users from going to the document imaging system and not locating records on a patient. This would be frustrating. Once there is a strong repository of data, the access would be rolled out throughout the organization. The actual scanning can be performed by the facility or it can be outsourced to a vendor. If the healthcare facility decides to scan the records themselves, additional staff would be needed to manage the current workload and to add backscanning medical records to their tasks. Many facilities overcome this need by hiring temporary employees to cover the difference in workload. Facilities that choose vendors to scan because of their high productivity and experienced staff enable the scanning to be completed quicker. Their charges are usually based on the number of images scanned and the actual tasks performed. These tasks may include preparation of the record for scanning, indexing, and quality control.

Many hospitals implement the document imaging system by scanning the current emergency department patient records and gradually working up to inpatient records. Emergency department records are smaller, more controllable, and easier to manage than the inpatient records. An average inpatient medical record can have 75 to 100 pages or more for a 3- to 4-day day stay on a regular nursing unit whereas an emergency department record may be 5 to 15 pages.

Justification of Cost of System

Healthcare facilities justify the cost of document imaging systems from the savings that occur from decreasing the operating costs of the HIM department and the organization as a whole. The savings come from reductions in clerical staff, improvement in accounts receivable, and increased revenue. The expenses will probably increase in the short term until problems with the new processes are worked out and the productivity improvements are realized (Mahoney 1997). Staffing may actually increase at first as both the existing paper record and the imaging system must be managed, but over time staffing can be reduced. Operating costs of the HIM department include elimination of the file folder and other supplies related to processing the paper record. Because costs may actually go up in the short term, the return on investment may be calculated on a five- to ten-year period. When the file area is eliminated, the organization can reallocate that space to a revenue-generating department, thus potentially generating revenue. Productivity is also increased, thus reducing the cost of staffing. For example, the release of information coordinator no longer has to stand in front of a copy machine and the coder does not have to wait on charts to be assembled and analyzed in order to code them.

Forms

Forms management is a key implementation issue that must be addressed. At least 6 months prior to implementation of the document imaging system, forms should be evaluated and redesigned to facilitate the scanning process. The weight of the paper used should be appropriate for use in a scanner. Paper that is too heavy or too light may jam the automatic feeder. White paper is recommended for all forms because the color of the document is scanned along with the content of the form. This significantly increases the size of the computer file and the quality of the printed document. The forms should be standardized 8.5 × 11 in size where possible. The redesign should include the addition of barcodes to each form. The **barcode** makes indexing more efficient because the barcode can enter data automatically. Standards for the use of barcodes must be established to facilitate scanning. These standards should include the size of the barcode, the standardized location of the barcode, and the amount of white space between the barcode and any text. The new forms with the barcode should be in use at the time of implementation. The recommended barcode **symbology** or format is **Code 39**, also known as Code 3 of 9. These barcodes should be placed on the form in a standardized location on the form (Dunn 2006).

Staffing Changes

With the transition of employees from filing paper to scanning, indexing, and quality control, new job titles and job descriptions will be required. For example, the file clerk role will disappear and the scanning clerk and quality control clerk roles will be created. There will be differences in skill level because the scanning clerk and quality control clerk will need more skill in order to use the computer. These changes in job titles and job descriptions must be in place at the time of the system implementation. With the changes in job skills, the compensation level may change. These changes would be decided after discussions with administration and the human resources department. The HIM department and other affected staff must be trained on the system prior to implementation to prevent backlogs from immediately occurring, which would impact user satisfaction.

Process Redesign

The implementation of an imaging system will have a tremendous impact on the workflow of a HIM department. As a result, the HIM department will have to reengineer workflows to adapt to an electronic environment and review and update policies and procedures, among many other tasks to aid in the transition. The HIM department will no longer have to assemble the medical record; they will prepare the medical record for scanning instead. The way the traditional discharge processing such as coding and chart analysis is done will also drastically change (AHIMA e-HIM Work Group on Electronic Document Management as a Component of the EHR 2003):

- Analysis will be performed online
- Physician completion of records can be performed in the HIM department or other location such as the physician's office
- Electronic signatures may be used to complete charts

See figure 6.1, which shows how document imaging changes the HIM department.

Figure 6.1.   How imaging changes the HIM department

How does department imaging implementation change the structure of a department? Here's an illustration of how some HIM positions might evolve during this transition.

Position	Preconversion	Transition Period	Postconversion
HIM Clerk, Level I	Yes (file clerks) • filed records, loose reports, pulled charts • some assembly	Yes (gradually decreasing)	No
HIM Clerk, Level II	Yes • ROI clerk • outsourced ROI • discharge analysis • physician/physician • incomplete combined with physician	Yes	Yes • ROI clerk handles most requests; outsourcing reduced significantly • discharge analysis (streamlined—process incomplete)
Follow-up Clerk	No	No	Yes • ensures the documents are flowing appropriately along workflow thread
Forms Coordinator	No	No	Yes • ensures all forms go through the proper process for approval and implementation into the imaging system
Imaging Specialist/ Scan Clerk	No	Yes	Yes • prepping, scanning, and indexing documents • quality control • many "Clerk Level I's" able to move into this position
Implementation Specialist	No	Yes • temporary position for implementation tasks	No
Lead Clerk (evenings)	Yes • handle scheduling and work direction for evening clerks	Yes	No (functions taken on by evening supervisor)
Supervisor(s)	Yes	Yes	Yes • Professional staff available for training, troubleshooting, and other projects.
Director/ Manager	Yes	Yes	Yes

Based on: McCarthy, T. and M. Johnson 2002 (September). "The HIM Department in Transition" in "Document Imaging, Workflow Restructure Department." *Journal of AHIMA* 73:8

Source: Rhodes and Dougherty 2003

Check Your Understanding 6.3

1. Document imaging eliminates which of the following function(s)?

   A. Scanning
   B. Assembly
   C. Analysis
   D. Coding

2. The term used to describe scanning all existing records when implementing a document imaging system is:

   A. workflow
   B. backscanning
   C. backlogs
   D. scanning

3. The most common form of barcode format used in imaging is called:

   A. Code 39
   B. OCR
   C. automated forms processing
   D. indexing

4. A disadvantage of document imaging is:

   A. fear of change
   B. data quality
   C. workflow
   D. forms redesign

5. Which of the following statements is true?

   A. Online accessibility of patient information can reduce productivity of staff
   B. Online accessibility of patient information can improve quality of patient care
   C. Online accessibility of patient information reduces the security of the record
   D. Online accessibility of patient information does not change the HIM department

When Should the Chart Be Scanned?

Ideally, scanning should be performed as documents are created to allow immediate online access to orders, progress notes, and other written documentation. Typically, however, the medical record is not scanned until after discharge. Some facilities scan the medical record immediately following discharge and use workflow technology to facilitate the record discharge processing. Other facilities complete the medical record and then scan the chart.

Immediately Following Discharge

Many facilities scan the medical record immediately following the patient's discharge from the hospital. There are a number of advantages to scanning charts at this point. This timing allows coding and analysis to be performed remotely if the facility so chooses. It also allows immediate access to the chart for patient care, coding, analysis, and other healthcare operations. In the traditional paper environment, the discharge processing of the medical record is a linear process. One step has to be completed before the next because only one employee can access the medical record at a time. With document imaging and workflow technology, coders, analysts, and other users no longer must wait for other steps in the discharge process to be complete before accessing the chart because imaging allows concurrent access. This speeds up the discharge processing function. Many patients are readmitted to the facility immediately after discharge, so having the recent discharged medical record scanned and available to the emergency department or other patient care areas improves the quality of care provided.

There are also disadvantages to scanning immediately after discharge. Not only do facility staff members have to be trained to use the document imaging system as part of their discharge processing, but physicians must also be trained on how to complete medical records online. In addition to retrieval of images, the physician would need to know how to use the annotation tools discussed later in this chapter and how to sign the documents electronically. The physician would also need to know how to complete forms electronically and to dictate discharge summaries and other documents.

The facility must have sufficient staff and equipment in place to ensure that the scanning is performed quickly so that the records are available to HIM staff, physicians, and other users in a timely manner. If scanning is not done promptly and the records are not available to physicians and other users in the appropriate time period, these users quickly become disillusioned with the document imaging system and do not want to use it. This is especially important in the early days of the system when everyone is getting used to it and learning about its benefits.

Scanning Upon Completion

Some facilities choose to scan the medical record after the completion of the medical record discharge processing. With this method, the physician is not impacted by the imaging system to complete charts and it does not allow coding and analysis to be performed remotely. The users of the chart in the immediate discharge period still must wait for the chart to be processed in the traditional linear method. There are expenses related to the management of the paper record during the discharge process, such as the cost of folders and space for record completion.

Components of a Document Imaging System

A document imaging system is a database that is made of many components such as a scanner, jukebox, magnetic storage, and file server. All of the components work together to scan, store, and retrieve the medical record documents. The following are descriptions of many of the components associated with a document imaging system and the role each plays.

Scanner

The **scanner** is the hardware that is used to transform the paper document into a digital image. Scanners are rated based on the number of pages per minute (ppm) the scanner can process. High-powered scanners used to accomplish high-volume scanning, usually found in HIM departments, resemble a copier with an automatic document feeder. Departments with only light scanning duties may only need a flatbed scanner. Scanning can be a slow process. To overcome time restraints, the scanner chosen should be fast enough to accommodate the volume of scanning that needs to be accomplished. Large facilities may need scanners with 90 to 140 ppm or other high-speed capabilities (Abdelhak 2007). The scanner should be able to adjust the density and contrast of the scanning automatically based on the type of the form being scanned. The need to adjust density and contrast automatically comes from the fact that some forms or their documentation are lighter or darker than others, thus they will need to be scanned darker or lighter accordingly—just as when a document is copied on a copy machine. The scanner is able to identify the type of form and make needed adjustments because of barcodes either on the form or the target sheets. **Target sheets** are pages that are blank except for a barcode that will tell the scanner and ultimately the computer the content of the pages that follow. The barcode may tell the form name, the patient name, or some other piece of information. If the scanner cannot scan both sides of a two-sided document, the operator must identify these documents and scan the other side manually. Because of the movement of the scanner and the dust that collects from the paper movement through the scanner, scanners must undergo frequent preventive maintenance. There will be times that even with preventive maintenance, the system will become inoperable. This must be considered when selecting the number of scanners and ppm ratings needed.

Scanning Workstation

The **scanning workstation** is the personal computer (PC) that controls the scanner. Once a document is scanned, the workstation compresses the bitmap (.bmp) file created by the scanner. Bitmap is a graphical file format that is often used in scanning images. Another common format that may be used is a tagged image file (tif). The file is compressed to save space for storage of the file. Another step performed by the scanning workstation is to give each document scanned an individual file name. The name is used to store the image and is ultimately used when the file is retrieved.

Abstracting/Quality Control Workstation

The abstracting/quality control workstation is also a PC. Rather than scanning, this workstation is used for indexing and quality control. Indexing is the abstracting of data that will be used to retrieve the image. The facility determines the data elements to be indexed based on their needs. During the quality control process, the clerk views every image to check for the quality of the image and verifies indexing is accurate and patient demographics are correct.

File Server

The file server is a large PC that is extremely powerful and has a large amount of memory and magnetic hard drive. When the user performs an inquiry on their PC to retrieve a patient's medical record, the file server receives the request for the document images, retrieves the document images, and sends the document images back to the requester. When documents are scanned into the computer, the files created are stored on the file server's magnetic hard drive. Images are typically stored on magnetic storage for 30 to 60 days. While images are stored in magnetic media, the records can generally be retrieved in three to five seconds (Mahoney 1997).

Long-term Storage

When a document image is ready to be moved from magnetic disk to long-term storage, the facility has a number of choices. These choices include DVD, CD, Blu-Ray, optical disk, magneto-optical disk, and more. Generally the document image is "burned" into the surface of the chosen media by a laser beam. In order to be used to store medical records, the platter must utilize **WORM technology**. WORM is an acronym for write once, read many. The use of this technology prevents the user from altering what is stored, but the data can be viewed as many times as necessary. There are also rewritable storage media, but these cannot be used for the medical record because it is a legal document. With the use of rewritable technology, the facility would face questions about whether or not the documentation had been altered—if the medical record was ever needed in court. The life expectancy of digital media is long, but CDs, DVDs, and other media do become unusable from time to time. Duplicates should be made and stored off site to prevent destruction of both copies in the event of a disaster.

Jukebox

A **jukebox** holds and retrieves the individual disks just as the traditional jukebox holds records or CDs. There are many sizes of jukeboxes and as the facility grows, jukeboxes may be linked together to accommodate expansion. When the user requests a patient's record, the file server identifies what disk the information is stored on. The jukebox then retrieves the disk and places the disk in a drive that will read the information and send it to the user. Because the disk has to be inserted into a reader, access is slower than accessing the information from the hard drive. The system should be set up so that the information is available to the user within 20 to 30 seconds (Mahoney 1997). The time required for the jukebox to locate the disk and access it is called exchange time (Abdelhak 2007). Anything longer than that will result in user dissatisfaction. The retrieval time is lengthened when the patient's record is spread over multiple disks. Some facilities solve this problem by copying all of the patient's information from the old disk to a new disk. The problem with copying the data to another disk is that the information stays on the old disk, creating redundant information. Another solution is to leave some space on all platters just in case one of the patients returns. This allows for room to expand if patients return. This method wastes space on some disks and other disks may still fill up.

Retrieval Workstation

This is the workstation used by the physician, HIM staff, or other users to retrieve patient information and view document images. If the workstation is used to access few records, a standard size monitor will work. With a standard size monitor, the entire image will not fit on the screen. The user will have to scroll to see the entire page. If the workstation is heavily used to view document images, it is better on the user's eyes and in the display of the image to have an oversized monitor. It is important to evaluate what size monitor is needed because there is a significant cost difference between the two.

Printers

The facility will need to determine who has the rights to print reports from the document imaging system. The size of the printer will be based on the volume of printing performed by that area. For example, in HIM a high-quality, high-speed laser printer is needed in order to print large volumes of information. The print server controls the location where documents are printed and controls the work queue or order in which a document prints. The fastest way to print is to use a print file server to control and facilitate the printing process.

Uninterruptible Power Supply

An uninterruptible power supply (UPS) is a battery backup to keep the system operational in the event of a power outage. The UPS should control key components of the document imaging system such as the file server and key users such as the emergency department. It would not be necessary to place all workstations on the UPS. Interruptions in electrical power can happen—a tree falls on power lines, hurricanes blow down power lines, or transformers blow out. Without UPS, the document imaging system would be inoperable, preventing access to critical patient care information.

Fax Technology

With fax technology, documents can be sent from the facility to another location such as a physician office without printing, thus saving time and paper. This method is frequently used with high-volume applications such as in transcription. A fax server may be necessary to manage this process by controlling the order of the faxes.

Check Your Understanding 6.4

1. To keep the document imaging operational when the power is out, what should be utilized?

    A. Automatic forms processing
    B. Retrieval workstation
    C. Server
    D. UPS

2. Scanners are rated on

    A. pixels
    B. pages per minute
    C. file type
    D. quality of scan

(continued on next page)

Check Your Understanding 6.4 (continued)

3. Images should be stored on what type of media?

   A. Magnetic media
   B. WORM technology
   C. Rewritable media
   D. Blu-Ray

4. Which of the following is a benefit of scanning after the chart is complete?

   A. Online chart completion
   B. Immediate access in case of readmission
   C. Do not have to train physicians to do online chart completion
   D. More benefits are realized

5. Pages that tell the scanner information about the page(s) that follow are called:

   A. barcodes
   B. automatic forms processing
   C. target sheets
   D. indexing

Imaging Process

Preparation

When a patient is discharged from the hospital, the medical record is generally removed from the folder that protects it during the patient's stay. During the patient's hospitalization, the documents contained within the medical record (the active medical record) were treated in a manner that was successful to the concurrent care of the patient, but would not be successful for the scanning process. For example, paper clips and staples may have been used to hold pages together. The medical record must be properly prepared before scanning can begin. The preparation process includes a number of steps:

- Remove all staples and paper clips

- Repair torn pages

- Verify pages to ensure accuracy in the proper medical record and proper admission

- Insert target sheets

- Ensure pages are in the right order (according to facility) and are all facing the proper direction. The organizing of the documents may be performed by the imaging system.

Indexing

After preparation, the documents are fed through the scanner's automatic feeder. Once digitized, the individual documents are indexed. Common data elements found in document imaging indexing are patient name, medical record number, document type, billing number, and discharge date; however, there may be other data fields such as physician name, diagnosis codes, and procedure codes to enhance the search capability. Indexing a number of data elements is good for retrieval of patient records, but indexing is a time-consuming process. To combat the time requirements, automatic indexing should be used whenever possible. A target sheet at the beginning of the stack of medical record documents can automatically index the patient's name, discharge date, and other basic information that applies to all of the documents in the batch. A batch is a stack of documents that are scanned at one time.

Scanning is not the only way to populate documents into the document imaging system. **Enterprise report management (ERM)**, also known as **computer output to laser disk (COLD)** technology is frequently used in place of scanning. ERM/COLD is the transfer of data from a computer directly into the document imaging system. This technology is frequently used for documents such as discharge summaries, laboratory reports, radiology; anything that is stored in a computer can be placed in the imaging system via ERM/COLD. Facilities try to use ERM/COLD as much as possible in order to save time in the scanning process and reduce delays in getting information to the users. Approximately 60 percent to 75 percent of the medical record may be captured by the EDMS through a COLD feed. This not only saves time in the data capture process, but also saves storage space as COLD documents consume about ten percent of the storage space used by a scanned document (Mahoney 1997).

Another method of automatic indexing is the placement of barcodes on forms. Barcodes identify the form, thus eliminating the need for HIM staff to enter the document type on every form. Facilities need to establish standards regarding the use of barcodes, such as format, size, and location on the form. When barcodes are used, the computer looks for them in the standard position, thus speeding the scanning process. The scanner reads the barcode and interprets the data into the data elements, thus automatically indexing the document. If a form does not have a barcode on it, a target sheet could be used to identify the document. The target sheet would act as a message that says the following document is a progress note or physician order.

Optical character recognition (OCR) is yet another method of indexing, in which the computer reads machine-generated characters and converts them into computer-processable code. OCR should be able to identify imperfect characters by deskewing and correcting superfluous and imperfect characters. OCR can index documents in a document management system or it can scan an entire page of text.

Another way to save time indexing is downloading information from the hospital information system to index the patient name, medical record number, and any other basic demographic information; all the indexer has to do is index data not available in the hospital information system, such as document type.

Quality Control

The final step is the quality control (QC) process. The QC clerk inspects every document to ensure that it has been scanned appropriately. For example, the QC clerk would confirm that each document was readable, not upside down or crooked and that no documents were missing. If the QC clerk identifies a problem, the clerk corrects it by usually deleting the problem image and rescanning it. This step can also serve as a final check to ensure that the documents all belong to the same patient and the same admission.

Magnetic Media Storage

The magnetic disk drive is physically located in the file server. When documents are scanned or transferred via ERM/COLD, the created file is stored on the magnetic disk where it remains for a predetermined time before being transferred to a long-term storage media like CD, DVD, optical disk, Blu-Ray, or other media. There are multiple reasons for keeping data on magnetic storage for a period of time. The first is that as long as the document is on magnetic media, documents that were poorly scanned or indexed incorrectly can be deleted and corrected. Another reason is that documents are often received from the nursing unit or other areas of the facility long after the medical record is scanned. If the document images were transferred to long-term storage immediately, additional documents that arrive may be stored on a different disk, which will then slow down retrieval. Fragmentation results because the file server has to retrieve two, three, or more disks in order to compile all of the patient information on the discharge. Storing recent discharges on magnetic disk is recommended because recent discharged medical records are the most active and magnetic storage provides quicker access than long-term storage or paper records. During this time, patients are readmitted and the HIM department staff needs access to the medical record for coding, analysis, and other functions. The patient may also frequently return to the facility for admission or follow-up care. On the other hand, because of the amount of data and the risk of alteration/loss, document images should not remain on magnetic media long term. The amount of time left on magnetic storage will be determined by the facility, but may range from 3 to 6 months.

Figure 6.2 provides an example of how the workflow of the document imaging process might work.

Workflow Technology

A document imaging system has a significant impact on the processes of the HIM department. If using workflow technology, this impact is even greater. **Workflow technology** is software that allows the facility to incorporate procedures and processes into the system based on criteria established by the organization. Workflow, while not limited to document imaging, frequently is a component of it. When a patient is discharged, there are a lot of processes that must be done to the medical record including coding, analysis, quality audits, documentation audits, and so on. With the traditional paper record, the record goes from station to station until all the steps are completed There are frequently delays such as employees being out on vacation or resigning, or higher than expected volume of work. The other employees down the queue cannot proceed until the previous steps are finished. With workflow technology, any task that does not have a prerequisite can be done at any time so the user does not have to wait for other tasks to be completed. For example, coding does not have to be performed before the chart can be analyzed. In fact, they could be performed at the same time. If the user has a question or needs additional information, the user can "pend" the chart so that it automatically returns to the work queue when the information is available or when the question has been answered by the appropriate person. For example, if the discharge summary or pathology report is missing from the chart, the coder could "pend" the chart. In other words, place the chart into a "hold" status until the missing reports are complete. When the missing form is available, the system knows to route the chart to the user for review. The HIM staff would no longer have to wait for physicians to come to the department to complete charts—the chart can be completed from their office, home, or other location.

Figure 6.2.   Document imaging process flow

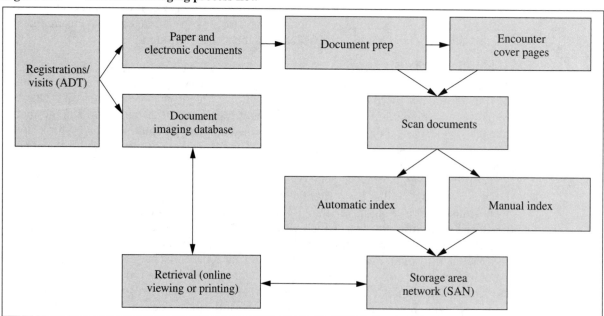

Source: Adapted from Myjer and Madamba 2002

There are two types of workflow technologies. These are automatic and manual, also referred to as push and pull technologies. Automatic or preprogrammed technologies send the work out to the user automatically. For example, when a coder completes coding a chart, a new chart is automatically available for coding. The coder does not have to choose which chart is to be coded. The chart is automatically directed to the user based on criteria set by the supervisor. The supervisor can make changes to the criteria as needed. For example, the regular criteria may be that the oldest discharge is sent to the coders first. If there are discharges with extremely large charges, the supervisor could change the criteria so that the coder codes these discharges first. With manual workflow technology, the user must select which chart is to be coded; although it does not take a lot of time to select the chart, the users may select the easiest charts to process or select charts based on some factor that is different from the supervisor's preference. With manual workflow technology, there is the risk that coders will try to get the "easy" charts to code such as hysterectomies, cholecystectomies, and other short stay charts, leaving the extended admissions for the other coders.

Workflow technology is not limited to routing charts through HIM functions. Other departments can also be involved. For example, if the coder identifies a risk management concern from the medical record document, the chart can be automatically routed to the risk manager for review. or if a chart meets criteria for current or ongoing reviews, the coder could route it to utilization review or other departments accordingly.

Check Your Understanding 6.5

1. The first stage in the scanning process is:

   A. Assembly
   B. Indexing
   C. Quality control
   D. Document preparation

2. The supervisor is controlling what charts are sent to the coders. This is called

   A. Automatic workflow
   B. Manual workflow
   C. Scheduling
   D. Routing

3. Which of the following is a true statement?

   A. Workflow only involves the HIM department
   B. Workflow cannot be easily changed once it is established
   C. Workflow is useful only for discharge processing
   D. Workflow technology can be used by the HIM department and other departments

4. The term used to describe how indexing can be performed without data entry is:

   A. Auto-indexing
   B. Scanning
   C. OCR
   D. Barcodes

5. Documents are moved from magnetic data to long-term storage:

   A. Immediately after scanning
   B. Immediately after chart is complete
   C. Never
   D. At a time period determined by the facility

Productivity

As with any task, the HIM staff should record their productivity each day. Some of the productivity can be captured electronically, but not all. For example, the scanner can capture the number of images that it scanned, but there is not an electronic means to capture the number of documents prepared for scanning. The HIM staff member who prepares the records for scanning should record their productivity in inches. The department should have a standard for the number of inches or number of documents in an inch expected from the employees preparing the charts for scanning. Each facility should determine their own productivity standards based on factors such as equipment, condition of charts, use of barcodes, and other factors. Table 6.1 gives examples of what the productivity standard could look like.

Annotation

One of the functions of a document imaging system is the ability to annotate the images. **Annotation** is the ability to alter the image in some way. Because the images may be a legal document, the image itself cannot be altered; however, an overlay to the document will show the annotation. These annotations are useful to call attention to some data on the form and to enhance viewing. There are a number of different annotations that can be used (Rhodes and Dougherty 2003).

Note

The note tool will allow the physician or other user to add a note to the image. This may be useful if additional data has come available that the physician wants to call to the reader's attention.

Highlighting

The highlighting tool works like a highlighter on paper. The purpose is to call the reader's attention to specific test results or other documentation.

Drawing

The draw tool can be used to draw circles, arrows, or other markings. This is another way to draw the reader's attention to specific data, or in the case of radiology imaging, the anomaly.

Zoom/Reduction

The zoom/reduction tool enlarges or reduces the size of the image to enhance viewing. This is helpful if the writing is small or there is a lot of writing on the page that is difficult to

Table 6.1.   Examples of productivity standards

Function	Expectations per Work Hour	Factors Affecting Production
Prepping	340–500 images	Tears; staples; lack of patient identification on each page; assembled or not
Scanning	1,200–2,400 images	Speed of scanner; age of scanner; scanner maintenance; size of batches
Quality control	1,700–2,000 images	Lack of attention to detail by the prepping and indexing staff; size of viewing screen
Indexing	720–800 images	Presence of barcodes on forms; presence of barcoded patient labels

Source: Dunn 2007

read. It is very helpful in the interpretation of radiologic reports because the radiologist can enlarge portions of the image to better see any anomalies.

Rotate

The rotate tool allows the user to flip an image. This is useful if a document has been scanned upside down or sideways.

Retrieval of Images

To retrieve and view document images stored in the document imaging system, one must be an authorized user with the proper permissions. A user would enter one or more of the indexed fields such as a patient's medical record number to retrieve the appropriate medical record and its associated document images for review. Figure 6.3 shows an example of document imaging and retrieval software.

In the event of audits, research projects, patient appointments, or other reviews of a number of medical records, the images may be moved to magnetic storage, also known as cache memory, in order to speed access time to the records. This reduces network traffic and improves user satisfaction. It is important to note that the files remain on long-term storage media; they are simply copied to magnetic storage temporarily. After a specified period, the information is purged.

Future of Imaging

Imaging systems are often seen as a temporary measure between the paper medical record and the EHR. It is unlikely, however, that imaging itself will go away anytime soon because there will continue to be paper documents brought by the patient or from an outside source that that will need to be scanned into the appropriate medical record.

Figure 6.3.   An example of document retrieval using HealthPort's software

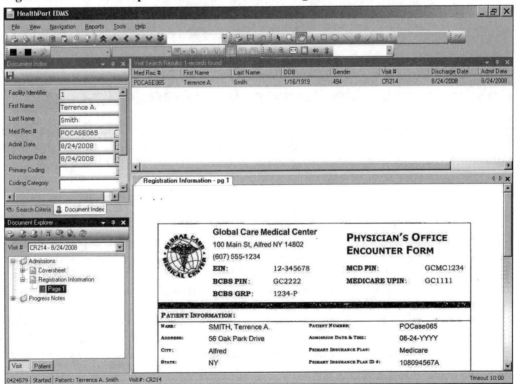

Source: HealthPort. Reprinted with permission.

Check Your Understanding 6.6

1. The reason for copying documents from long-term storage to magnetic storage would be:

   A. backup
   B. purging
   C. faster access to chart
   D. scanning

2. Which of the following statements is true?

   A. Document imaging will disappear when the EHR becomes widespread
   B. Document imaging will have a role in the EHR environment
   C. Document imaging is obsolete technology
   D. Document imaging does not allow for the annotation of documents

3. Which annotation tool allows the user to make comments on the imaged document?

   A. Note
   B. Zoom
   C. Highlighting
   D. Drawing

4. Productivity standards for imaging processes should be based on:

   A. speed of scanner
   B. national standards
   C. attributes of facility, such as equipment
   D. national average size of chart

5. When annotation is used, the document:

   A. is changed forever
   B. remains the same; however, an overlay displays the annotation
   C. is duplicated and both are stored in the system
   D. is deleted and a new document is scanned into the system

---

Maintenance and Monitoring of Data Storage Systems

Problems with computers such as hardware failure and viruses can result in data being lost or destroyed. Media can also be lost or stolen. To protect the facility from the lost or destroyed data, magnetically stored data should be backed up at least once a day, and maybe more often if the criticality of the data warrants it. Full backup copies everything on the hard drive whereas incremental backup only copies files that have changed since the last backup (Quinsey 2004).

Before relying completely on backup tapes or other media, it is important to test the backup utility to make sure that the data is on the tape as expected. The restore utility must also be tested to ensure that if data are lost or damaged, tape or other media can be used to reload the data without any problems. The backup tapes or other media should be stored in a different location to prevent total loss in fire, flood, or other disaster. For instance, if a hospital had a backup of their system document imaging system stored about 15 feet from the original and damage had been caused by tornado, flood, or other disaster, the data would have been completely lost. When determining how the data will be stored, the facility should consider the archival quality of the source, the length of time to be stored, and the amount of data.

Routine maintenance on information systems includes upgrading software and replacing failing hardware components. Software upgrades include patches to resolve errors in the software, updating data, and adding or revising system functionality. The software vendor provides these releases routinely as part of the support fee that the healthcare facility pays annually. This routine maintenance is usually done at low volume times such as the middle of the night to have as little impact on the organization as possible. Software upgrades should be loaded in the test system before they are loaded into the production environment. The use of a test system allows errors to be made without impacting the production system with the live patient data.

A number of technical maintenance tasks must be routinely performed. Examples of these tasks are (Hebda et al. 2005, 188):

- Performing problem solving and debugging

- Maintaining a backup supply of hardware such as monitors, printers, cables, trackballs, and mice for replacement of faulty equipment in user areas

- Performing file backup procedures

- Monitoring the system for adequate file space

- Building and maintaining interfaces with other systems

- Configuring, testing, and installing system upgrades

- Maintaining and updating the disaster recovery plan

In spite of the efforts of the information systems staff, there are times when emergency downtime is unavoidable such as when a piece of hardware fails unexpectedly. As a preventative measure, information system staff are constantly monitoring the system for signs of a system crash. Signs that a system is in trouble include a slowed response time.

When a user identifies a problem with the information, there should be a centralized reporting center. This reporting center is generally called a help desk. The help desk in a healthcare environment is usually available 24 hours a day, seven days a week. The help desk staff assists users with simple issues and refers more complicated issues to the specialized staff required to resolve the problem.

Monitor Available Storage

Hard drives, jukeboxes, CDs, and other storage media can only store a finite amount of data. The facility must monitor the available space on the system in order to plan for expansion. Computers slow down as their hard drives fill up. To prevent the system from slowing down, the facility must manage the storage effectively to ensure that the needed storage space is always ready and available.

The size of the individual files from an imaging system will vary based on the factors such as dots per inch (DPI) used during scanning, use of color in the form, and size of the form. The industry standard for a scanned black and white image is 50 kilobytes (kb) (Rhodes 1997). If the expected number of documents is known, the number of documents × 50 kb will identify the amount of storage space needed for the period of time. For example, if there are 750,000 documents, the amount of space required is roughly 37,500,000 kb, which is 37.5 gigabytes if the pages are single-sided. More space would be required for double-sided documents.

A 700-MB CD can store up to 14,000 standard 8.5 × 11-inch documents, depending on the size of the file (Twin Imaging Technology, Inc. 2008). If the number of documents expected was 750,000 and these were all single-sided documents, it would take approximately 54 CDs to store the images.

See table 6.2 for size of digital storage terms.

The vendor can help the facility determine the amount of storage needed for the patient volume expected. Imaged data is not the only data to be stored. Administrative and clinical information systems collect data that must be stored. Each character is a byte of data, so if memory has 2 million bytes, it can hold 2 million characters of data.

Data Retention

Each facility must decide how long patient-specific data will be retained. This decision must be made based on the needs of the organization, regulations, and laws. The needs of the facility to be considered are the amount of research performed, patient care, and available resources such as record storage and staff. Each state has laws specifying the length of time that patient information must be maintained and stored. Generally this time frame ranges from 7 to 10 years, although the records of minors must be maintained until the age of majority plus a specified period of time. Both the American Health Information Management Association (AHIMA) and the Medicare Conditions of Participation recommend a 10-year retention (Fletcher and Rhodes 2002). Once this time has passed, the data should be destroyed as per standards discussed in Chapter 12.

Patient information is not the only retention issue to address. HIPAA mandates the retention for 6 years of various other documentation including disclosure logs, authorizations, policies and procedures, and forms. Although HIPAA does not mandate that these documents be retained electronically, many facilities choose to do so. Policies and procedures must also address how long administrative and financial data should be retained. Some data, such as that contained within the master patient index, should be retained permanently. Other data can be destroyed after a specified period of time based on laws, regulations, needs of the facility, accreditation standards, and professional guidelines. Please see table 6.3 for recommended retention.

Once a decision has been made on the retention time, a media to store the medical record and other documents must be chosen. The media must be durable and permanent enough to retain the data for the specified time period. The durability of newer computer media has not been proven at this time and it is because of this that some facilities copy their backup files periodically to ensure the longevity of their data.

Table 6.2.   Digital storage terms

Byte	1 Character of Data
Kilobyte (K)	1,024 bytes
Megabyte (MB)	1,024 K
Gigabyte (GB)	1,024 MB
Terabyte (TB)	1,024 GB

Source: Kroenke 2008, 73

Table 6.3.   AHIMA's recommended retention schedule

Health Information	Recommended Retention Period
Diagnostic images (such as x-ray film)	5 years
Disease index	10 years
Fetal heart monitors	10 years after the age of majority
Master patient index	Permanently
Operative index	10 years
Patient health/medical records (adults)	10 years after the most recent encounter
Patient health/medical records (minors)	Age of majority plus statute of limitations
Physician index	10 years
Register of births	Permanently
Register of deaths	Permanently
Register of surgical procedures	Permanently

Source: Fletcher and Rhodes 2002

The Optical Storage Technology Association (OSTA) reports that the life expectancy of a CD is impacted by a number of factors including the manufacturer quality, physical handling, and storage. According to OSTA, manufacturers claim that the CDs will last for 50 to 200 years; however, only time will tell how accurate this prediction is. The manufacturers test the media to try to simulate time passing but because digital storage technologies currently used are significantly newer than 50 to 200 years, no one knows for sure (OSTA 2001).

The healthcare facility should develop a retention schedule to control when data should be destroyed. Please see Chapter 12 for more information on destruction of digital data.

Check Your Understanding 6.7

1. Retention of patient health information and birth registers should be maintained for the same period of time.

   A. True
   B. False. Patient information should be maintained permanently and birth registers for 10 years after the most recent encounter
   C. False. Birth registers should be maintained permanently and patient information for 10 years after the most recent encounter
   D. This is up to the facility because there are no guidelines regarding retention

2. The average size of a black and white scanned document is:

   A. 50 kb
   B. 75 kb
   C. 100 kb
   D. 100 mb

3. Incremental backups:

   A. copy only files that have changed since the last backup
   B. copy all files on the hard drive
   C. consume more resources than full backups
   D. are automatic

4. When a hard drive is filling up, what might a user notice?

   A. Change in the media used for backup
   B. More frequent backups
   C. Slower response time
   D. Testing of backup processes

5. Routine maintenance should be performed:

   A. daily
   B. at off-peak times
   C. when a full staff is on-site
   D. at least weekly

Business Continuity Planning

A **business continuity plan (BCP)** must be developed in order to prepare the facility for an unexpected failure of the computer system. This failure can be from hardware failure, software errors, sabotage, floods, tornados, and other events. Some failures occur as a result of intentional actions such as hacking and viruses. Other failures are unintentional, such as a hard drive failure, a network failure, or flood. Regardless of the cause for failure, the business of providing patient care must continue.

BCP includes policies and procedures on how the operations of the organization will function while the system is down. It should also include policies and procedures on how the facility will restore the information system and get it ready for use after the problem has been resolved. The BCP should also provide instruction and guidance on how paper forms will be used, manual processes, and how the system will be brought up-to-date when it is operational again. The forms needed would include test requisitions, test results reporting, and other reports needed to operate the healthcare facility during downtime. If the system is down for longer than a few minutes, patients will be admitted to the hospital while the system is down. The BCP should have a mechanism in place to look up the patient's medical record number while the system is down as well as a system in place to issue a medical record number.

Backup

Data in the information system must be routinely backed up. The frequency of the backup depends on the criticalness of the data. Some systems can be backed up daily or even weekly. Others are backed up with every transaction. The tapes, CD, or other media should not be stored near the original data because the same disaster that affects the original files may affect the backup files. For example, the tapes should be sent to a site in another state.

There should be a redundant backup server that mirrors the system. This hot site would be an identical system with regard to software, specifications, and data. If the EHR or other system crashes, the system can be up and operational in a short period of time. For more information on system backup, please see Chapter 12.

Report Generation/Data Monitoring

Healthcare facilities collect a tremendous amount of data. The facility must be able to convert this data into information and use it to improve the efficiency of the organization and the quality of care provided. The organization must have quality data so that the information created is accurate. Data entered into the system is used to create reports. Every effort should be made to ensure the information used to create these reports is accurate so that valid, informed decisions can be made.

Reports use four operations in order to create information from the data in the information systems (Kroenke 2008, 493):

- Filtering data
- Sorting data
- Grouping data
- Calculations

Filtering data is when the report extracts data based on specific criteria. For example, the report could list all patients discharged from the facility on July 1, 2009. Sorting data is when the data is manipulated in some way. The type of data controls the sorting method. For example, a list of patients discharged from the hospital would be sorted in alphabetical order by last name, or a list of medical records to be pulled may be sorted in terminal digit order. Grouping data requires the pulling of data together based on criteria. An example of grouping would be data grouped together by ICD-9-CM code. Data can be used to calculate simple statistics, totals, or other measures. For instance, the list of admissions to the hospital could have a total identifying the number of patients admitted for a certain day. Another example of a calculation is the average length of stay or the average daily census. These four operations are not mutually exclusive. A report may have two or more of the operations. For example, the diagnosis register would group diagnoses by code number and then sort the patients alphabetically.

Reports fall into two report types (Kroenke 2008): static and dynamic. The contents of a static report do not change. A large number of the routine reports created are static. For example, a report that calculates the number of patients discharged in May 2009 would not change. Another example of a static report is the birth register for a specific day. Dynamic reports change as the data change. An example of a dynamic report is the current number of delinquent medical records or the current census report showing the number of patients currently in the hospital.

The healthcare facility can provide the reports to the users in two different ways—automatically or manually. An automatic or preprogrammed report is provided to the user at a predetermined time, whereas a manual report is initiated by the user. Automatic reports may be set to be printed in the information system department or any other department within the facility. They can also be electronically submitted via e-mail or other electronic means. These reports are usually those needed daily, weekly, or at other routine periods. Manual reports are probably those reports that are needed periodically and not necessarily at prescribed periods of time. The user generates these reports when necessary.

A reporting system involves report authoring, report management, and report delivery. Report authoring is the development of the report by connecting to the data in the database, creating the report structure, and formatting the report. During report authoring the title of the report, headers, footers, column headings, and other formatting is performed. Report management controls who receives the reports and when and how the report is distributed.

Data vs. Information

Data are raw facts and figures, whereas information is data that has been converted into some meaningful format. Data does not help management and other users to make decisions. For example, a list of patient names and the services they received does not tell the user anything about the average patient or the most common services. There are times when data are adequate. For example, when generating the patient's bill, data such as patient name, date of admission, and other data elements may be just what is needed.

To obtain useful information, data need to be turned into information. For example, a list of all patients and their services does not tell the users anything, but a list of the top five services tells the user something about the types of patients treated at the facility. However, knowing that the top five services are medical, general surgery, obstetrics, newborns, and cardiology may or may not be adequate, and more detailed information may be needed, such as the specific procedures performed by the general surgeons.

Structure and Use of Health Information

Information retrieved can be in four formats: patient-specific, aggregate, comparative data, and knowledge-based. Patient-specific information identifies the patient. When executing a query, the user generally retrieves a single patient's information such as discharge summary, laboratory tests, and list of patients who had blood transfusions. Patient-specific data are generally connected through the use of a medical record number or other unique identifier. Aggregate reports retrieve information about multiple patients such as in a diagnosis or procedure index. Aggregate data are grouped together in a way that the individual patients, employees, or others are not identifiable. Examples of reports that use aggregate data include top ten diagnosis-related groups or the monthly statistical reports on patient volume. Aggregate data frequently come from secondary data sources such as the cancer registry. Comparative data do not identify the patient, but rather use facility-specific data and compare them to national data or those of another similar facility. Examples of data that may be compared are the complication/comorbidity rate, number of advanced beneficiary notices awarded, charges, and costs. Knowledge-based data are data combined with one's knowledge and then used to make decisions.

Health information is used by many different users and in many different formats. The Joint Commission has identified five different uses for health information: clinical decision making, organizational decision making, research, performance improvement, and education. In clinical decision making, data are used for patient care and administrative purposes. The primary users are the healthcare providers such as physicians and nurses who use the medical record to document the care they provide, justify the care provided, and to communicate with other healthcare providers. Health information is also used for administrative purposes such as coding, qualitative analysis, quantitative analysis, risk management, quality improvement, utilization review, and case management. These administrative tasks fall into several of Joint Commission's uses of data including clinical decision making, performance improvement, and organizational decision making. Without analysis of data, administration would not know what services should be expanded into a new building under consideration, physicians would not know the best drugs to use, and health information managers would not know if they were in compliance with HIPAA, Joint Commission accreditation standards, and other rules and regulations. Researchers use aggregate data to learn about the best treatments and about risk factors and life expectancy. Managers can learn about the type of patients they treat, what services make money, and where they need to expand. Health information managers use aggregate data to monitor chart deficiency rates, productivity rates, and coding errors.

Data Quality

Because data collected and stored in the information systems are used to generate reports and calculate statistics that in turn are used to make management decisions, quality data is critical. Despite all efforts to build data quality on the front end, inaccurate data sometimes is entered into the system. The phrase garbage in, garbage out (GIGO) is a very true idiom. Every effort must be made to ensure that the quality of the data is high. Data cleansing, the process of looking at the data and taking the necessary steps to correct any problems with quality, may be needed. Data cleansing may require transforming data from one format to another, filling in missing data, and looking for data that are obviously incorrect. Face validity is a type of data cleansing that involves looking at data to determine if it makes sense. Just because something makes sense does not mean it is right, but there are some data that just cannot be accurate, such as a patient having a temperature of 157°F. For an example of face validity, see figure 6.4.

For a full discussion of data quality, refer to Chapter 3.

Data Retrieval Tools

The purpose of data retrieval is to identify and extract (retrieve) data from a database. Retrieval can be as simplistic as looking up one piece of data such as a medical record number for a patient. When looking up a medical record number, data such as the patient's name are entered. All of the patients with that name will be listed along with additional information such as date of birth. The correct patient is selected and the patient's medical record number and other information are retrieved. Other data retrieval needs require accessing data across systems and displaying that data on a single screen. There are a wide range of tools that can be used to retrieve data. See figure 6.5 for an example of a search screen.

When retrieving data, color, animation, icons, and sound may be used to guide the navigation process. Although color is frequently used, some users are color-blind and without some other cue may miss out on the benefits of color. Whatever navigation tools are used, they should be consistent across the system.

Figure 6.4.   Example of face validity

- Number of bassinets: 10
- Number of discharges for January: 3,421

That equates to 342 discharges per bassinet in 31 days. This just is not possible.

Figure 6.5.   Example of search screen

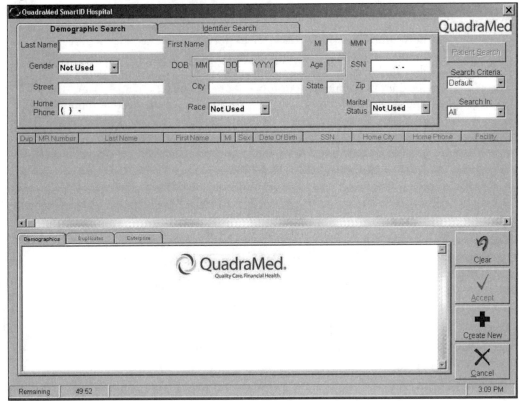

Source: Copyright 2009 QuadraMed® Corporation. All rights reserved.

Screen design is important to data retrieval. Different types of users need different types of views. For example, cardiologists will want to access something different than nurses; or, Dr. Smith, a cardiologist, may want to view things a little differently than Dr. Jones, also a cardiologist. With the user input, the screens can be customized to show the desired view.

When designing screens in an information system application, the data elements on the screen should have a logical flow and design. The screen should follow the traditional left to right and top to bottom formatting (Williams 2006). The screens should be designed with the needs of the user in mind, providing instructions to the user where needed to facilitate data quality and data collection. There should also be consistency throughout all of the screens with regard to terms used, abbreviations, and overall look and feel of the system (Williams 2006). New screens can be created to meet user needs where existing screens fail, but these screens should not be created just for the sake of creating a screen. Default entry should be used when possible to eliminate the need to enter data and reduce error. Recording today's date without entering it is an example of a default entry.

Unlike paper documents, which are controlled by the size of the paper (generally 8.5 × 11 inches), the screen is controlled by the size of the computer monitor. Terminals vary on the number of characters per line and the number of lines per screen. The general rule is that only what would be one third of a form will show on a screen at any given time. Screens can use color, blinking lights, and other special features to alert the user to important information such as allergies.

A common retrieval tool is **structured query language (SQL)**. SQL was developed by IBM in the 1970s. It was designated as an American National Standards Institute (ANSI) standard in 1986. It is the standard language for the relational database. SQL defines data elements, and manipulates and controls data. The data definition components of SQL allow the user to create tables, delete tables, and show how something is viewed. Data definition also allows the user to define the fields with regard to characteristics such as number of characters, alphanumeric, and so on. **Data manipulation** allows the user to add and delete rows in a table and to sort, find, and compare ($>$, $<$, $=$). Other functions of the data manipulation component are to update data. The control command limits access and what the user can do. It also controls aborting incomplete transactions. Examples of SQL commands are: CREATE TABLE, SELECT, WHERE, COUNT, and UPDATE PATIENT (Oppel 2004).

These are all examples that assume a table with the name Patients and the columns ID, FirstName, LastName, DateAdded:

To retrieve all the records and all the columns
    Select * from Patients

To retrieve all the records and only the FirstName column
    Select FirstName From Patients

To retrieve all the records and all the columns ordered by LastName Descending
    Select * From Patients Order By LastName desc

To retrieve all the records and all the columns that were added before 1/1/2008
    Select * From Patients Where DateAdded < '1/1/2008'

To select only the records where the FirstName is equal to Mark
    Select * from Patients Where FirstName = 'Mark'

Query by example (QBE), like SQL, is a data manipulation language. QBE does not require the use of structured formats and statements but rather uses a graphical user interface to query the database. This type of language makes it easier for the general user to develop his or her own reports (Oppel 2004).

A **Boolean search** uses Boolean operators to control search results. Boolean operators are "and," "or," and "not." They are used to refine the search to ensure that only the information needed is identified. For example, a search of "EHR" and "implementation" would find all references to EHR implementation but would not include articles on EHR evaluation, EHR selection, or other terms. A search of "EHR" not "implementation" would identify all articles on EHRs excluding those on EHR implementation.

Before the user can access anything, the system must be designed in such a way as to facilitate retrieval as needed for the facility. For example, the user could not run a report on all of the patients from Georgia if the city and state are in the same field. Because the names of cities vary in length, you could not say that the state started X characters in. To solve this problem, the data would need to be stored in separate fields for city and state. This process is called normalization. See Chapter 4 for more information.

Ad hoc vs. Routine

Routine reports are those that are needed repeatedly. These reports may be daily, weekly, monthly, semiannually, or annually. Examples of these reports are daily discharge list, discharged not final billed report, and monthly discharge statistics. **Ad hoc reports** are needed only once. They may be used for a special report, a research program, or other purpose.

Routine reports are developed during the system implementation process and may be revised and added to at any time. The ad hoc reports can be created at any time. Who writes the ad hoc reports or prints out the routine reports depends on the software and the policies of the hospital.

Check Your Understanding 6.8

1. Ad hoc reports are run:

   A. when needed
   B. monthly
   C. routinely
   D. quarterly

2. Storing data in such a way to facilitate retrieval is called:

   A. query by example
   B. ad hoc
   C. maintenance
   D. normalization

3. SQL is the standard language for which type of database?

   A. object-oriented
   B. relational
   C. network
   D. object-oriented, relational, and network models

4. Reviewing a report to determine if the data makes sense is called

   A. data quality
   B. face validity
   C. ad hoc reporting
   D. Boolean search

5. Which of the following terms would be seen in a Boolean search?

   A. select
   B. sort
   C. print
   D. and

References

Abdelhak, M., S. Grostick, M.A. Hanken, and E. Jacobs. 2007. *Health Information: Management of a Strategic Resource.* St. Louis, MO: Saunders Elsevier.

Amatayakul, M.K. 2007. *Electronic Health Records: A Practical Guide for Professionals and Organizations.* 3rd edition, Chicago AHIMA.

Agency for Healthcare Research and Quality. 2009a. Nationwide HCUP Databases. http://www.ahrq.gov/.

Agency for Healthcare Research and Quality. 2009b. Overview of HCUP http://hcupnet.ahrq.gov/HCUPnet. jsp?Id=6D133B27E4926DD6&Form=MAINSEL&JS=Y&Action=%3E%3ENext%3E%3E&HCUPnet%20 Overview.x=1.

AHIMA e-HIM Work Group on Electronic Document Management as a Component of EHR. 2003. Practice brief: Electronic document management as a component of the electronic health record. *Journal of AHIMA* 74(9). http://library.ahima.org/xpedio/groups/public/documents/ahima/bok1_022141. hcsp?dDocName=bok1_022141.

AHIMA e-HIM Work Group on the Legal Health Record. 2005. Update: Guidelines for defining the legal health record for disclosure purposes. *Journal of AHIMA* 76(8):64A–G.

Centers for Disease Control. 2009. About CDC. http://www.cdc.gov/about.

Dunn, R. 2006. Quick scan of bar coding. *Journal of AHIMA* 77(1):50–54.

Dunn, R. 2007. Benchmarking imaging: making every image count in scanning programs. *Journal of AHIMA* 78(6):42–46.

Fletcher, D.M. and H.B. Rhodes. 2002 (June). Practice brief: Retention of health information (Updated). *Journal of AHIMA* (Web extra).

Hebda, T, P. Czar, and C. Mascara. 2005. *Handbook of Informatics for Nurses & Health Care Professionals.* Upper Saddle River, NJ: Pearson Prentice Hall.

Joint Commission. 2009. Facts about ORYX. http://www.jointcommission.org/AccreditationPrograms/Hospitals/ORYX/facts_oryx.htm.

Kroenke, D. 2008. *Experiencing MIS.* Upper Saddle River, NJ: Pearson Prentice Hall.

LaTour, K.M. and S. Eichenwald Maki, eds. 2006. *Health Information Management: Concepts, Principles, and Practice.* Chicago: AHIMA.

Mahoney, M.E. 1997. Document imaging and workflow technology in healthcare today. *Journal of AHIMA* 68(4):28–36.

Myjer, D. and R. Madamba. 2002. Implementing a document imaging system. *Journal of AHIMA* 73(9): 44ff.

National Center for Health Statistics. 2008. http://www.cdc.gov/nchs/.

Oppel, A. 2004. *Databases DeMYSTiFieD: A Self-Teaching Guide.* Emeryville, CA: McGraw-Hill Osborne.

Optical Storage Technology Association. 2001. Understanding CD-R and CD-RW disc longevity. http://www.osta.org/technology/cdqa13.htm.

Quinsey, C.A. 2004. In case of a crash…Computer backups. *Journal of AHIMA* 75(5):60–61.

Rhodes, H. and M. Dougherty. 2003. Practice brief: Document imaging as a bridge to the EHR. *Journal of AHIMA* 74(6):56A–G.

Rhodes, H. 1997. Implementing the wireless computerized patient record. *Journal of AHIMA* 68(7):44–46.

Twin Imaging Technology, Inc. 2007. Document imaging. http://www.twinimaging.com/ourservices.html.

Williams, A. 2006. Design for better data: How software and users interact onscreen matters to data quality. *Journal of AHIMA* 77(2):56–60.

Chapter 7
Computers in HIM

Objectives

- Identify the systems needed to support efficient operations in the HIM department.
- Differentiate between the various software products used in the HIM department.
- Improve the quality of the data within the health information management systems.

Key Terms

Automated codebook encoder
Birth certificate information
   system
Cancer registry information
   system
Chart deficiency system

Chart locator system
Data quality indicator
   information system
Dictation system
Disclosure management system
Encoder

Expander
Grouper
Release of information system
Rules-based encoder
Trauma registry software
Transcription system

Introduction

Computers are critical to the health information management (HIM) department. Many of the department's processes depend on computers to function efficiently and effectively. Many systems used by the HIM department staff, such as the master patient index and the financial information system, are available to authorized users throughout the organization.

Other information systems are designed specifically for HIM functions, which may limit the usage to the HIM department, or for other departments to use to support the HIM department or the medical record. Facilities vary widely in their organizational structure; as a result, some of these systems may be technically used by other departments but all support HIM. For example, the birth certificate software may be solely used by the HIM department to create and report births occurring in the facility, whereas the dictation system may be purchased and managed by the HIM department but used by physicians. All of these HIM systems greatly improve the efficiency and effectiveness of the HIM department. The HIM systems include:

- Release of information system/disclosure management
- Encoder/grouper system
- Cancer registry system
- Chart locator system
- Birth certificate system
- Chart deficiency system
- Transcription system
- Data quality indicators system
- Dictation system

The purpose of this chapter is to present an overview of the information systems that support the HIM functions and their functionality, common data elements found in these systems, and reports.

Release of Information System/Disclosure Management

The HIM department receives requests for copies of patient records on a daily basis. These requests for copies of records must be logged into the system to allow for tracking on the status of the request. The **release of information** (ROI) system is designed to manage all aspects of requests for protected health information received and processed by the HIM department. Use of the system begins when a new request is entered into the system. It continues to track the request as it is processed and acts as a historical database of all requests processed and ultimately used to generate reports. For an example of an ROI system, see figure 7.1.

A **disclosure management system** tracks the disclosures made throughout the healthcare organization. This tracking is required by the Health Information Portability and Accountability Act (HIPAA). The covered entities must provide the patient with accounting of disclosure upon request. The disclosure management system may be part of the ROI system or it may be a separate system used by HIM and non-HIM departments. In addition to disclosures, a disclosure management software system may also track requests for amendments to protected health information as well as restrictions to disclosures. If a separate disclosure management system is used, it would also have a link to the hospital information system to populate basic patient demographic information. It would keep up

Figure 7.1. **Sample ROI interface: HealthPort eSmartLog's "New Request" screen**

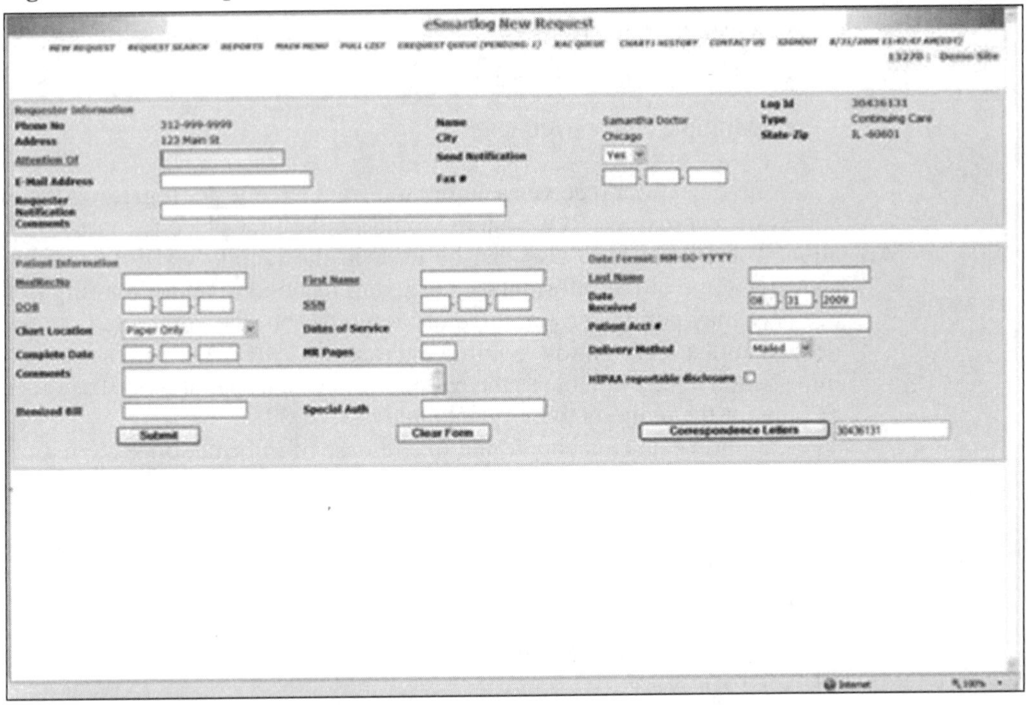

Source: HealthPort. Reprinted with permission.

with who received information, what information was provided, date of release, any charge for accounting of disclosures, and more.

Functionality

The ROI system is a valuable tool for the ROI staff. Once the requests for copies of records are entered into the ROI system, the data can be used for many different purposes to support the workflow.

The ROI staff also can use the system to check on the status of requests. The staff will be able to determine where in the process the request is and to whom the request has been assigned. The patient's name or medical record number can be entered and the appropriate request opened to identify status and personnel responsible.

Throughout the release process, the status of a request must be updated and kept current by ROI staff at all times. The status can include details about issues encountered, a need for review by risk management, a need for a medical record or microfilm to be pulled, or other action required. Once the record has been copied or reports printed, the request should be marked as complete. Completed requests generally include an indicator showing the request is the complete status, the date processed, and specifically what has been sent. The individual reports and dates of reports would also be entered. Based on the number of copies and other activities, the ROI staff would also record any changes that were applied.

The ROI system provides a number of reports and statistics for the HIM management team. Some of the data provided to the management team include:

- Requests that have not been processed

- Requests that have been processed

- Turnaround time of requests

- Revenue collected

- Accounts receivable

- Productivity by individual staff members
- Overall productivity
- List of frequent requesters
- Multiple customized letters

If the supervisor receives a complaint from a requester regarding the inability to obtain copies of records, the ROI system would be the first place to start investigating the situation. The ROI system also can be used in the facility's HIPAA compliance because it provides some of the information needed to respond to an accounting of disclosure. Management may periodically archive old requests, but the completed requests should not be deleted until after retention requirements are met. HIPAA requires accounting of disclosure information to be available to the patient for 6 years, so that would be the minimum amount of time for the requests to be maintained (3M 2009).

Common data elements found in a release of information system are:

- Patient name
- Medical record number
- Patient type
- Date request received
- Type of requester
- Name of requester
- Name of contact at requester
- Address of requester
- Type of request (for example, insurance, patient, attorney, or patient care)
- Assigned to
- Action taken (request completed, type of letter sent, records requested, and more)
- Date action taken
- Date request completed
- Information sent (specific documents and dates of reports)
- Charges
- Amount paid
- Amount due
- Comments

The basic patient information such as name and medical record number are frequently populated in the ROI system by an interface from the admission, discharge, transfer system, thus eliminating the need to enter this information. This link also improves the data quality. The requests can typically be retrieved by items such as patient name, medical record number, or requester name.

Tables are an important part of the ROI system. Some tables are a default within the system while others can be set up and customized by the facility. For example, the user only has to enter the name and address of a requester once, thus managing time wisely. After the initial entry, the user is able to select the requester from a drop-down box or other graphical user interface tool. If the requester is from a large organization such as Blue-Cross BlueShield, there can even be a table listing individuals in that organization so that the copies are forwarded to the correct person. Tables also may be used to record charge information such as charge per copy, microfilm, certification, and other chargeable actions. Another use of tables is identifying all of the individual forms or groups of forms that may be released. The table may list discharge summary, history and physical examination, operative report, pathology report, laboratory report, and other forms individually. The ROI system may have requests for common groupings of reports, such as the entire medical record or the discharge summary and history and physical examination. Tables help to save the user a significant amount of time because they do not have to individually type each document released. Drop-down boxes or check boxes containing the individual documents or sets of document also allow for consistent data entry.

The ROI software can perform many other tasks. The ROI system reminds the ROI staff of the need to perform maintenance tasks on the information system. The maintenance can include backups, deletion of old requests, or archiving of completed requests to speed processing.

The ROI system will allow ROI staff to pull up a work queue showing the requests that need to be processed. With the use of the electronic health record (EHR), more of the requests can be fulfilled without the need for the paper record. ROI staff just need to print or fax the requested documents from the appropriate system. Once the number of pages and other chargeable actions are known, the ROI coordinator can post the charges into the system and once received, post payment.

Reporting

Reporting is an important part of a ROI system. The reports are used by ROI staff or HIM management and to communicate with requesters (McKesson Corp. 2009).

In a paper environment, the ROI coordinators are able to generate a list of medical records to be pulled so the appropriate contents of the record can be copied. This list can be sorted into terminal digit or other numeric or alphabetic order to facilitate the retrieval process. Depending on the structure of the department, the ROI staff or file area staff can use this list to retrieve the paper records.

Customized letters are critical to the ROI system. Customized letters and forms may be used to communicate with the requester for many purposes, including to:

- Notify requester that the facility does not have a record of the patient being treated at the facility and/or on that date

- Remind requester that they have an outstanding balance for copies of records

- Request that copies of records be paid prior to their release

- Provide cover letter for records being sent

- Notify requester that the authorization is invalid

- Notify requester that an authorization is needed

- Notify requester that there will be a delay in the release of the information

- Notify requester that the records will be released as soon as the facility has received prepayment for copies

- Generate invoices for the copies of the record copied

- Generate reminder invoices when payment is not received timely

HIM department staff monitor the efficiency of the ROI staff through a multitude of management reports. These reports provide information on various functions including turnaround times, productivity, backlogs, revenue, and accounts receivable, to name a few. Depending on the information contained in the report, the report can include requests by employee, by requester type, by specific requester, or all requests. For example, a report on the average turnaround time for all requests or for BlueCross BlueShield requests can be obtained. The manager also is able to track the turnaround times by employee, which can be used in performance evaluations and other management monitoring. Many of these reports come prepackaged with the software, but many systems allow the user to develop and customize their own routine and ad hoc reports.

Encoder/Grouper

The **encoder** is used by coders to select the appropriate code for the diagnosis(es) and procedure(s) supported by the medical record. There are two types of encoders. **Rules-based encoders** require the user to type in the name or portion of the name of the diagnosis or procedure. This entry into the encoder generates a list of suggestions from which the coder selects. For example, if the coder types in pneu-, the encoder may suggest: pneumonia and pneumonitis. From there the coder scrolls down until the proper code is selected. The **automated codebook encoder** looks much like the alphabetic index located in the International Classification of Diseases, Ninth Edition, Clinical Modification (ICD-9-CM) and Current Procedural Terminology (CPT) codebooks. This similarity eases the transition from the book to the encoder. For an example of a rules-based encoder, see figure 7.2.

For an example of an automated codebook encoder, see figure 7.3.

The **grouper** assigns the codes entered into the encoder into the appropriate Medicare severity diagnostic related groups (MS-DRG) or other diagnosis-related group (DRG). The grouper uses the appropriate grouping software for the insurer assigned to the patient. The most common grouper is the MS-DRG grouper; however, other insurers, including some Medicaid programs, have developed their own groupers for use in determining payment to the healthcare facility.

For an example of a grouper, see figure 7.4.

Figure 7.2.   Example of a rules-based encoder—3M's Coding and Reimbursement System

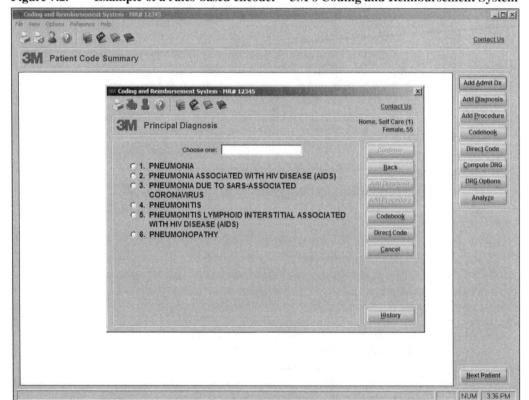

Copyright © 2010 3M Health Information Systems. Reprinted with permission. All rights reserved.

Figure 7.3.   Example of an automated codebook encoder

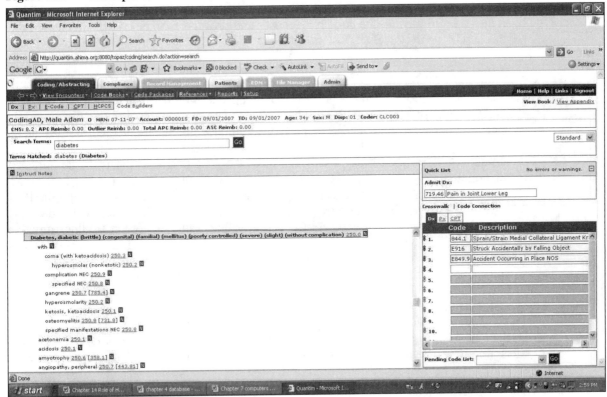

Source: Copyright 2009 QuadraMed® Corporation.

Figure 7.4.   Example of a grouper—3M's Coding and Reimbursement System

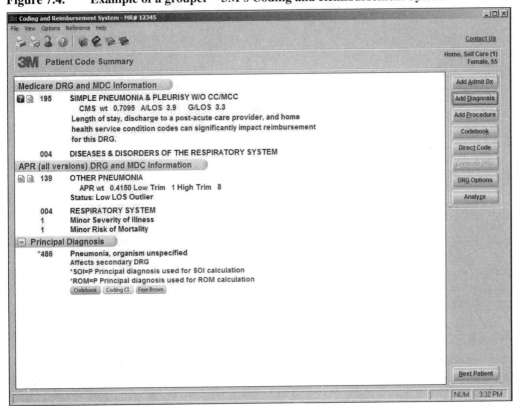

Copyright © 2010 3M Health Information Systems. Reprinted with permission. All rights reserved.

Coding quality and DRG assignment are not ensured by the use of an encoder because the code selected is only as good as the data entered into the system. It is the responsibility of the coder to identify the correct diagnoses and procedures to be coded and entered into the encoder appropriately.

Functionality

One of the biggest advantages in the use of an encoder/grouper is the prompts. For example, if a higher-paying MS-DRG can be assigned with the addition of a specific diagnosis, specific procedure, complication/comorbidity, or major complication/comorbidity, then the computer will ask the coder if any of them are present. The grouper allows the coder to resequence the principal diagnosis when more than one diagnosis meets the definition of the principal diagnosis. The coding guidelines allow the facility to choose any of the diagnoses as the principal as long as it meets the definition. The encoder can assign the ICD-9-CM, CPT and HCPCS codes required on the patient claim. These assigned codes must be validated through the Medicare Code Editor, the National Correct Coding Initiative, and other edits. These edits will look for invalid codes, illogical codes, nonspecific codes, and other possible errors. For example, the coder cannot give a newborn code to an adult and cannot assign a hysterectomy code to a male. These edits are designed to catch errors before they can be submitted on a claim improperly and to improve the quality of the code assignment.

Coders are also permitted to manually enter codes into the system rather than looking them up each time. For the more frequent diagnoses such as diabetes or dehydration, this is a more efficient method. Once entered, the system will then confirm and validate the code.

Common data elements in an encoder/grouper are:

- Admitting diagnosis

- Principal diagnosis

- Secondary diagnoses

- Principal procedure

- Secondary procedure

- Age of patient (or date of birth)

- Discharge disposition

- Gender

- Patient name

- Medical record number

- Account number

The encoder/grouper is usually linked to the hospital's financial information system so that the codes can be automatically transferred to that system for billing. Without this link, the coder would have to reenter codes into the financial information system. This double entry leaves room for data entry errors, which would in turn cause problems with billing and reimbursement.

Reporting

The encoder/grouper does not rely heavily on reporting. Rather, the system is more about assigning codes and DRGs using edits to assist the coder in proper assignment of codes and other information transferred to the hospital financial system. However, if needed, the system may print out a report listing all of the codes and respective DRGs assigned.

Check Your Understanding 7.1

1. I need to provide an accounting of disclosure. Which of the following systems should I use?

   A. Disclosure management
   B. Release of information
   C. Encoder
   D. Grouper

2. I have been hired to design and implement the HIM for a new hospital under construction. One of my tasks is to select systems that traditionally are used solely by the HIM department. Which one of these would I have to purchase?

   A. Chart deficiency system
   B. Master patient index
   C. Picture archival communication system
   D. Admission, discharge, transfer system

3. I need a computerized system to help me assign the proper code. The system that I need is a(n):

   A. grouper
   B. release of information
   C. disclosure management
   D. encoder

4. The system used to notify requesters of invalid authorization is called:

   A. grouper
   B. release of information
   C. disclosure management
   D. encoder

5. The software application that assigns the MS-DRG is:

   A. grouper
   B. release of information
   C. disclosure management
   D. encoder

Cancer and Other Registries

There are many types of registries currently found in healthcare. These registries track conditions such as cancer, diabetes, trauma, and transplants. Although registry software across these different diseases and situations has similarities, each has its own unique characteristics. All registries are designed to record data on patients who meet criteria for inclusion in the registry. These registries would generally require basic demographic information, reporting, treatment, description of condition, and frequently long-term patient tracking. Commonly found data elements across registries include:

- Patient name

- Medical record number

- Dates of service

- Physician

- Date of birth

- Date of diagnosis

Two common registries will be discussed in more detail—cancer (tumor) and trauma registry.

Cancer (Tumor) Registry

Functionality

- The **cancer registry information system** tracks information about the patient's cancer from the time of diagnosis to the patient's death. The cancer registry information systems are extremely complex and track very detailed information regarding diagnosis and treatment. Some of the common data elements unique to the cancer registry include (CDC n.d.):

- Site of cancer(s)

- Type of cancer

- Treatment received

- Date of last contact

- TNM (tumor, node, metastasis) stage

- Number of lymph nodes involved

- Behavior type

- Date of death

- Grade of neoplasm

- Size of mass

- Physician name

- Physician address

- Physician phone number

- Facility name

- Facility address

- Facility phone number

- Clinical trials

- Accession number

- ICD-O code

The cancer registry can electronically submit a file containing the data required for state cancer reporting. As the patient's treatment and clinical follow-up progress, this information is entered into the system so that it reflects the patient's treatment and current status regarding their cancer.

Edits assist the cancer registrar in the data entry and staging. These edits are key to ensuring the quality of the data in the registry. Edits vary widely. For example, an edit can show the user how to enter data such as the discharge date. It should be entered in MMDDYYYY format. An edit could also be a list of valid state abbreviations or cancer sites from which the cancer registrar can choose. An edit may also verify that a code number is valid. For more on data quality, see Chapter 3. When data entered has passed all of the edit checks, it is ready for analysis. (CDC 2009). Of course, the data provided could pass an edit check and still be incorrect, so ongoing monitoring of the abstracting process is still necessary.

Cancer registry software can also assist the registrar in the patient follow-up process. The software tracks the last contact date, and manages letters and other activities related to the follow-up process (Impac Medical Systems, Inc. 2009).

Figure 7.5 shows the Centers for Disease Control and Prevention's (CDC's) free software, National Program of Cancer Registries.

Cancer registry software typically provides many functions for the registry staff. Some examples of this functionality are:

- Check Social Security Death Index to see if patient died

- Transfer data to the state registry

- Perform edit checks on data entered

- Perform collaborative staging

- Perform TNM staging

- Provide links to SEER (surveillance epidemiology and end results) manuals

- Reference previous versions of staging systems such as Facility Oncology Registry Data Standards (FORDS)

- Assign accession number

- Suspend records for abstracting when the documentation is incomplete

- Provide list of disclosures made for compliance with the HIPAA accounting of disclosure

- Validate ICD-O code

Figure 7.5.   CDC's National Program of Cancer Registries

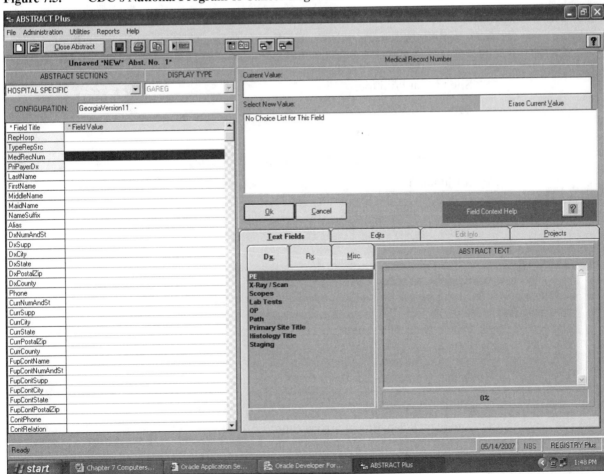

Source: Center for Disease Control and Prevention © 2009.

Reporting

Reporting is a key role of the cancer registry system. The system can provide management reports such as productivity as well as reports on the content of the registry. Common reports include (CDC 2009):

- Life expectancy
- Follow-up rate
- List of patients due for follow-up
- Patients lost to follow-up
- Follow-up letters to patient and physicians

The registry will also allow the reporting of patient-specific information such as

- Patient abstracts
- Accounting of disclosures

Ad hoc reporting would be an important part of a registry. These reports would be designed specifically for the research project or other purpose for which the report is being run. For example, these reports could be based on site of cancer, cell type of cancer, or treatment modalities.

Trauma Registry

Functionality

Trauma registry software tracks patients with traumatic injuries from the initial trauma treatment to death. Data elements would include (Lancet Technology, Inc. 2005):

- Site of injury/injuries
- Type of injury
- How injury occurred
- Length of time between injury and first treatment
- Residual(s)
- Date of injury
- Time of injury
- Work-related
- ICD-9-CM code
- ICD-9-CM E-code
- Protective devices used
- Emergency medical services deployment
- Registry number
- Autopsy performed
- Emergency department arrival time

The data collected is far more rigorous than the list above. The National Trauma Data Bank (NTDB) has identified a minimum data set that a hospital-based trauma registry software package should meet or exceed. These data are reported to the state and ultimately the NTDB. Although the NTDB has established a minimum data set, each state has its own rules related to data collection (American College of Surgeons 2009).

The system also tracks care provided to the patient before hospitalization and during hospitalization, as well as posthospital care. The trauma registry allows the registrar to code ICD-9-CM codes to the injuries. The data abstracted into the system is used to calculate the Injury Severity Scores (ISS), Revised Trauma Scores (RTS), and Probability of Survival (Ps) (Lancet Technology, Inc. 2005). The ISS is used for patients who have multiple trauma to indicate the severity of the injury to the various anatomical locations. The higher the ISS score, the more severe the injury and less likelihood of survival. The RTS is considered to be a physiological scoring system that predicts the probability of death through the use of the Glasgow Coma Scale, the patient's blood pressure, and the patient's respiratory rate. The Ps score is calculated by using the ISS and the RTS along with his or her age. (Trauma.org 2009).

This registry, like the cancer registry, requires follow-up of patients.

Reporting

Trauma registry software packages generally have report writers for ad hoc reporting. The common reports for the trauma registry would be similar to those of the cancer registry, such as outcomes, follow-up rates, and best practices for patient care. The system would provide statistics on cause of injuries, types of injuries, frequency of injury severity score, and other descriptive statistics. The software can generate a report identifying the most common times trauma patients are admitted to the emergency department, which could be used in staffing decisions (Lancet Technologies, Inc. 2005).

Chart Locator

The **chart locator system** is designed to track the paper medical record. This tracking is important because paper records are moved from place to place for patient care, quality reviews, coding, and many other purposes. The Joint Commission regulations require medical records to be readily accessible for patient care. The chart locator supports that mandate. Figure 7.6 shows an example of chart locator software.

Functionality

The purpose of the chart locator is to provide the ability to change the location of the patient record from one location to another. All of the functions of this system support this objective. The chart locator is valuable to both HIM department staff and management. The chart locator tracks a medical record as it moves from each location. The data in the system identifies where the record is currently physically located, how long it has been in that location, when the record is due for return to the HIM department, when a record is overdue to be returned, and to whom the record was checked out. These data are used to generate a list of records checked out to a location for auditing to ensure that the data in the system is accurate.

The emergency department and other locations may need one record or 50 records. When checking out multiple records to one location, the user only has to enter the location once and then enter all of the records being relocated. This entry of records into the system is frequently supported by barcodes, which, at a minimum, contain the patient's medical record number and volume number of the record. Barcodes speed the data entry process and improve the quality of the data entered, thus improving the efficiency and effectiveness of checking in and out records.

Figure 7.6.   Sample of the ATHENS Tracking function

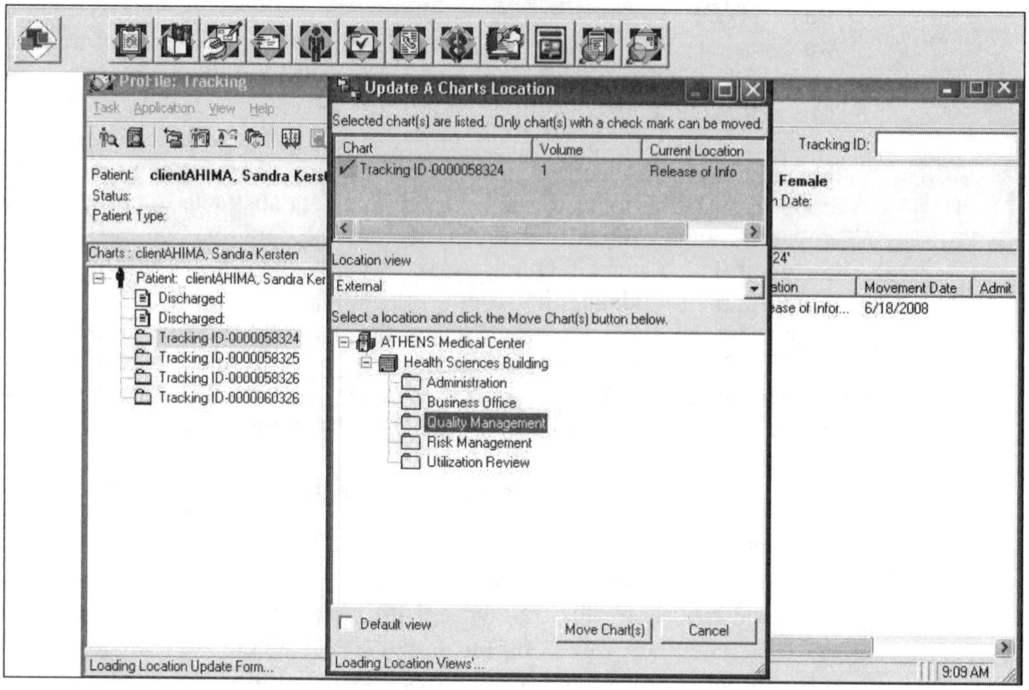

Source: © Cerner Corporation. AHIMA has restricted permission to reproduce and distribute this copyrighted work. Further reproduction or distribution is strictly prohibited without written consent of Cerner Corporation.

Common data elements in the chart locator are:

- Patient name

- Medical record number

- Volume

- Location to which the record is checked out

- Date record checked out

- Date record returned

- Who checked out/checked in the record

The system may provide the last five or so locations of the record. This may be helpful in locating lost records because it can help the user determine where in the process the record has been and where it may have gone. Past locations may also be useful in privacy incident investigation or other risk management investigations to know who has had access to the record. For example, if an employee has been accused of improperly disclosing a patient's protected health information, it would be important to know if the record has been in a location to which that employee would have had access.

Data quality is important because a significant amount of time can be wasted looking for records when the paper medical record is not where the chart locator indicates. Tables, which are preprogrammed lists and options for a user to select from, can be used to save time and improve data quality. For example, only approved locations would be programmed into the "Locations" table. As a result, the user would choose the location desired from a drop-down box.

These tables are generally user defined during the implementation. The user can update the tables as needed to keep the content of the data current. To keep the chart location system accurate, routine audits should be conducted. These audits would confirm that records checked out to a location are actually at that location. It would also identify records located outside of the permanent file that had not been checked out at all.

Reporting

Management uses the chart locator reporting for multiple purposes, including identification of most user requests of records, productivity tracking, identification of trends in the volume of record retrievals, and identification of areas of the facility for which records are not returned in a timely manner (3M 2009).

Check Your Understanding 7.2

1. The term used to describe messages that let the user know there is a problem when abstracting a cancer patient into the cancer registry system is called a(n):

    A. reporting
    B. alert
    C. abstract
    D. staging

2. Which type of registry software tracks patients who have been injured?

    A. Cancer registry
    B. Implant registry
    C. Trauma registry
    D. Transplant registry

3. Which system tracks the paper medical record?

    A. Chart deficiency
    B. Chart locator
    C. Release of information
    D. Disclosure management

4. Barcodes are key to the efficiency of what type of system?

    A. Chart deficiency
    B. Chart locator
    C. Release of information
    D. Disclosure management

5. Life expectancy is information that would come from the:

    A. chart locator
    B. disclosure management
    C. release of information
    D. cancer registry software

Birth Certificate

For years, birth certificates were typed on a typewriter and manually sent to the local health department. Now birth certificate data is entered into a state-approved **birth certificate information system**. This software reports births occurring in the healthcare facility to the state health agency. The birth certificate information system software may be developed by the state or by a vendor. Birth certificate software will capture the minimum data set established by the National Center for Health Statistics and any state-required data.

Figure 7.7 shows the standard content of a U.S. birth certificate.

Functionality

Functionality common in birth certificate information systems typically includes (Brookins Communications, Inc. 2009):

- Collect data mandated by the National Center for Health Statistics

- Automatically report standard information such as name of facility

Figure 7.7.   Content of U.S. birth certificate of live birth

Child's Information
Child's name
Time of birth
Sex
Date of birth
Facility (hospital) name (if not an institution, give street address)
City
County

Mother's Information
Current legal name
Date of birth
Mother's name prior to first marriage
Birthplace
Residence (state)
County
City
Street number
Zip code
Inside city limits?
Mother married?
If no, has paternity acknowledgment been signed in the hospital?
Social security number (SSN) requested for the child?
Mother's SSN
Father's SSN
Education
Hispanic origin?
Race

Father's Information
Current legal name
Date of birth
Birthplace
Education
Hispanic origin?
Race

Certifier's Information
Certifier's name
Certifier's title
Date certified
Date filed by registrar

Figure 7.7.   Content of U.S. birth certificate of live birth *(continued)*

Medical and Health Information
Date of first prenatal care visit
Date of last prenatal care visit
Total number of prenatal visits for this pregnancy
Number of previous live births
Mother's height
Mother's pregnancy weight
Mother's weight at delivery
Did mother get WIC food for herself during this pregnancy?
Number of other pregnancy outcomes
Cigarette smoking before and during pregnancy
Principal source of payment for this delivery
Date of last live birth
Date of last other pregnancy outcome
Date last normal menses began
Risk factors in this pregnancy
Infections present and/or treated during this pregnancy
Obstetrical procedures
Onset of labor
Characteristics of labor and delivery
Method of delivery
Maternal morbidity

Newborn Information
Birth weight
Obstetric estimate of gestation
Apgar score (1 and 5 minutes)
Plurality
If not born first (born first, second, third, etc.)
Abnormal conditions of newborn
Congenital abnormalities of the newborn
Was infant transferred within 24 hours of delivery?
Is infant living at time of report?
Is infant being breastfed at discharge?

Source: National Center for Health Statistics 2003

- Allow users to choose from list of obstetrical physicians
- Capture demographic information from hospital information system
- Prevent omissions of required data before birth certificate is sent to the state
- Submit birth certificate data
- Submit parent's request for social security number
- Print out data captured for parent(s) to proof
- Create birth log, eliminating need for paper log in labor and delivery
- Use drop-down boxes to improve data consistency
- Use edits to improve data quality
- Allows parent(s) to order copy of birth certificate

Some electronic birth registration systems have incorporated the preparation of fetal death reports as well. Additionally, some systems allow the facility to download the data on their births to an Excel spreadsheet so that they can create their own reports.

Many birth certificate fields have check boxes for completion. For example, the field for infections present and/or treated during this pregnancy lists gonorrhea, syphilis, chlamydia, hepatitis B, hepatitis C, and none of these. The birth certificate coordinator would click all infections that apply (Brookins Communications, Inc. 2009).

Figure 7.8 shows an example of an entry screen in Electronic Vital Events Registration Systems (EVERS), the birth certificate information system used by the Alabama Center for Health Statistics and Computer Systems Center.

Reporting

The birth certificate systems used may be developed and provided to the facilities by the state or may be purchased from a vendor. State facility systems are designed more to capture and report birth certificate data. Vendor products may have more management tools than the state systems, such as productivity and turnaround times.

The system may also generate statistical reports such as cesarean section rate or trending births rates. The key reporting capability, however, is the ability to report the births to

Figure 7.8.   Family screen in Electronic Vital Events Registration Systems (EVERS)

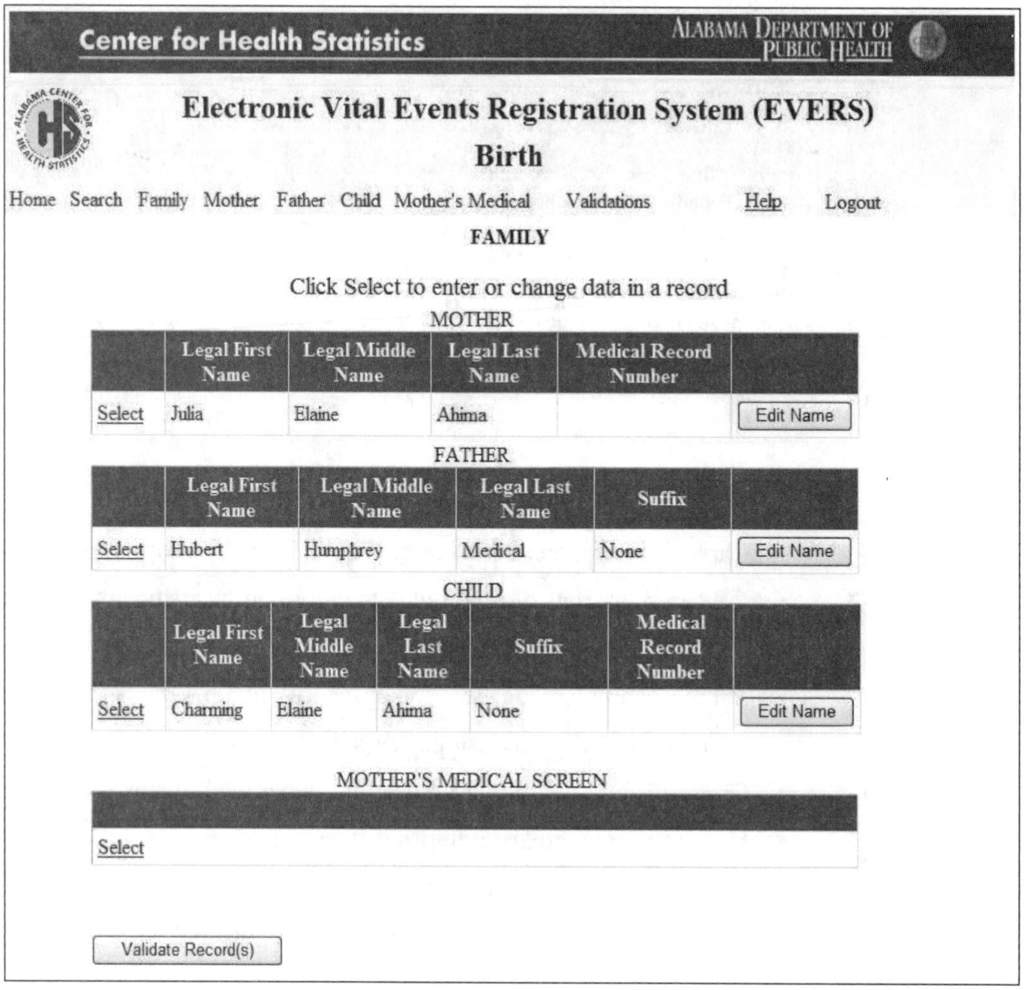

Source: Alabama Center for Health Statistics and Computer Systems Center, Alabama Department of Public Health. Used with permission.

the state in the approved format. The state may use the birth certificate data reported via the birth certificate system to feed other databases, such as immunization registry to enhance tracking of childhood immunizations (Brookins Communications, Inc. 2009).

Chart Deficiency

Physicians and other clinicians have certain documentation requirements mandated by facility policy and medical staff rules and regulations. Documentation requirements are based on Joint Commission regulations, state licensure regulations, and other standards or regulations that the facility is subject to. The specific documentation requirements mandate when reports such as the history and physical examination should be dictated or written. It should also mandate the content of the various reports analyzed, and the deadline in which the entire medical record should be complete. This deadline would include the presence of all required documents and the authentication of these documents. If the medical record comes to the HIM department with a deficiency, then the documentation omission is recorded and tracked in the **chart deficiency system**. The deficiencies can be in paper, imaged, and/or electronic records depending on the system used. With imaged or electronic records, the physician can complete the deficiency from his or her office, home, or other location. With paper records, the physician must come to the designated area in the facility. The chart deficiency system should be linked to the hospital information system so that patient name, discharge date, and other demographic information are maintained and automatically populated.

Figure 7.9 shows McKesson's chart deficiency system, Horizon Patient Folder.

Figure 7.9.   McKesson's chart deficiency program, Horizon Patient Folder, showing all deficiencies for a patient encounter assigned to a specific doctor

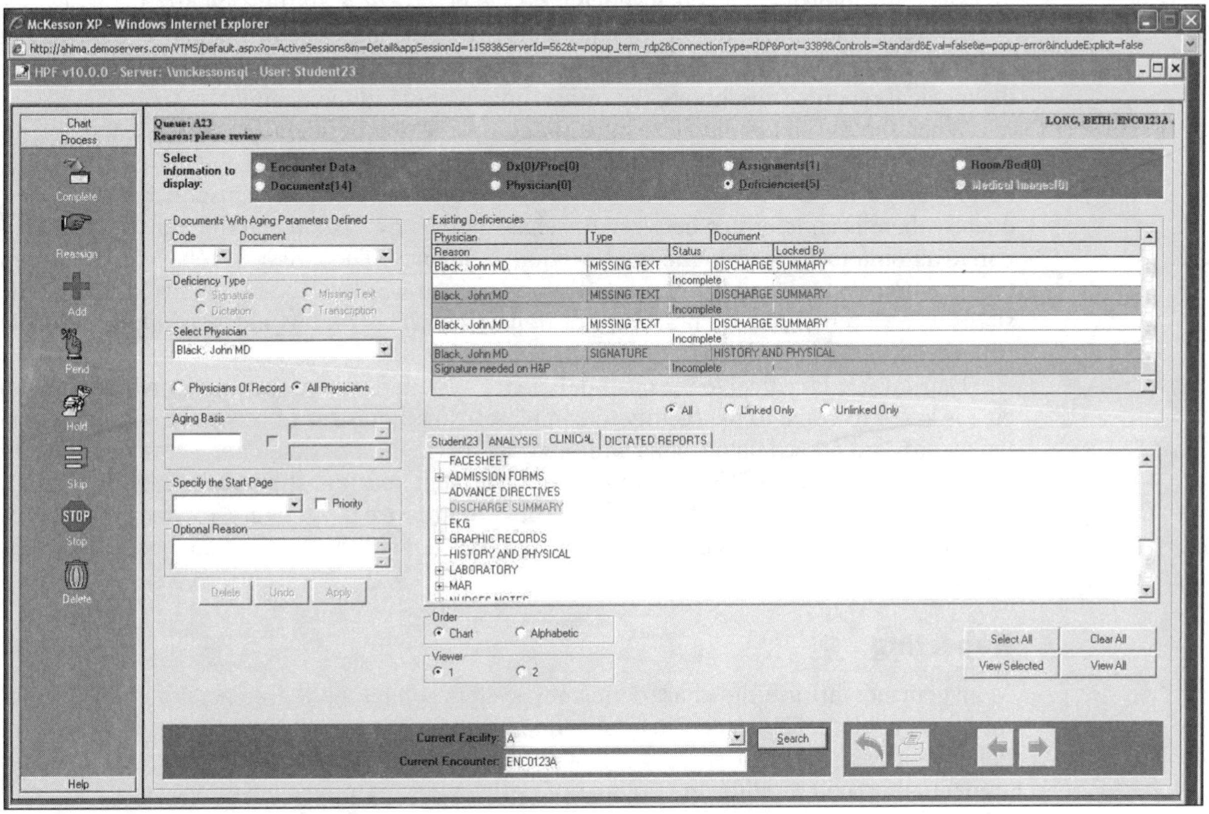

Source: McKesson Horizon Patient Folder

Functionality

The chart deficiency system is utilized by both staff and management. The chart deficiency system is used by staff to record what deficiencies a physician, or other clinician, has on specific records. When these deficiencies are completed by the physician, the chart deficiency system is updated to reflect the change. The chart deficiency system will identify the incomplete records by physician so the physician can be notified for completion. Common data elements include:

- Patient name
- Discharge date
- Physician needing to complete deficiency
- Type of document with deficiency (for example, history and physical examination, discharge summary, or progress note)
- Type of deficiency (for example, sign or dictate)
- Date of surgery
- Comments
- Date physician last worked on records

When a patient is discharged from the hospital, the medical record is automatically reviewed for deficiencies. When a deficiency is identified, the analyst is generally able to retrieve basic demographic information of the patient from the chart deficiency system. The analyst then enters other pertinent information such as discharge date, physician, document type, type of deficiency, date of surgery, and any other information needed into the system. In a paper environment, sticky tabs or flags are frequently posted on the medical record to indicate to the physician where a signature is needed. In an electronic environment, a work queue would route the deficiencies automatically to the assigned physician. The physician could then automatically complete all needed deficiencies. The physician could complete the medical records from home, the office, or anywhere in the hospital.

When the physician dictates, signs, or completes the deficiency, the analyst is able to delete or update the status of the deficiency. An example of updating the deficiency would be to change the deficiency from dictated to transcribe or from transcribe to sign. Frequently there is an interface between the chart deficiency system and the transcription system to automatically update the transcription deficiency. There may also be a link between the dictation system, and the chart deficiency system would also automatically update the status when a report had been dictated or transcribed. This link would also help staff locate paper records for completion.

Data quality is critical to the chart deficiency system. Instances can occur where a physician is asked to come to the facility to complete a small number of records and upon arrival the records are not available. This will be upsetting to the physician and show poor quality in the use of the system. Records inappropriately entered into the system can also have a negative impact on Joint Commission statistics. To improve data quality, routine audits of the records should be conducted to ensure that records are still incomplete and available to the physician.

Reporting

Management staff use the chart deficiency system to age the deficiencies for Joint Commission tracking. The system can generate a report listing all physicians suspended for delinquent medical records, track when physicians are suspended for use in medical staff credentialing, and monitor the volume of deficiencies by physician and service. A list of all records in the system can be printed out for use in auditing the quality of the data in the system (3M 2009).

The chart deficiency system also has customizable letters. These letters can be used for many purpose such as notifying physicians that they have a deadline to complete records, been suspended for delinquent medical records (or other penalty for noncompliance with medical staff rules and regulations), or to thank physicians for completing medical record(s).

Transcription

Physicians and other appropriate clinical staff dictate into the facility's dictation system. The transcriptionist then types the actual report using the **transcription system**. The transcription system is used by the transcriptionist to type the various documents dictated by the physicians. The transcription system should be interfaced with the hospital information system so that the patient name, medical record, and date of service are already populated within the system.

Functionality

The transcription system works much like any word processor in that the transcriptionist is able to type, edit, and spell-check a document, but there are many features in the transcription systems that are not found in the word processor. Basic information is collected about every document. This information can include:

- Patient name

- Medical record number

- Date of admission

- Date of discharge

- Date of surgery

- Dictating physician

- Date of dictation

- Date of transcription

- Report type

- Name of transcriptionist

The transcription system typically has user-defined templates for each report type. The template prevents the transcriptionist from having to type headings (such as history of present illness or review of systems) every time a history and physical examination is dictated. The system typically uses expanders, which may also be called macros. **Expanders** allow transcriptionists to type an acronym such as "CHF" and the full phrase "congestive heart failure" will automatically be spelled out, thus saving keystrokes and time. The expanders can typically be controlled by the facility (3M 2009).

The spell-checking capabilities are able to handle both the English language as well as medical terminology. Medical terminology includes not only terms such as esophagogastroduodenoscopy but surgical instruments, medications, and other terms specific to healthcare.

In the event of a request or error, the document may need to be retrieved. The transcription system allows the transcriptionist to search for the document by patient name, medical record number, date of dictation, dictator, document type, document number, and transcriptionist.

The transcription software products in use today are designed to work seamlessly with dictation systems and voice recognition to promote efficiency in the entire process. These products also are designed for transcriptionists to work from home if desired (Nuance Communications, Inc. 2009).

Figure 7.10 shows a screen from Nuance's transcription software displaying the available jobs waiting for the user to transcribe.

Figure 7.10.   Nuance's transcription software, EXText Editor

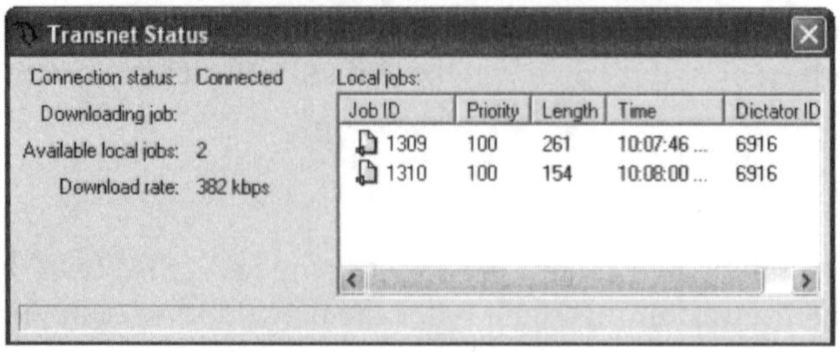

Source: Nuance

Reporting

Once a document is transcribed, the transcription system is able to route reports to a departmental printer, fax, or other location. The routing of the report is based on settings established in the system. This routing enables reports to reach the physician and/or patient care area faster. The report may also be available in the electronic health record.

The transcription system is used by management for many purposes. One purpose is to track productivity, which is critical because transcriptionists usually are paid based on it. Another purpose would be for incentive pay. Many systems can calculate incentive pay automatically based on criteria established by the facility. Management may also use reports to monitor overall volume by report type to help identify trends and needs.

Data Quality Indicator

The **data quality indicator system** is an abstracting system that records information about the patient and the care provided to the patient. This software may be used by the HIM department or other department performing this function. HIM staff or nurses are the typical users of the data quality indicator system, and it is included in this chapter because of its limited usage. Users in the HIM department may be the coders or a separate group of employees with the necessary skills and qualifications to read, understand, and abstract information from the medical record into the quality indicator system. Abstracting and reporting are two critical aspects of the quality indicator systems. Information on the patient's care is entered into the system to be in the facility quality improvement program. The data is then turned into information to evaluate the quality of care provided to the patient, patient safety, utilization review, and more. For example, the hospital could use information from the system in the physician credentialing process. Problem areas would be identified and resources assigned in order to investigate and resolve the quality problems (Cardinal Health, Inc. 2009).

Functionality

The system may be interfaced to the hospital information system to obtain demographic information. Data abstracting is the key functionality to the quality indicator monitoring system. Examples of data collected would include:

- Units of blood
- Nosocomial infections
- Physician
- Nursing unit
- Apgar score

The information abstracted can be used in reports and can be trended. The information can then be used to make changes in how care is provided. Some data would be collected on all patients. Other fields required for data entry may change based on data entered previously. For example, the user may be required to enter estimated blood loss for a surgical patient, but would not be asked for this information when abstracting medical patient data. Another example would be to enter the Apgar score of a newborn, but not of other patients.

Some of the data in the data quality indicator system may be downloaded from other systems used in the facility, saving time and improving data quality. These systems could be the hospital information system with the demographic information, the laboratory information system with the laboratory results, and other clinical systems.

Reporting

Because the data from this system will be used in performance improvement, reporting is a key part of this system. Reporting must be flexible so that the user is able to create the report needed for the study being conducted. The reports will include statistics and graphs to facilitate the identification of trends. Reports may include monitoring facility infection rate, number of deaths by physician, blood incompatibility, surgical errors, maternal deaths, and outcomes, for example.

Dictation System

The **dictation system** is used by physicians to dictate various medical reports such as the operative report, history and physician, and the discharge summary. The dictation system is included in this chapter because of the limited use of the system outside of the HIM department. The physician dictates history and physical examinations, discharge summaries, radiology reports, autopsy reports, catheterization reports, and other designated reports into the dictation system. Most systems allow physicians to use dedicated dictation units or any telephone. The dictation is typically transcribed by a transcriptionist, but if the facility utilizes voice recognition, then the system would be used by an editor rather than a transcriptionist. The transcriptionist utilizes the transcription system to type the document. A document editor would use the appropriate software to correct any errors that the system made in the translation of voice to text. Please see voice recognition in Chapter 11 for additional information.

Functionality

When dictating the report, the physician is expected to enter the patient's medical record number or encounter number as well as the document type. The physician also may indicate that the dictation should be transcribed immediately. The date and time of dictation is automatically captured by the system. The transcriptionists utilize the dictation system to listen to the dictation for transcription. The dictation system will route priority reports to the transcriptionists ahead of other dictated reports in the work queue. Priority status may be assigned to the report by the physician because of patient transfer or other reasons. HIM managers use the dictation system to route dictated reports to the various transcriptionists. For example, the transcription supervisor may need to assign another transcriptionist to type history and physical examination information to meet turnaround time. The HIM manager also uses the system to monitor backlogs and trends on volume.

Figure 7.11 shows Nuance EXText's Transcription Menu after a user has logged in.

Reporting

The key reporting focus is on workload. The system is able to track the volume of work dictated and how much is remaining to be transcribed.

Figure 7.11.   Nuance's dictation system, EXText, showing the Transcription Menu

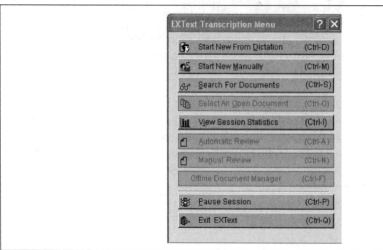

Source: Nuance

Check Your Understanding 7.3

1. Which system would tell a physician that she needs to sign an operation report?

   A. Dictation
   B. Chart locator
   C. Chart deficiency
   D. Quality indicator monitoring

2. A physician speaks into a phone and gives a summary of the patient's care, which is later transcribed. What type of system is the physician using?

   A. Dictation
   B. Chart locator
   C. Chart deficiency
   D. Quality indicator monitoring

3. I am entering the number of units of blood that a patient received during the recent hospitalization. I must be using the:

   A. dictation
   B. chart locator
   C. chart deficiency
   D. quality indicator monitoring

4. I am entering the Apgar score. I must be using the:

   A. birth certificate software
   B. chart locator
   C. chart deficiency
   D. quality indicator monitoring

5. I type out the abbreviation EGD and the term esophagogastroduodenoscopy is spelled out. I am using a(n)

   A. abstract
   B. bar code
   C. expander
   D. template

References

3M. 2009. What we do: Health information management. http://solutions.3m.com/wps/portal/3M/en_US/3M_Health_Information_Systems/HIS/What_We_Do/Health_Info_Management/.

American College of Surgeons. 2009. National Trauma Data Bank (NTDB). http://www.facs.org/trauma/ntdb.html.

Brookins Communications, Inc. 2009. Birthtype™ Electronic Birth Registration Software. http://www.birthtype.com/.

Cardinal Health, Inc. 2009. MediQual's Atlas. http://mediqual.com/products/atlas.asp.

Center for Disease Control and Prevention. (n.d.). *Program Manual: National Program of Cancer Registries Version 1.0*. http://cdc.gov/cancer/NPCR/npcrpdfs/program_manual.pdf.

Center for Disease Control and Prevention. 2009. Registry Plus™ Software Programs for Cancer Registries. http://www.cdc.gov/cancer/npcr/tools/registryplus/.

Impac Medical Systems, Inc. 2009. Hospital Registry. http://www.impac.com/productsNEW/cancer-registry/hospital-registry.html.

Lancet Technology, Inc. 2005. TraumaOne. http://lancettechnology.com/products/traumaone.shtml.

McKesson Corp. 2009. Paragon Release of Information. http://www.mckesson.com/en_us/McKesson.com/For+Healthcare+Providers/Hospitals/Community+Hospital+Solutions/Paragon+Modules/Paragon+Release+of+Information.html.

National Center for Health Statistics. U.S. Standard Certificate of Live Birth, revised November 2003. www.cdc.gov/nchs/data/dvs/birth11-03final-ACC.pdf

Nuance Communications, Inc. 2009. Dictaphone Enterprise Express. http://www.nuance.com/dictaphone/products/enterpriseexpress/voicesystem.asp.

Trauma.org. 2009. Scoring Systems. http://trauma.org/index.php/main/category/C16.

Chapter 8
Administrative Information Systems

Objectives

- Determine what administrative information system is needed for a particular task.

- Differentiate between administrative information systems.

- Differentiate between a decision support system and an executive information system.

- Describe how administrative systems impact health information management practices.

Key Terms

Administrative information
    systems
Admission, discharge, transfer
    (ADT)
Chargemaster
Decision support system
Deterministic algorithm
Enterprise master patient index
    (EMPI)

Executive information system
    (EIS)
Financial information system
Hospital information system
Human resources information
    system
Materials management
    information system
Master patient index (MPI)

Patient registration
Practice management system
Probabilistic algorithm
Registration-Admission,
    discharge, transfer (R-ADT)
Revenue cycle
Rules-based algorithm
Scheduling system

Administrative systems were the first information systems to be utilized in healthcare. Their purpose is to manage the business of healthcare. The data collected in **administrative information systems** are mainly financial or administrative in nature, rather than clinical. The administrative information systems perform many tasks throughout the organizations. Some administrative systems, such as the **master patient index**, are utilized by many departments and employees throughout the organization. Others, like the **decision support system**, are utilized by a select group of authorized users. The **hospital information system** is the major system utilized by a healthcare facility. This system is made up of many administrative systems such as the **financial information system** and the master patient index. The major administrative information systems are listed and summarized below. Each of these components will be discussed separately.

- Financial information systems monitor and control the financial aspects of the healthcare facility.

- Human resources information systems track and manage people within the organization.

- Decision support systems assist management in making decisions.

- The master patient index provides a permanent record of patients treated at the facility.

- **Patient registration** systems collect information on patients receiving treatment.

- **Scheduling systems** allow the facility to make efficient use of resources such as operating rooms.

- **Practice management systems** combine a number of applications required to manage a physician practice.

- **Materials management information systems** manage the supplies and equipment within the facility.

- Facilities management systems allows physical plant operations to control the automated systems within the facility for patient safety and comfort—that is, heating and air systems, automated key control, and preventive maintenance on computerized systems on many software applications used in the facility.

Financial Information System

The financial information system is critical to the fiscal health of the facility. The facility must receive accurate financial information in a timely manner to monitor and manage the finances of the facility. This information can be used to plan and control the expenses of the day-to-day operations as well as long-term investments.

The management of the accounts receivable and the accounts payable on a daily basis by the facility is known as the **revenue cycle**. The revenue cycle is a very complex process involving several departments and many employees who perform tasks of reviewing services provided for claims submitted as well as reviewing outstanding claims, returned claims, denials, missing accounts, bill holds, and other claims involving the revenue of the facility (Johns 2007, 315). Many HIM professionals are involved in working with the revenue cycle in their facilities and some work for vendors who specialize in the area of revenue cycle management and cleanup as a business.

Functionality

The financial information includes functions related to:

- Patient accounting
- Accounts receivable

- Accounts payable

- General ledger

- Investment management

- Contract management

- Payroll

The patient accounting module collects all of the charges related to patient care. Some charges, such as the patient's room charge, are automatically generated but others are created when nurses, respiratory therapists, and other staff enter charge information either through the financial information system or a clinical information system. These charges come from the chargemaster. The **chargemaster** (see figure 8.1) automates the coding process for routine procedures such as laboratory tests and radiology examinations. Attached to each of these codes is the charge associated with the service. This amount and other charges recorded are used to determine the amount of money charged to the patient's account. The system then generates the bill and submits it to the third-party payer. The patient accounting system also generates the discharged not final billed report, which lists the patient accounts that have not been billed.

Updating the chargemaster codes is of utmost importance. These codes, such as the relative point value and user area, must be updated annually and sent to each facility to be uploaded into their computer system's chargemaster software application. HIM professionals must be aware of these coding updates and ensure that their respective chargemaster updates are completed annually by the facility's information systems (IS) department when the software is received. Otherwise, charges billed can mean a loss of revenue to the facility. Once the updates are performed on schedule, the facility is reimbursed the amount owed them for their particular geographic region of the country.

Accounts payable records what the facility owes to others. This amount may be a refund to a patient or an insurance company, or it may be payment to companies that provide supplies and equipment to the hospital.

The general ledger records debits and credits to the various accounts managed by the financial information system. All of the financial transactions are recorded for the time frame. These transactions include receipt of payment, payroll, and disbursements.

Figure 8.1.   Example of Chargemaster screen showing basic data fields

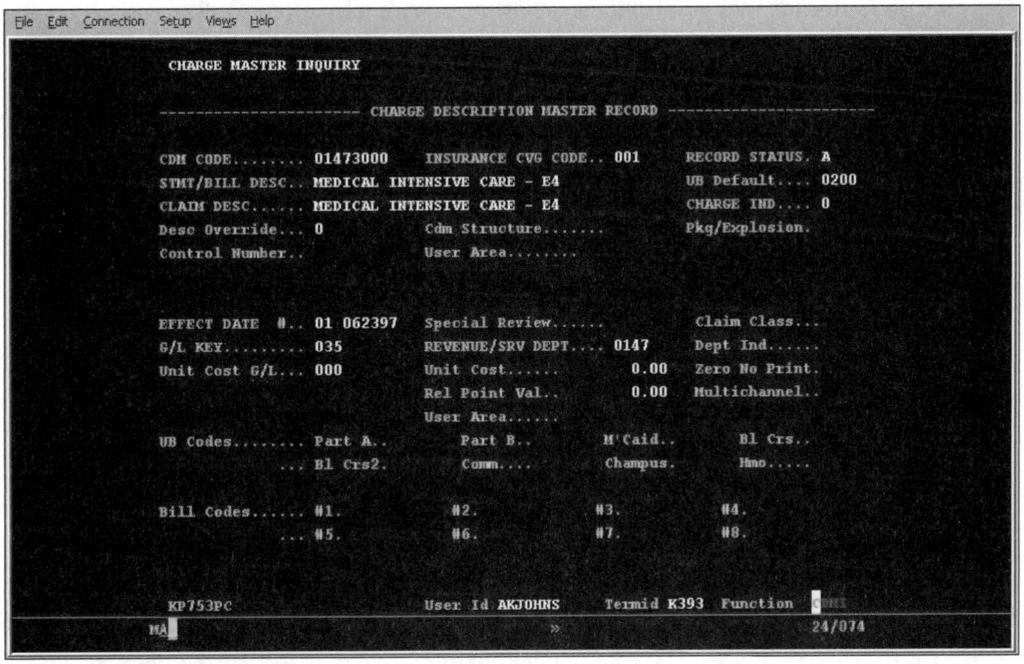

Source: Healthquest system by McKesson

Healthcare facilities invest their excess cash. The investment management features of the financial information system track the investment accounts and analyze the return on the investments. Changes to the investment portfolio can be made according to the findings.

Healthcare facilities sign many contracts, including those with software vendors, insurance companies, businesses that purchase healthcare services, and other companies. The contract management portion of the financial information system can track particulars such as who the contract is with and expiration dates. The information that comes from the financial information system is used to negotiate managed care contracts and monitor the impact of the contract based on information such as the number of patients, amount of revenue, cost of care, and whether or not the facility is making money on the contract.

The last module of the financial information system to be discussed is the payroll functions. Payroll functions include tracking employees, salaries, taxes to be deducted, taxes to be paid, heath insurance deductions, life insurance deductions, and direct deposits. The payroll functions would need to track salary increases and changes in deduction from one year to another.

The information is also used to generate financial reports that are needed by the facility's management staff. The financial information also provides the balance sheet, statement of revenue and expense, and cost reports and illustrates cash flow. These financial reports can assist in the pricing of services rendered, control inventory, analyses of productivity of staff, and other purposes.

Impact on HIM

The coding staff will populate the diagnosis and procedure codes either through direct data entry or from an interface to the encoder. The encoder is discussed in chapter 7. HIM professionals should also be involved in the development and management of the chargemaster. The codes and charges would have to be updated at least annually. Services would be added and subtracted as the services provided by the facility change.

Human Resources Information System

A healthcare facility requires many staff members in order to operate. Many operate 24 hours a day, 7 days a week. Because of staffing requirements, payroll expenses make up a large part of the operating budget. This large outlay of cash demands strong management of the human resources department within the organization.

Functionality

The **human resources information system (HRIS)** tracks employees within the organization. This tracking includes promotions, transfers, performance appraisal due dates, and absenteeism, for example. The individual data elements collected include:

- Employee name
- Employee number
- Department
- Title
- Salary
- Benefit information
- Hire date
- Results of performance appraisal
- Previous titles

- Termination date
- Certifications
- Disciplinary actions
- Eligibility for rehire

These and other data are used to create a permanent record for the healthcare facility. This information is used to manage staff while employed and to verify that employees worked at the facility. The HRIS data will track the benefits that an employee has selected, such as family healthcare plan, dental insurance, long-term disability insurance, or retirement. The HRIS will be able to track the utilization of staff by department, job title, or other grouping. The human resources staff would have access to the records of all employees, whereas the various department directors should have access only to those employees reporting to that director. Figure 8.2 shows a sample timecard in the Kronos Workforce Central program.

Department managers may use an automated timekeeping system for their employees when staff clock in and out. This system tracks the hours per week worked by pay period. Human resources as well as management can then use the system to determine sick time, vacation time, and benefit time per employee.

The HRIS can also assist with the hiring process. For example, the HRIS can track resumés and applications submitted by potential employees. The system can compare the skills and education of the candidate with those of the other applicants, thus speeding up the hiring process.

Reporting is important in the HRIS. Reporting features can be used to track items such as turnover rate, open positions, labor costs, benefits, budget, or overtime. The facility may also track employee satisfaction and report on the findings of the surveys (Glandon et al. 2008). Many facilities offer in-house educational opportunities to employees and attendance at these events is tracked within the HRIS software. These might include optional educational seminars to advance managers with training and development skills. Other

Figure 8.2.   Example of human resources information system screen—TimeKeeper for use by department managers

Date	Pay Code	Amount	In	Transfer	Out	In	Transfer	Out	Shift	Daily	Cum...
Sun 3/08			10:16AM		5:39PM				7.0	7.0	7.0
Mon 3/09			8:04AM		5:40PM				9.25	9.25	16.25
Tue 3/10			8:21AM		5:11PM				8.5	8.5	24.75
Wed 3/11			8:25AM		5:02PM				8.0	8.0	32.75
Thu 3/12			8:50AM		4:49PM				7.5	7.5	40.25
Fri 3/13			7:48AM		3:43PM				7.5	7.5	47.75
Sat 3/14											47.75
Sun 3/15											47.75
Mon 3/16			8:15AM		1:27PM	2:20PM		5:41PM	8.5	8.5	56.25
Tue 3/17			8:04AM		5:17PM				8.75	8.75	65.0
Wed 3/18			7:41AM		5:41PM				9.5	9.5	74.5
Thu 3/19			8:05AM		4:53PM				8.5	8.5	83.0
Fri 3/20			9:01AM		5:49PM				8.25	8.25	91.25
Sat 3/21											91.25

Account	Pay Code	Amount
...001000348/04/0000/0000/00000000/0	Diff10	7.0
...001000348/04/0000/0000/00000000/0	OT	11.25
...001000348/04/0000/0000/00000000/0	Grand Total	91.25
...001000348/04/0000/0000/00000000/0	REG	80.0

Source: Kronos Workforce Central by Kronos

workshops might include optional cardiopulmonary resuscitation (CPR) training classes for staff. The HRIS software may also track mandated classes for all employees that require annual attendance such as fire and safety classes, OSHA standards, HIPAA training, etc. Department directors can then easily use the reporting function to assess the attendance within their own departments as well as results of these educational classes by their employees annually.

Impact on HIM

HIM department staff do not use the HRIS; however, the HIM director may use HRIS to generate reports, perform queries, review applications, and perform other tasks related to the HIM department staff.

Check Your Understanding 8.1

1. Which administrative system tracks investments?

   A. Financial information system
   B. Human resources information system
   C. Scheduling system
   D. Master patient index

2. Which component of the financial information system tracks the amount of money that the facility owes a vendor?

   A. Patient accounting
   B. Account payable
   C. Account receivable
   D. General ledger

3. Which of the following tasks is one for which the HIM professional uses the financial information system?

   A. Manage chargemaster
   B. Manage account receivable
   C. Manage investment
   D. Manage general ledger

4. Which of the following statements is true?

   A. The HRIS is available to all employees of the facility
   B. The HRIS does not track resumés and applications
   C. The HRIS stores data only for the period of time that an individual is employed at the facility
   D. The HRIS can track turnover and open positions

5. Which of the following data elements would be found in an administrative information system?

   A. History of present illness
   B. Charge for complete blood count
   C. Laboratory test results
   D. Vital signs

Decision Support System

The decision support system (DSS) takes data collected by the healthcare facility, turns them into information, and uses this information to make decisions about the healthcare facility (Hebda et al. 2005).

Functionality

LaTour and Eichenwald Maki (2006) define the DSS as "a computer-based system that gathers data from a variety of sources and assists in providing structure to the data by using various analytical models and visual tools in order to facilitate and improve the ultimate outcome in decision-making tasks associated with non-routine and non-repetitive problems" (LaTour and Eichenwald Maki 2006, 920). Note the requirement for non-routine and non-repetitive problems. This means that the DSS is not used to schedule staff, determine inventory levels, or perform other routine decisions, but rather to make decisions about whether to open a new women's health center or a geriatric center. Other decisions that may be candidates for the DSS are whether or not to add new examination rooms in the emergency department or to open new operating rooms. To make these decisions, the DSS utilizes the data in the data repositories and data warehouses described in chapter 4. The DSS use models to run analyses such as "what if" to determine what would happen if certain decisions were made or to forecast the future.

Executive Information System

The **executive information system (EIS)** is a type of decision support system that is designed to be used by healthcare administrators. As such, it must be easy to use and have access to a wide range of data. With the EIS, a lot of graphs and charts generally are used as part of the results. Advantages of the EIS include:

- Improved competitiveness of the organization

- Knowledge of the organization

- Information is available to authorized users throughout the organization

- Assistance in making strategic decisions about the facility

The EIS assists the administrator and other top administration staff in making quick decisions. To generate the data manually that the EIS generates with a few clicks of the mouse would take days, if it is possible at all. Figures 8.3 and 8.4 show examples of various data displayed in the EIS dashboard.

A dashboard report gives administration data to make intelligent decisions for the future. In this example, administration can view the dashboard report and see from the diagnostic related groups (DRGs) and the length of stay (LOS) what the facility was actually reimbursed and what it actually cost the facility. The last columns give administration an idea of the profit that was expected versus the actual profit made. This type of report is useful to administration in planning for the future to make decisions. Would this be a good idea with the balance as given on this report to have enough cash flow to add on to the vascular laboratory? If you were the administrator, what would you decide based on this data?

Figure 8.4 shows an example of an EIS dashboard report. Administration can view detailed data by types of graphs that are selected, depending on the software used. For this example, a pie chart is used.

Administration can easily view the pie chart of these ten physicians on this DRG example and see that the physician highlighted by the slice that is 3-D is not one of the larger problems in comparison. There are two other slices or physicians with a larger percentage of the pie (larger slices) that represent a greater problem. Administration must focus priority on the largest percentage first and then the second-largest percentage next, and so on. The data from this DSS planning tool is a visual representation to administration of where the problem is greatest and where the priority should be focused.

Impact on HIM

The HIM department is not a user of the DSS.

Figure 8.3.   Example of EIS dashboard: DSS showing profit actual vs. profit expected

Date Range: January 2000
Patient Type Selection: IN -
Additional Criteria: InsGroup   MC; BC; MD

Year	IN DIS	OUT	Total LOS	Average LOS	Charges	Average Charges	Reimb Actual	Total Cost	Profit Actual %	Profit Expected	Balance
Jan 99	307	0	1Total LOS	5.6	$1,556,402	$5,070	$967,127	$178,917	81.50%	$1,122,910	$9,460
Jan 00	379	0	5599	14.8	$2,350,780	$6,203	$1,520,057	$1,604,684	-5.28%	$419,750	$20,508

Drg	IN DIS	OUT	Total LOS	Average LOS	Charges	Average Charges	Reimb Actual	Total Cost	Profit Actual %	Profit Expected	Balance
5	1	0	2	2.0	$6,486	$6,486	$5,519	$4,954	10.23%	$65	$00
12	2	0	2003	1001.5	$149,279	$74,639	$24,273	$83,478	-70.93%	-$58,936	$224
14	2	0	10	5.0	$15,139	$7,570	$9,122	$9,694	-5.90%	$5,445	$00
15	1	0	2	2.0	$3,194	$3,194	$2,833	$1,916	32.35%	$1,278	$00
20	2	0	13	6.5	$20,355	$10,177	$9,988	$11,721	-14.79%	$5,617	$00
24	1	0	6	6.0	$8,583	$8,583	$3,507	$6,507	-46.12%	$2,076	$00
25	2	0	5	2.5	$7,073	$3,536	$4,616	$6,009	-23.18%	$1,064	$00
53	1	0	3	3.0	$4,620	$4,620	$4,749	$4,167	12.25%	$453	$00
78	1	0	10	10.0	$13,060	$13,060	$5,305	$7,612	-30.31%	$5,448	$00
79	2	0	11	5.5	$15,742	$7,871	$12,594	$11,440	9.16%	$4,302	$00
87	4	0	40	10.0	$52,961	$13,240	$20,917	$26,710	-21.69%	$26,210	$00
88	21	0	80	3.8	$93,924	$4,473	$66,606	$68,860	-3.28%	$21,705	$773
89	37	0	131	3.5	$156,914	$4,241	$117,994	$103,907	11.93%	$33,825	$2,916
90	4	0	7	1.8	$8,414	$2,103	$8,849	$5,569	37.06%	$2,845	$00
91	2	0	7	3.5	$6,600	$3,300	$3,201	$5,902	-45.76%	$575	$00
96	4	0	13	3.3	$13,647	$3,412	$9,091	$10,255	-11.35%	$1,182	$00
97	2	0	4	2.0	$4,380	$2,190	$3,820	$2,351	38.45%	$2,024	$00
98	1	0	7	7.0	$6,307	$6,307	$1,226	$5,177	-76.32%	$1,129	$00
99	1	0	2	2.0	$1,668	$1,668	$2,611	$00	0.00%	$1,668	$00
116	1	0	3	3.0	$22,498	$22,498	$9,405	$5,812	38.20%	$15,882	$00
121	13	0	59	4.5	$80,804	$6,216	$61,200	$54,828	10.41%	$21,456	$04
122	2	0	5	2.5	$10,969	$5,484	$4,867	$7,463	-34.79%	$3,506	$00
127	19	0	152	8.0	$106,854	$5,624	$84,482	$74,232	12.13%	$32,622	$02

EXTRACRANIAL VASCULAR PROCEDURES   110 Drgs

Source: Copyright © AHIMA 2010. All rights reserved.

Figure 8.4.   Example of EIS dashboard: DSS showing comparison of 10 physicians on DRG 127 with pie chart

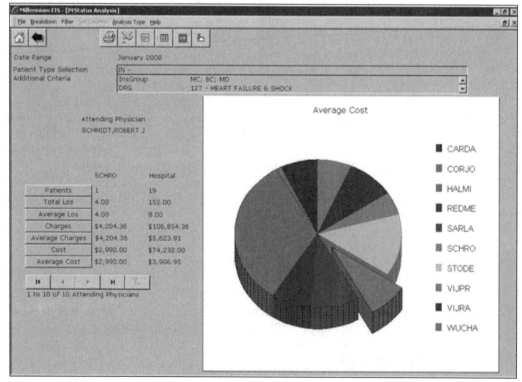

Source: Copyright © AHIMA 2010. All rights reserved.

Master Patient Index

The master patient index (MPI), also known as the master person index, is part of the hospital information system. The MPI identifies every patient who has been admitted to the facility, and it is the key to locating all patient records. The MPI lists patient names and health record numbers and cross references them. An MPI is to be kept permanently as mandated by legal statutes. The information contained within the MPI was originally limited to demographics that could readily distinguish between any two patients as not having the same record. These data include both demographic data and visit-specific information. The demographic information will include data such as the patient name. The visit information will include items such as discharge date. The data contained in the MPI include (AHIMA MPI Task Force 1997):

- Last name
- First name
- Middle initial
- Social security number
- Medical record number
- Admission date
- Discharge date
- Physician
- Patient type (inpatient, outpatient, emergency department, and others)
- Date of birth
- Former names
- Billing number
- Gender
- Race
- Emergency contact
- Discharge disposition
- Marital status

Other data may be collected depending on the needs of the facility.

The example master patient index screen in figure 8.5 shows the available fields of data that must be collected and entered into the MPI by the abstractor. This person could be an admissions staff member who interviews the patient upon entering the facility at the time of the visit encounter. Once data is entered into the MPI, data is easily transferable into other screens and other systems within the software for other users.

Functionality

Information on patients can generally be retrieved using many of the previously mentioned data elements. The most commonly used are patient name and medical record number. The MPI usually has soundex capabilities, which allow the user to retrieve patients based on the sound of the name. Soundex is a phonetic-based indexing system that is easily incorporated into computer software for searching surnames that sound alike but are spelled differently. Soundex "has been adopted by the U.S. Census Bureau to organize master patient index (MPI) cards in communities with large populations of foreign-sounding names" (Green and Bowie 2005, 199). The soundex search is useful when there are multiple ways to spell a last name, such as Burger, Burgur, and Burgher.

There are times when a patient is issued one or more duplicate medical record numbers. When the duplication is identified, the MPI must have the capability to combine these

Figure 8.5.   Example master patient index of data collection screen

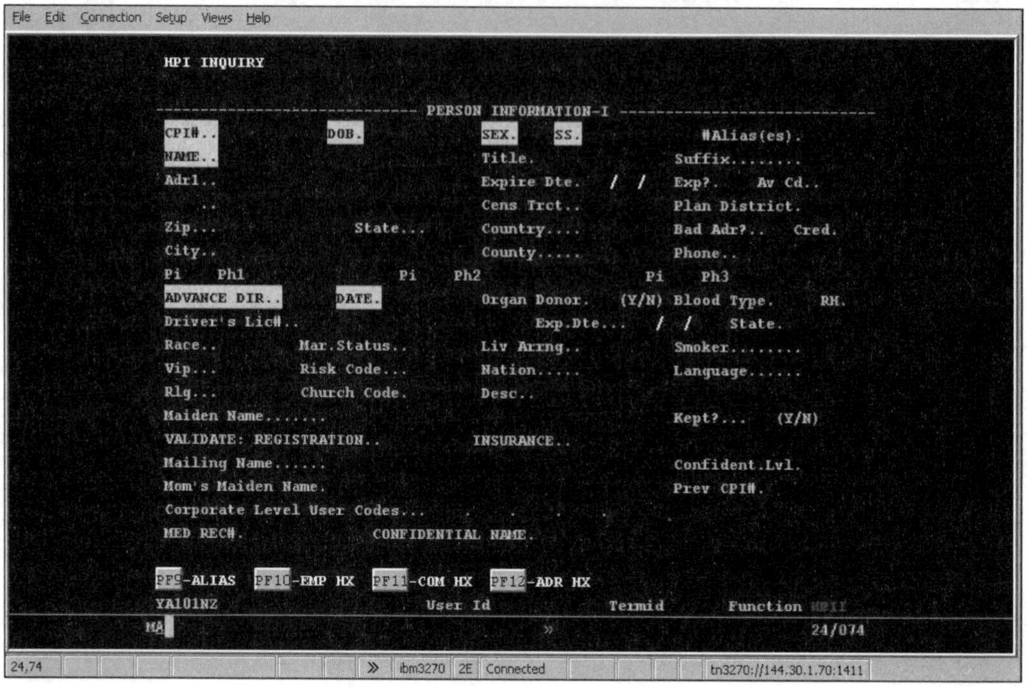

Source: Healthquest by McKesson

records under one medical record and keep record of the medical record number eliminated. The MPI must also be able to address overlays. Overlays are instances where two patients are assigned the same medical record number because of the incorrect assumption that they were the same patient. Duplicate medical record numbers and overlays cause problems with data quality and ultimately can create a quality of care risk because the patient information is either fragmented or two patients' records are intertwined.

The MPI is often hard to imagine for a novice as it is a database of every patient visit from the opening of the facility's doors. This includes inpatient, ambulatory, emergency, outpatient, and other types of visits that the facility includes within its visit types. There could be hundreds or thousands of patient visits depending on the age of the facility (when it began treating patients). To aid in a visual look of an MPI, a snapshot of a subset might include a few patients of a certain physician or those with a certain diagnosis. If these could be queried and sorted, then printed for viewing, a possible subset of an MPI might look like the example in table 8.1.

As mentioned earlier, the MPI is the data storehouse of patient information which by legal statutes must be maintained permanently. The information stored in the MPI is also vital to the administrative functions of the facility's database system. When a patient is admitted, discharged, or transferred, the **registration data of the admission, discharge, transfer (R-ADT)** application is "used to initiate or update basic demographic data, establishes and tracks the location or service of the patient, and feeds data to other systems such as billing or the laboratory" (Abdelhak et al. 2007, 163). Because the MPI and **admission, discharge, transfer (ADT)** systems are both part of the hospital information system, sophisticated algorithms can be used to help prevent duplicate medical record numbers when admitting a patient. When the user enters a patient's name and other identifying information into the ADT and there is a patient with the same or similar information, the system notifies the user. Essentially the system asks the user if the patient being admitted is one of the patients listed. If so, duplication of the medical record number has been avoided. Not only can these algorithms identify exact matches based on name, social security number, and other identifying information, but they can identify patients whose information is almost identical. Maybe the social security number or date of birth is one character off. Maybe the patient's last name has changed because of marriage or divorce since the last visit. The sophisticated algorithms

Table 8.1.   Subset of a master patient index table

MRN	Last Name	First Name	Middle Name		DOB	Payment Type	Zip Code
096543	Jones	Georgia	Louise		11/21/1957	Self	29425
065432	Lexington	Milton	Robert		08/12/2000	Private	29425
467345	Lovingood	Jill	Karen		10/14/1992	Medicaid	29401
467345	Martin	Chloe	Mary		05/30/1978	Private	29465
234719	Martin	John	Adams		06/22/1961	Private	29401
786543	Nance	Natalie	JoAnn		11/27/1922	Medicare	29464

Source: Latour and Eichenwald Maki 2010

can catch these items. Many systems utilize a ranking system to identify the amount of confidence that the system has in the match. Exact information would receive the maximum score. A potential match with almost everything identical would be a high score but not a perfect score. A potential match where very little, if anything, is a perfect match will be a low score. The type of scale varies by system but could be 1 to 10, or 0 to 100, or some other scale.

Algorithms take a variety of forms and have varying degrees of sophistication. The algorithms discussed above can be grouped into three different types utilized by the various MPI systems. These types are (AHIMA MPI Task Force 2004):

- Deterministic

- Rules-based

- Probabilistic

Deterministic algorithms look for exact matches. The algorithm looks at data elements such as name, birth date, gender, and social security number. The accuracy rate of identifying potential duplicates with this type of algorithm is only 20 to 40 percent. Another problem with deterministic algorithms is a high percentage of false matches. The deterministic algorithms, because they look for exact matches, do not identify matches with transpositions of letters or numbers, and name changes (AHIMA MPI Task Force 2004).

The **rules-based algorithms** may also be called fuzzy logic. It is the rules-based algorithms that utilize the weights described above. Rules-based algorithms may use phonetic searching in order to identify potential duplicates. With this type of algorithm, 50 to 80 percent of the potential duplicates are identified (AHIMA MPI Task Force 2004).

The most sophisticated type of algorithms are probabilistic, which have the highest rate of success in identifying potential duplicates, at 90 percent or even higher. Sophisticated mathematical formulas are used to identify the potential duplicates. It takes into consideration the frequency of the patient's name when applying the probabilities of a match. For example, Smith would be much less certain a match than Burchfield. **Probabilistic algorithms** are able to identify transpositions and name changes and can use phonetic search capabilities (AHIMA MPI Task Force 2004).

Enterprise Master Patient Index

Integrated delivery systems (IDS) typically have an **enterprise master patient index (EMPI)**. An EMPI allows all of the components of the IDS to share information about the patient. The medical record number assigned may be the same for all hospitals, ambulatory settings, and other components of the system. There may also be an enterprise medical record number with each component issuing its own medical record number to the patient. The EMPI would identify all patient visits to the IDS and the data stored would include the facility that the patient visited.

Impact on HIM

The HIM department is a key user of the MPI. The HIM staff is responsible for the data quality of the system, so they perform the various tasks to maintain quality such as combining duplicate medical records and correcting overlays, along with other data quality issues. The HIM staff also uses the MPI to:

- Look up medical record numbers
- Identify discharge dates
- Confirm that the medical record contains all patient visits
- Look up when the patient was last seen in the facility
- Merge duplicate medical record numbers
- Unmerge overlays

Although this list of activities is not long, the amount of time spent using the MPI is significant. For example, the release of information staff must look up the medical record number on every authorization to release information that comes into the department. Depending on the number of requests, this could take hours.

With computerized records, the MPI is seen as an electronic database that serves this purpose but can also perform other functions. An MPI can link to other databases within the facility. Duplicate health record numbers can easily be assigned by other departments such as admissions, clinics, and the emergency department. It is extremely important that the MPI be routinely maintained and updated for accuracy and data control.

Check Your Understanding 8.2

1. The type of algorithm that utilizes weights is called:

   A. rules-based
   B. probabilistic
   C. deterministic
   D. all-use weights

2. How would an HIM professional utilize the MPI?

   A. Admit patient
   B. Generate bill
   C. Determine when the patient was last treated at the facility
   D. Purge the data on an annual basis

3. Decision support systems are used for what types of decisions?

   A. Routine
   B. Repetitive
   C. Clinical
   D. Nonroutine

4. The system designed to be used for top-level administration is:

   A. decision support
   B. executive information system
   C. master patient index
   D. enterprise master patient index

5. The most sophisticated algorithm is:

   A. rules-based
   B. probabilistic
   C. deterministic
   D. no difference in level of sophistication

Patient Registration (Admission, Discharge, Transfer)

Patient registration systems are frequently known as ADT. This system collects data on the patient from preadmission to discharge. The data collected include (Hebda et al. 2002):

- Basic demographic information
- Insurance information
- Information about the stay

Functionality

The basic demographic information includes patient name, address, and other typical identifying information. The insurance information includes the insurance company, policy number, and group number. Information about the stay includes data such as date admitted, date discharged, attending physician, room, and service. If a patient needs multiple tests or services performed on the same day such as laboratory, physical therapy, and x-ray, the registration system should be able to schedule all of these tests with one phone call. The ADT system issues the medical record number assignment to the patient folder

The ADT system generates some key reports used by many departments within the facility. These include the daily:

- Admission list
- Discharge list
- Census report
- Transfer list
- Bed utilization reports

The facility may also generate monthly, quarterly, yearly, and ad hoc reports to show type of patient treated, number of discharges, number of admissions, occupancy rates, and other information needed.

The ADT system may also print out routine documents, such as general consent form, notice of privacy practices acknowledgment, and advance directives that the patient needs to sign. This system can also alert the provider to link patient services provided by others to aid the facility in avoiding duplicate services to patients, which improves productivity, decreases costs, and decreases chances of fraud to third-party payers (Green and Bowie 2005, 229).

Impact on HIM

Although the HIM department does not generally register patients, the HIM department utilizes the reports that come from this system. For example, the discharge list is often used to confirm that all discharged records arrive in the HIM department after discharge.

Scheduling System

Scheduling systems are used to control the use of resources throughout the organization (Hebda et al. 2002). These resources can include staff, equipment, rooms, and more. Scheduling systems may be centralized or independent. Centralized scheduling allows the scheduling of all services of the facility where one call can make multiple appointments. The independent system utilizes the scheduling features of the radiology and other systems that may be used, so calls would have to be made to more than one location to schedule multiple tests.

Functionality

Healthcare facilities need to keep expensive equipment and other resources generating revenue rather than allowing them to remain idle. The scheduling system can help with this by scheduling tests, beds, operating rooms, staff, and other resources wisely. For example, if Dr. Smith needs to perform an appendectomy on a patient, the scheduling system knows what operating rooms are available, how long the operating room will be needed, the staff required, and what equipment will be required. This scheduling of the patient and resources ensures that everything is available when needed, thus preventing unnecessary cancellation of surgeries.

To schedule a patient for admission, tests, or other services, the physician office may call the hospital or other healthcare facility to make the necessary reservations.

In a typical appointment book scheduling system (see figure 8.6), a patient appointment can be made by the month and date by clicking on the month and date that is desired for the next appointment follow-up.

The patient's name is then entered onto the timeline of the hour that the appointment time is made. Physician offices use these types of appointment books for routine patient visits in their offices. Clinics and ambulatory surgical facilities may also use these software applications. In some cases, the patient is able to log in and schedule routine tests, such as an annual mammogram.

The scheduling system can assist with many management functions. The reporting capabilities of the scheduling system can track cancellations, resource utilization, patient volume, and other topics important to management. The reservations can also be used as part of the preadmission process to collect data such as insurance information and precertifications.

Impact on HIM

The HIM department is not a user of the scheduling system.

Figure 8.6.   Example of scheduling system—Appointment Book

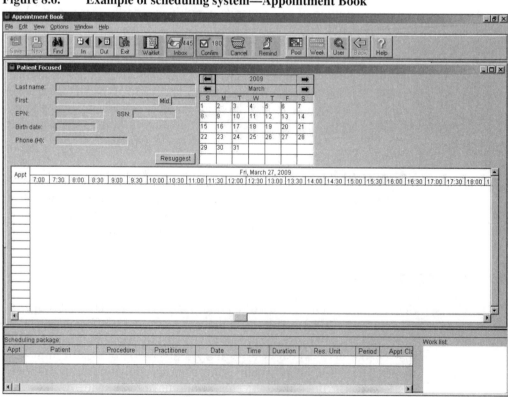

Source: Pathways Healthcare Scheduling by McKesson

Practice Management

Practice management systems are used by physician practices. With the practice management system, scheduling, patient accounting, patient collections, claims submission, appointment scheduling, human resources, and other functions all are built into a single system.

Functionality

The practice management system may be fully functional systems, or the physician practices can select from a variety of modules as needed by the practice. A sample of a physician office program is shown in figure 8.7.

    The practice management system can automate prescription renewals and other routine tasks. The practice management system may also connect to administrative information systems at the healthcare facility. Some physician practices started out with a single billing system but many offices rely on external labs and radiology satellites for diagnostic testing on patients. Physician offices now must rely on practice management systems to communicate externally with these other clinics and hospitals for patient data and billing systems (LaTour and Eichenwald Maki 2006, 216).

Figure 8.7.   Example of physician office software

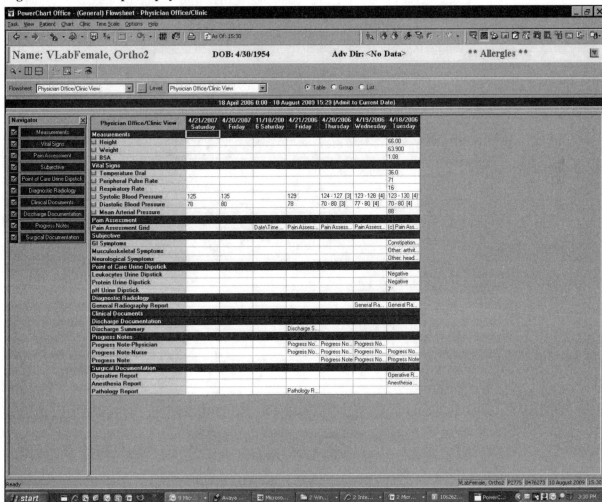

© Cerner Corporation. AHIMA has restricted permission to reproduce and distribute this copyrighted work. Further reproduction or distribution is strictly prohibited without written consent of Cerner Corporation

Impact on HIM

The HIM professional in a physician office manager role will utilize the practice management information system in many of the same ways as the financial information system, master patient index, and other administrative systems. These tasks include chargemaster management, entering codes for billing, and tracking patient visits.

Materials Management System

Healthcare facilities must manage a large amount of equipment and supplies. The typical materials management system automates the:

- Purchasing process
- Inventory control
- Menu planning
- Food service

Functionality

Requisitions for nonroutine purchases can be made, checked against budget, and approved by the proper level of authority. An example of SAP's materials management system is shown in figure 8.8.

Creating purchase requisitions online to order supplies is performed in every department. In doing so, costs are contained by keeping control of supply and demand throughout the facility (Glandon et al. 2008). The materials management system is able to automatically

Figure 8.8.   Example of materials management system—ordering supplies

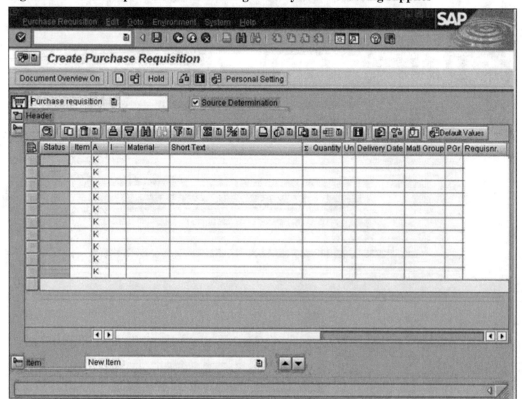

Source: SAP America, Inc.

order supplies and equipment based on predetermined thresholds for inventory supplies, allowing for just-in-time inventory controls. For example, if the healthcare facility wants to keep at least 200 bedpans in stock, the system automatically triggers an order for bedpans with the preferred vendor when the inventory drops to 250 bedpans. The materials management system can notify the financial information system when the supplies arrive so that the vendor can be paid.

The materials management system can generate barcodes to be applied toward supplies to be used and charged to the patient correctly. The use of "materials management systems include cost savings, reductions in inventory, greater efficiency, fewer lost charges, and lower labor costs" (Johns 2007, 804).

The dietary component of the system tracks the patient's dietary needs, food inventory, and costs. The system should have a variety of menus available from which to choose. The system may be designed to provide choices to the patient (Glandon et al. 2008).

Impact on HIM

The HIM department is not a typical user of the materials management system. However, purchase requisitions may be used to order office supplies for HIM departments. This is dependent on the setup of the materials management and ordering system of each facility.

Facilities Management

The physical plant will require maintenance and upgrades over the years. A facilities management system is used by a healthcare facility to manage the physical plant (Glandon et al. 2008). A facilities management system will track routine maintenance such as elevator inspections, fire extinguisher inspections, and equipment preventive maintenance. Preventive maintenance will enable the equipment to last longer, so tasks such as filter changes, inspection of electrical cables, and other tasks will save the facility money. The facilities management system will track the preventive maintenance tasks and other inspections that can be used in risk management investigations as well as inspections from outside sources, such as accreditation and state licensing. It is critical to provide "high-quality patient care and a safe, comfortable environment for the patient and their families" (Johns 2007, 804). With the focus by the Joint Commission on patient safety, the physical plant is focused on providing equipment and a healthcare environment that is vital to the well-being of the guests, staff, and ultimately the patients within the facility.

Functionality

The facilities management software can control various features of the facility such as thermostat, key cards, or automatic locks. For example, the temperature provided by the air conditioner and heating systems can be controlled, making the facility more energy efficient. Doors can be locked and unlocked automatically at a prescheduled time and employees can be given access to or denied access to restricted areas.

From time to time, major renovations or new construction is necessary. The facilities management system can track and plan the project through the use of project management tools such as Project Evaluation and Review Technique (PERT) charts and Gantt charts.

Impact on HIM

The HIM department is not a direct user of the facility management information system. Indirectly, the HIM department may use key cards for entry into locked areas or doorways or use the automated HVAC system from the physical plant. The HVAC (heating, ventilation, and air conditioning) system is set by the physical plant, usually in zones for larger buildings to run at set temperatures during various seasons to make operating costs of heating and cooling more economical.

Check Your Understanding 8.3

1. The system that can monitor menus is:

   A. facilities management
   B. materials management
   C. practice management
   D. scheduling system

2. The census report would be generated by which system?

   A. Patient registration
   B. Financial information system
   C. Master patient index
   D. Scheduling system

3. The scheduling system knows which of the following:

   A. Amount of time needed to perform colonoscopy
   B. Physicians who are up for reappointment to the medical staff
   C. Census report
   D. The latest version of the notice of privacy practice

4. The system used by the physician office is called:

   A. patient registration
   B. facilities management
   C. scheduling system
   D. practice management

5. The facilities management system controls

   A. major construction
   B. scheduling
   C. patient registration
   D. practice management

References

Abdelhak, M., S. Grostick, M.A. Hanken, and E. Jacobs. 2007. *Health Information: Management of a Strategic Resource*, 3rd ed. St. Louis, MO: Saunders/Elsevier

AHIMA MPI Task Force. 2004. Practice brief: Building an enterprise master person index. *Journal of AHIMA* 75(1):56A-D.

AHIMA MPI Task Force. 1997 (July/August). Practice brief: Master patient (person) index (MPI)—Recommended core data elements. http://library.ahima.org/xpedio/groups/public/documents/ahima/bok1_000073.hcsp?dDocName=bok1_000073.

Glandon, G.L., D.H. Smaltz, and D.J. Slovensky. 2008. *Austin and Boxerman's Information Systems for Health Management.* Chicago: Health Administration Press.

Green, M.A. and M.J. Bowie. 2005. *Essentials of Health Information Management: Principles and Practices.* Clifton Park, NY: Thomson Delmar Learning.

Hebda, T., P. Czar, and C. Mascara. 2005. *Handbook of Informatics for Nurses & Health Care Professionals.* Upper Saddle River, NJ: Pearson Prentice Hall.

Johns, M.L., ed. 2007. *Health Information Management Technology: An Applied Approach.* Chicago: AHIMA.

LaTour, K. M. and S. Eichenwald Maki, eds. 2006. *Health Information Management: Concepts, Principles, and Practice.* Chicago: AHIMA.

LaTour, K.M. and S. Eichenwald Maki, eds. 2010. *Health Information Management: Concepts, Principles, and Practice*, 3rd ed. Chicago: AHIMA.

Chapter 9
Clinical Information Systems

Objectives

- Differentiate between the various clinical information systems.

- Define clinical information system.

- Determine what clinical information system is needed to meet the needs of the facility.

- Determine what clinical information system is needed to meet the needs of the enterprise-wide organization.

Key Terms

Clinical information system (CIS)

Laboratory information system (LIS)

Nursing information system (NIS)

Pharmacy information system (PIS)

Patient monitoring system

Picture archival communication system (PACS)

Radiology information system (RIS)

Telehealth

Telesurgery

Smart cards

Clinical information systems (CIS) collect and store information related to patient care; therefore, data contained within the various systems are patient identifiable. The clinical data stored in the CIS are used to diagnose a patient's condition, make treatment decisions, monitor current condition, and manage overall care. The CIS discussed in this chapter are:

- Radiology information system (RIS)

- Laboratory information system (LIS)

- Nursing information system (NIS)

- Pharmacy information system (PIS)

- Patient monitoring system

- Telehealth

- Smart cards

Other CIS include computerized provider order entry (CPOE), electronic health record (EHR), and electronic medication administration system. These systems are discussed in chapter 10 of this text. CIS are frequently source systems for the EHR as they populate the database that serves as the foundation for the EHR.

Demographic information is collected in the hospital information system, which is an administrative information system. The demographic information is passed on to the CIS, eliminating the need for duplicate data entry, which saves time and improves the quality of the data. Some of the data elements generally passed to the CIS include:

- Last name

- First name

- Middle initial

- Date of birth

- Medical record number

- Social security number

The system may be designed so that any changes to demographic information in the CIS are fed back to the hospital information system to keep data in all systems consistent. Figures 9.1 and 9.2 illustrate communication between systems. Clinical data may be stored in a data warehouse or clinical data repository, as discussed in Chapter 4.

Clinical information systems are used to support patient care throughout the facility in many areas. The information provided within the system offers healthcare providers timely access to data, complete data regarding the patient, and a comprehensive view of the care given to the patient both in the past and during the current stay (Johns 2007, 801).

Radiology Information System

A **radiology information system (RIS)** is used to collect, store, and provide information on radiological tests such as ultrasound, magnetic resonance imaging, and positron emission tomography. The RIS also supports other radiological procedures performed in radiology such as ultrasound-guided biopsies and upper gastrointestinal series. A RIS is designed to assist the technician by identifying the steps required to prepare for each test or procedure.

Figure 9.1.   Diagram of hospital information system feeding clinical information systems

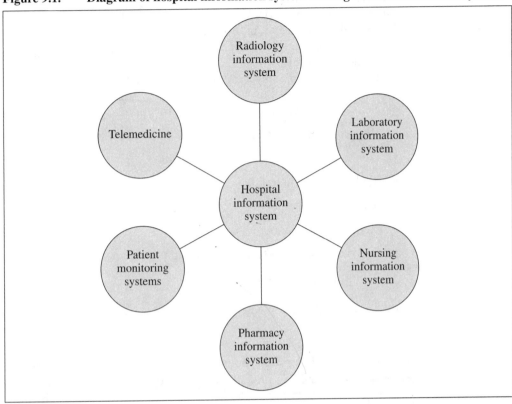

Figure 9.2.   Clinical information systems feeding EHR

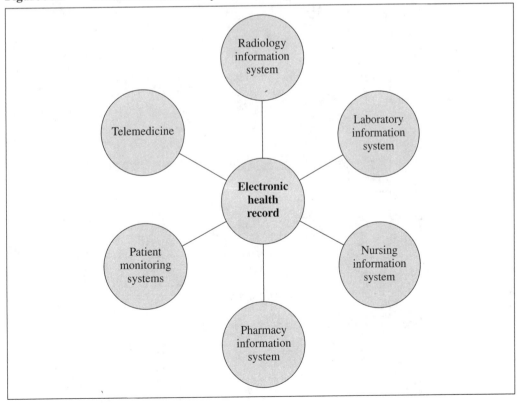

The RIS can also assist the technician with taking x-rays and other radiological examinations by controlling radiation exposure, positioning of the patient, and image quality. Ultimately, the RIS provides patients with follow-up instructions to take home after the procedure.

The RIS can be used to assist in the management of the radiology department as well as document patient care.

A RIS can perform many administrative tasks such as:

- Schedule patient examinations and procedures
- Report charges to the financial information system
- Generate reports
- Track nuclear materials
- Transcribe documents
- Retrieve test results
- Fax radiology reports to the ordering physician and other administrative tasks
- Monitor supply inventory

Figure 9.3 shows an example of an RIS.

Figure 9.3.   Radiology information system—charge adjustment/finance

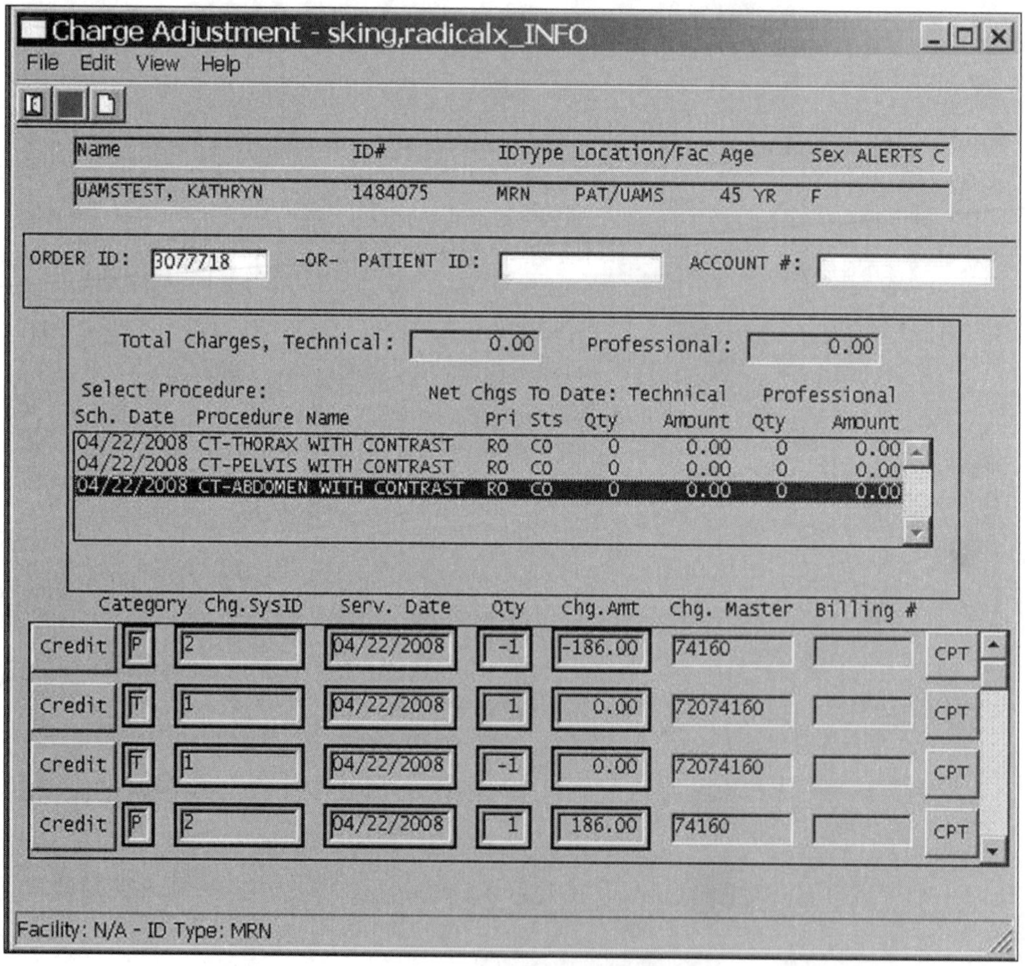

© Cerner Corporation. AHIMA has restricted permission to reproduce and distribute this copyrighted work. Further reproduction or distribution is strictly prohibited without written consent of Cerner Corporation.

Some of the reports generated by the RIS include number of tests performed, types of tests or procedures performed, productivity by technicians, and productivity levels for each radiologist.

Picture Archival Communication System

A RIS frequently has **picture archival communication system (PACS)** capabilities, as shown in figure 9.4. In a PACS, x-rays, magnetic resonance imaging, mammograms, and other radiological examinations are stored digitally, thus eliminating the need to store and manage the physical film. The digital image is immediately available for patient care, which is especially important in emergency department and intensive care situations. The filmless radiology department makes the facility more efficient by eliminating the need to pull and file radiology films and reports, make copies for patients, or purchase folders for storage. Eliminating these steps saves money and physical space for the facility. As such, radiology departments are able to provide improved customer service because there is no waiting for films to be pulled and copied. In addition, the PACS eliminates lost files.

The ability of these images to be viewed from any location by the radiologist and other users is called **teleradiology**. The images can even be viewed at multiple locations at the same time. A radiologist can read images from home in the middle of the night, or in the case of a rural hospital, from another city.

Figure 9.4.   **Example of picture archival communication system (PACS)**

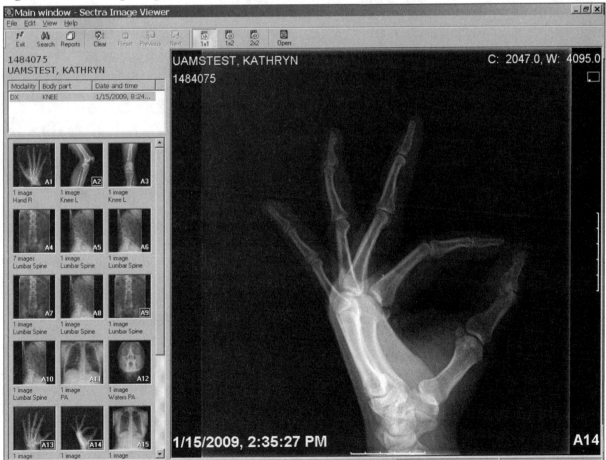

Source: Sectra System. Picture Archival Communication System (PACS). Vendor: Sectra; City: Shelton, CT. http://www.sectra.com/global/contact/medical/regional/na.html

Because of the required resolution of the image for it to be of diagnostic quality, the image must be compressed as it is transported across the network or Internet and then decompressed in a lossless manner to maintain its original form.

A PACS affords the radiologist many conveniences. He or she can easily compare previous films to current ones, zoom in on suspicious areas, enhance an image, move an image, and apply pointers to identify problem areas. Once the images are pulled up, the radiologist is able to magnify, rotate, measure, and use many other tools to view the images. The radiologist is also able to view previous images, compare the old images to the new ones, and, view the results from previous studies without having to go to the RIS or other system to read the results. When an image is read, the radiologist is usually able to dictate the report from within the system.

Laboratory Information System

The **laboratory information system (LIS)** collects, stores, and manages laboratory tests and their respective results. The LIS can speed up access to test results through improved efficiency from various locations, including anywhere in the hospital, the physician's office, or even the clinician's home. A LIS has the necessary functionality to be used in all areas of the laboratory, including blood chemistry, blood banks, microbiology, virology, and pathology. Figure 9.5 shows a sample LIS order entry screen.

Figure 9.5.   Example of laboratory information system—order entry

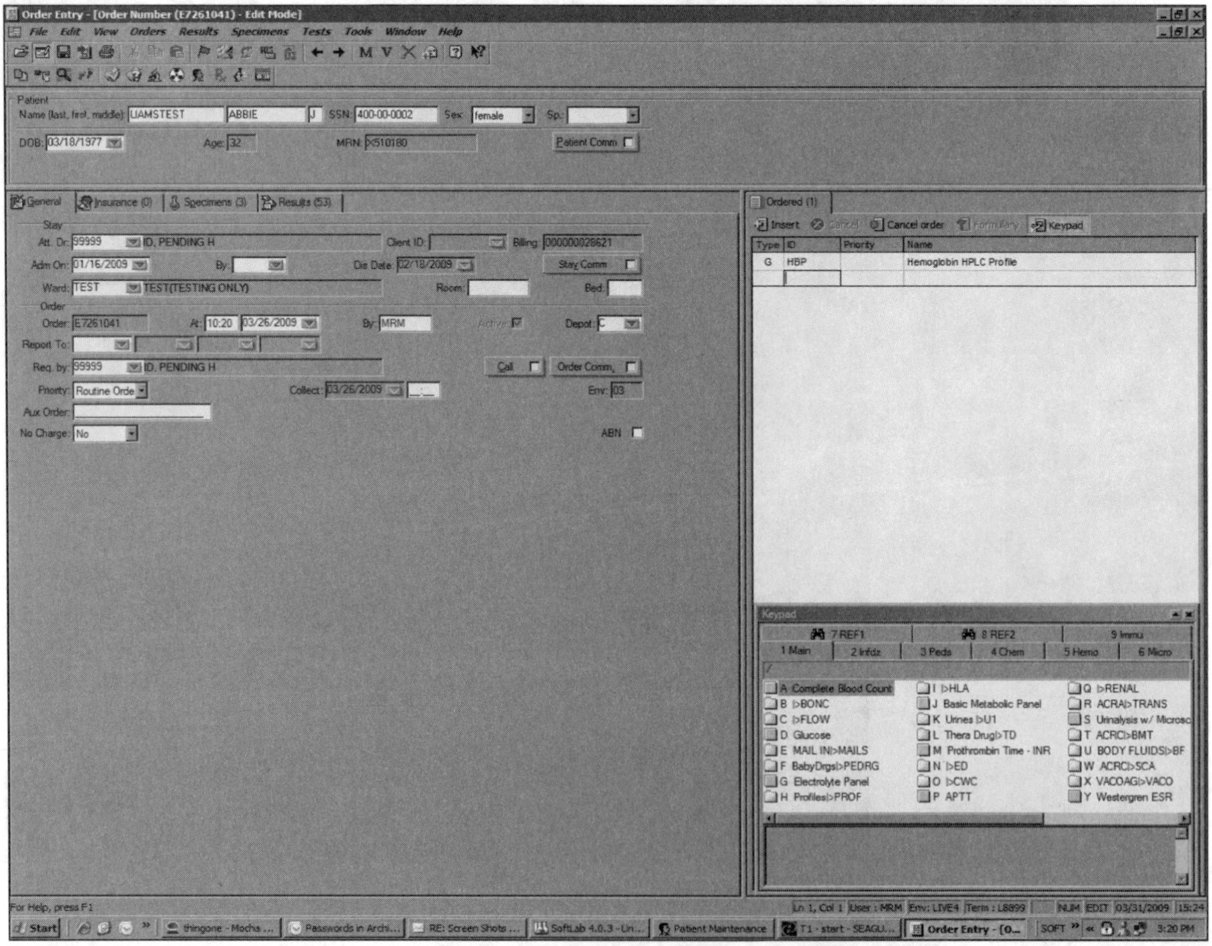

Source: SoftLab System. Laboratory Info System - Order Entry. Vendor: SCC Soft Computer; City: Clearwater, FL. http://www.softcomputer.com/contact-us/

The physician order for a laboratory test is generally received from a CPOE or other order entry system. The system lists what test(s) need to be run and then schedules the blood to be drawn. This list indicates where the patient is located and if the test is routine or urgent. Test results can be entered into the LIS manually or can be collected automatically from the instruments running the test. A LIS can also print out various laboratory reports needed, such as all of the tests performed on a single day or during the entire hospitalization. Other functions include:

- Printing out specimen labels
- Notifying laboratory staff and physicians of panic values
- Identifying normal ranges for each laboratory test
- Marking laboratory values as high, low, or panic level
- Printing barcodes to track specimens
- Recording quality control activities
- Generating reports
- Submitting charges to the financial information system

The LIS can assist management in running the laboratory department through the reporting capabilities. It should be able to generate reports such as the number of tests run per month and productivity reports on individual laboratory technicians.

Check Your Understanding 9.1

1. The radiology system that provides postprocedure patient instructions is:

   A. laboratory information system
   B. PACS
   C. radiology information system
   D. monitoring information system

2. How can the HIM professional utilize the radiology information system?

   A. Design and enter patient instructions
   B. Track nuclear materials
   C. Develop retention plan
   D. Determine procedures to be performed by department

3. Which of the following is a clinical information system?

   A. Hospital information system
   B. Radiology information system
   C. Financial information system
   D. Encoder

4. Demographic data:

   A. are generally obtained from the hospital information system
   B. are directly entered into the CIS
   C. are not required in the CIS
   D. are far more detailed than in administrative systems

5. The term used to describe viewing images from a remote location is:

   A. PACS
   B. e-health
   C. RIS
   D. teleradiology

Nursing Information System

Nursing information systems assist in the planning and monitoring of overall patient care. A **nursing information system (NIS)** will document the nursing care provided to a patient. There may be different systems available for the emergency department, intensive care areas, and other nursing areas because of the differing needs of each specialization. The capabilities of a strong nursing information system are flexible to accommodate the needs of the nurse. Conveniences such as efficient and quality documentation practices as well as easy access to quick reference guides are important.

Advantages to nursing information systems include:

- Reduction in costs of providing nursing care
- Improved patient care
- Immediate access to information on services rendered by the nursing staff
- Reduction in lost charges
- Reduced average length of stay
- Submitting charges to the financial information system

Many of these advantages result from the documentation of information at the time of care.

A NIS must be designed to support and promote quality documentation and practices through the use of protocols and vocabularies. Based on information entered into the system, such as the patient's diagnosis or procedure, the appropriate nursing protocol will be selected. Figure 9.6 shows a sample of a nursing information system.

The nurse will plan the patient's nursing care needs based on this protocol. Nursing documentation traditionally includes:

- Admission assessment
- Nursing activities
- Intake and output
- Graphic information
- Activities of daily living
- Nursing care plans
- Nurses' notes
- Medication administration record

The nursing information system can also assist in the overall management and daily operations of the nursing department by:

- Monitoring staffing allocation
- Scheduling nursing
- Generating performance improvement reports

Figure 9.6.   Example of nursing initial assessment screen—adult patient profile

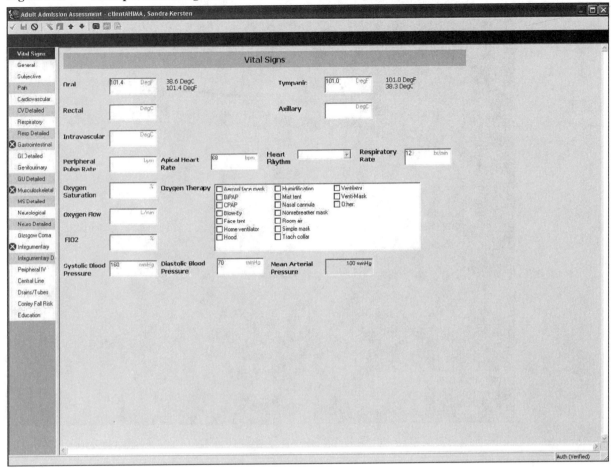

© Cerner Corporation. AHIMA has restricted permission to reproduce and distribute this copyrighted work. Further reproduction or distribution is strictly prohibited without written consent of Cerner Corporation.

Pharmacy Information System

A **pharmacy information system (PIS)** (see sample in figure 9.7) assists the care providers in ordering, allocating, and administering medication. With a focus on patient safety issues, especially medication errors, the pharmacy information system is a key tool in providing optimal patient care. The pharmacy information system stores demographic information, allergies, medication history, diagnoses, laboratory results, and other key information.

Data contained within the system and the functions of the system assist in reducing medication errors. The pharmacy system can be stand-alone or integrated with other systems in the facility such as CPOE. The greatest benefits, of course, come from the integration of data. For example, CPOE can record the medication order in the pharmacy system, which, in turn, can automatically update inventory levels—thus, automatically charging the patient.

Pharmacy information systems are used in hospitals, drugstores, and other healthcare settings. Functions will vary according to the needs of the facility. For example, a drugstore might need to track the number of refills remaining whereas this function would not be as important to a hospital.

Pharmacy information systems check for drug interactions, food and drug interactions, and other contraindications. When problems are identified, the pharmacy information system alerts the pharmacist or end user. It should also determine whether or not the dosage

Figure 9.7.   Example of pharmacy information system—initial menu screen

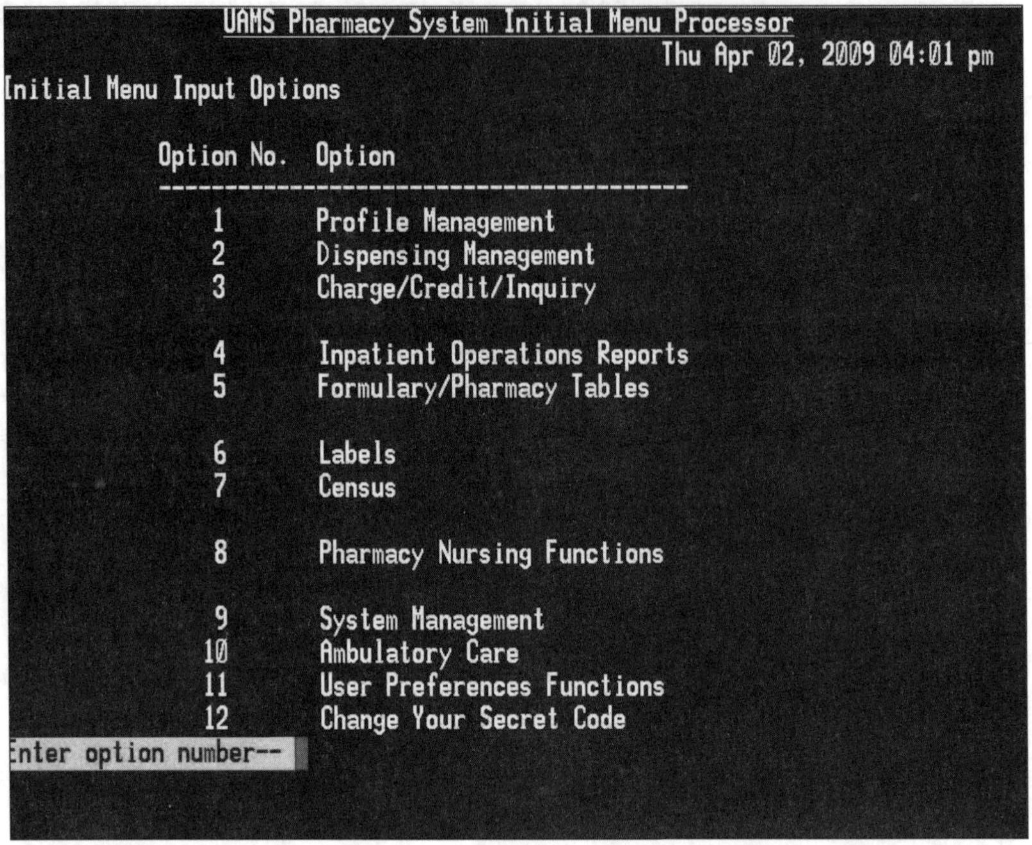

```
         UAMS Pharmacy System Initial Menu Processor
                                  Thu Apr 02, 2009 04:01 pm
Initial Menu Input Options

         Option No.  Option
         ----------------------------------------------
             1       Profile Management
             2       Dispensing Management
             3       Charge/Credit/Inquiry

             4       Inpatient Operations Reports
             5       Formulary/Pharmacy Tables

             6       Labels
             7       Census

             8       Pharmacy Nursing Functions

             9       System Management
            10       Ambulatory Care
            11       User Preferences Functions
            12       Change Your Secret Code
Enter option number--
```

Source: Star Pharmacy by McKesson

and administration method is appropriate for the size and age of the patient. The PIS can also manage the inventory of drugs in the pharmacy. This includes:

- Ordering drugs
- Inventory control
- Managing the formulary
- Tracking the costs of drugs
- Reporting on the usage of controlled medications

The pharmacy can analyze data stored within the system such as looking for patterns of drug usage and signs of abuse. These patterns may identify potential abuse by patients or physicians.

Pharmacy information systems can assist in the dispensing of medications in the pharmacy, which can help the nursing units in a number of ways:

- Creating individual dosages
- Use of secure storage systems
- Robotics
- Secure access to medications
- Documentation of medications administered, when and by whom
- Barcodes

Patient Monitoring Systems

Patient monitoring systems automatically collect and store patient data from various systems used in healthcare. These systems include:

- Fetal monitoring
- Vital signs
- Oxygen saturation rates

Patient monitoring systems are typically utilized in the intensive care units and other specialty areas such as the operating and recovery rooms.

A patient monitoring system must be able to capture the desired data automatically. The nurse or other user should be able to monitor a patient's condition from the nursing unit, physician office, or other remote location if necessary. This may require the use of the Internet to access the system. A nurse or other user must be able to create notes if needed to document and report variations in results, such as if the fetal monitor slipped out of position.

Vital signs and other data collected must be also reviewed and approved by the user regularly to ensure proper system functioning.

Telehealth

Telehealth is the use of telecommunications and networks to share information between a patient and a healthcare provider located at different sites. These locations can be across town or across the world. Most specialists are located in urban areas, leaving patients in rural areas without easy access to them. Telehealth allows a physician to examine and treat a patient without either party traveling. Telehealth can utilize video (see figure 9.8),

Figure 9.8.   **Example of use of telehealth by physicians**

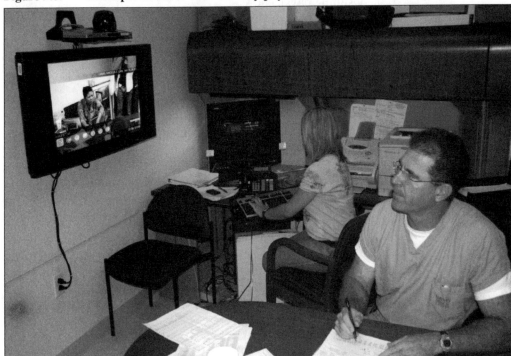

Source: Interactive Solutions, Inc.

telephone, computers, and other medical devices. A nurse may be required to interact directly with the patient in order to support the physician's evaluation and treatment.

Physicians find clinical telehealth a benefit in giving patients living in rural areas or those who are homebound medical consultations and monitoring. Telemonitoring is used at the patient's home to monitor cardiac rhythms, blood sugar, blood pressure, and other values to be submitted to the care provider. This type of monitoring can be performed through the use of the telephone or the computer. The data collected at the patient's home are digitally submitted into a CIS and thus made a part of the EHR.

Telehealth is a very sophisticated technology. Technology used includes virtual reality and robotics, which may be used to assist with the examination or treatment of a patient. The use of robotics to perform surgery is called **telesurgery**. This allows surgery to be performed on a patient in a different location.

Telehealth provides many advantages such as improved access to care, treatment provided via communication tools, and home monitoring. The problem is that the infrastructure is expensive and because physicians are licensed to practice medicine by state, the geographic range in which the physician can consult is limited.

Impact on HIM

Telemedical records must be managed as with any other patient care encounter. There are no differences in the documentation requirements between patient care provided remotely or at bedside, so the current documentation practices and forms are adequate. The American Health Information Management Association (AHIMA) recommends the minimum information of:

- Patient name

- Identification number

- Date of service

- Referring physician

- Consulting physician

- Provider facility

- Type of evaluation performed

- Informed consent

- Evaluation results

- Diagnosis/impression

- Recommendations for further treatment (Fletcher 1997)

The HIM professional must take the necessary steps to ensure that the privacy and security of the information is protected according to HIPAA requirements. The HIM professional may also be involved in the medical staff credentialing process to ensure physicians are indeed licensed and qualified to practice within the state. Finally, specific attention must be paid to the varying state laws and regulations to ensure they are met.

Figure 9.9 shows some common telehealth terms and their definitions.

Figure 9.9.   Some common telehealth terms

E-care:	The provision of health information, products, and services online as well as the automation of administrative and clinical aspects of care delivery.
E-health:	A broad term that is often interchangeable with the term telehealth to refer to the provision of health information, products, and services online.
E-medicine:	The use of telecommunication and computer technology for the delivery of medical care.
Telecardiology:	Transmission of cardiac catheterization studies, echocardiograms, and other diagnostic tests in conjunction with electronic stethoscope examinations for second opinions by the cardiologist at another site.
Teleconsultation:	Videoconferencing between two healthcare professionals or a healthcare professional and a client.
Telehomecare:	The use of telecommunication and computer technologies to monitor and render services and support to home care clients.
Telementoring:	Real-time advice is offered during a procedure to a practitioner in a remote site via a telecommunication system.
Telenursing:	The use of telecommunication and computer technology for the delivery of nursing care.
Telepathology:	Transmission of high-resolution still images, often using a robotic microscope, for interpretation by a pathologist at a remote location.
Teleprevention:	The use of telecommunication technology to provide health.
Telepsychiatry:	Variant of teleconsultation that allows observation and interviews of clients at one site by a psychiatrist at another site.
Telerehabilitation:	The use of interactive technology to facilitate exercise and rehabilitation activities.
Teleradiology:	Transmission of high-resolution still images for interpretation by a radiologist at a distant location.
Telesurgery:	Surgeons at a remote site can collaborate with experts at a referral center on techniques.
Teletherapy:	The use of interactive videoconferencing to provide therapy and counseling.
Teleultrasound:	Transmission of ultrasound images for interpretation at a remote site.

Source: Hebda et al. 2005, 357.

Smart Cards

Smart cards are plastic cards, similar in appearance to a credit card, with a computer chip embedded in it. Smart cards have been widely adopted for use in banking, retail, government, and other applications. The Smart Card Basics Web site identifies three uses of smart cards in healthcare:

- Rapid identification of patients; improved treatment
- A convenient way to carry data between systems or to sites without systems
- Reduction of records maintenance costs (Cardlogix Corporation 2009)

Smart cards enable portable storage of health and insurance information. They are relatively inexpensive and are able to protect the information stored within them from unauthorized access. In an emergency situation, smart cards can provide a physician with the critical information needed for proper care and treatment of a patient. The technology for smart cards "has a capacity of a microprocessor-based card (smart card) ranges from 8 to 128 K" (Degoulet and Fieschi 1997, 5). It is "based on the model of banking cards with a built-in microprocessor". . . and may serve as an instrument for identification and authentication "that authorizes access to medical computer files in hospitals" (Degoulet and Fieshchi 1997, 111). Data readers can easily be plugged into the USB port or other connections on the computer (Ross 2000).

There are three types of smart cards: straight memory cards, protected/segmented memory cards, and central processor unit/microprocessor unit (CPU/MPU) microprocessor multifunction cards. The straight memory cards are the most basic and can only store data; for this reason, they are the least expensive and look similar to a floppy disk. The protected/segmented memory cards have the ability to use logic and restrict a user's capabilities to view or edit the data. A password is the typical method used to protect this type of smart card. The most sophisticated option is the CPU/MPU microprocessor multifunction card. These cards are capable of segmenting and storing data. They also allow use with multiple functions and applications, thus reducing the number of cards that a patient must keep track of.

Although smart cards are useful tools, the patient must manage and maintain the accuracy of information on the card. Also, if a password or personal identification number is used, the patient must remember it for access (Deike 2000).

Impact of Clinical Information Systems on HIM

The health information management (HIM) professional is typically not a direct user of the various CIS discussed throughout this chapter. However, the HIM professional is the expert on the management of health records and input from this individual is important to ensure that accreditation, regulatory, and other requirements are met. The same is true for privacy and security issues. HIM professionals are highly recommended to be a part of the system implementation team to ensure that all HIM-related concerns such as quality documentation, confidentiality practices, and retention schedules are addressed up front. As each CIS submits charges to the financial information system, the HIM professional may be involved in developing the charges, similar to the involvement in the facility's chargemaster. Lastly, remember that every clinical information system (CIS) can populate the EHR with information that is ultimately managed and maintained by HIM professionals.

Check Your Understanding 9.2

1. The type of smart card that allow multiple purposes on one card is called

   A. generic smart card
   B. straight memory card
   C. CPU/MPU microprocessor multifunction card
   D. protected/segmented memory card

2. The clinical information system that records vital signs automatically is called a:

   A. patient monitoring system
   B. nursing information system
   C. telemedicine system
   D. e-health

3. Telehealth utilizes which two technologies to communicate between a patient and healthcare provider?

  A. Telecommunications and modem
  B. Telecommunications and networks
  C. Networks and modem
  D. Virtual reality and robotics

4. The two types of pharmacy information system are:

  A. stand-alone and EHR
  B. EHR and smart card
  C. interfaced and integrated
  D. stand-alone and integrated

5. Which of the following statements is true about telehealth?

  A. Documentation requirements are different from the typical face-to-face patient care.
  B. Documentation requirements are the same as the typical face-to-face patient care.
  C. Telehealth is not allowed by Joint Commission.
  D. Telehealth is a new technology and is not widely utilized.

References

Cardlogix Corporation. 2009. Smart card basics. http://www.smartcardbasics.com/.

Degoulet, P. and M. Fieschi. 1997. *Introduction to Clinical Informatics.* New York: Springer-Verlag, Inc.

Deike, K. 2000. Smart cards may make security a non-issue. *In Confidence* 8(6):7–8.

Fletcher, D. 1997 (April). Practice brief: Telemedical records.

Hebda, T., P. Czar, and C. Mascara. 2005. *Handbook of Informatics for Nurses & Health Care Professionals.* Upper Saddle River, NJ: Pearson Prentice Hall.

Johns, M.L. ed. 2007. Health *Information Management Technology: An Applied Approach*, 2nd ed. Chicago: AHIMA.

Ross, B. 2000. Smart cards for healthcare—A follow-up visit. *In Confidence* 8(2):8–9.

Chapter 10
Electronic Health Record

Objectives

- Participate in the development and implementation of an electronic health record (EHR).
- Explain the role of clinical vocabularies in the EHR.
- Support the need for the EHR.
- Address issues related to the EHR.
- Describe what the EHR is and what it is not.
- Educate the provider on benefits of the EHR.
- Prepare for the health information exchange.
- Justify the need for mapping.
- Identify the need for the multiple systems required to support the EHR.

Key Terms

American Health Information Community (AHIC)
American National Standards Institute (ANSI)
Centers for Medicare and Medicaid Services (CMS)
Classification systems
Clinical decision support system (CDSS)
Clinical messaging
Clinical provider order entry (CPOE)
Continuity of care record (CCR)
Current Procedural Terminology
Data content standards

Data repository
Data set
Data warehouse
Database
Digital Imaging and Communications in Medicine (DICOM)
Digital signature
Digitized signature
Electronic document management systems (EDMS)
Electronic health record (EHR)
Electronic medication administration record (EMAR)
Electronic signature

Health Level 7 (HL7)
Health Information Technology Standards Panel (HITSP)
Hybrid record
International Classification of Diseases, Ninth Edition, Clinical Modification
Interoperability
Logical Observation Identifiers Names and Codes (LOINC)
Mapping
MEDCIN
Messaging standards
National Council for Prescription Drug Programs (NCPDP)

National drug codes (NDC)
National eHealth Collaborative
   (NeHC)
National Health Information
   Network (NHIN)
Natural Language Processing
   (NLP)
Office of the National
   Coordinator of Health
   Information Technology
   (ONC)

Order entry/results reporting
Patient provider portal
Personal health record (PHR)
Population health
Presentation layer
Radiofrequency identification
   device (RFID)
RxNorm
Source system
Systematized Nomenclature of
   Medicine (SNOMED)

Standards development
   organizations (SDOs)
Structured data
Template-based entry
Unified Medical Language
   System
Unstructured data
Use case
Vocabulary standards

Introduction

The term **electronic health record** (EHR) means many different things to different people. LaTour and Eichenwald Maki (2006, 218) define the EHR as "a comprehensive system of applications that afford access to longitudinal health information about an individual across the continuum of care, assist in documentation, support clinical decision making, and provide for knowledge building." The Computer-based Patient Record Institute (CPRI) calls for the EHR to have three key criteria (Amatayakul 2007, 2):

- Integrates data from multiple sources

- Captures data at the point of care

- Assists the providers in their decision-making process

The term "longitudinal" used in LaTour and Eichenwald Maki's definition refers to the need for the EHR to collect data over time. The ultimate goal is to be able to access health information from birth to death. Expressions such as "cradle to the grave" and "womb to tomb" have been used to describe the concept of a longitudinal medical record. Access to the EHR should not be limited to the healthcare facility, but rather be accessible remotely for providers as well as the consumer.

The EHR is not about buying a software program, loading it on a server, and starting to use it the next day. It takes years to properly implement an EHR because of the number of components and the complexity of the system. The EHR is a collection of multiple technologies and systems that work together to create the EHR. **Source systems** are information systems that populate the EHR. These source systems include the electronic medication administration record, laboratory information system, radiology information system, hospital information system, and nursing information systems. These systems are used to capture data and feed it into the EHR. Source systems are not just clinical systems, but also include administrative and financial systems (LaTour and Eichenwald Maki 2006). To realize the full benefits of the EHR, data should be captured at the point of care. Data can be captured in a multitude of ways, which can include personal computers, personal digital assistants, voice recognition, handwriting recognition, and other methods of data entry.

The facility must have the necessary infrastructure to integrate data. Infrastructure includes the hardware, software, and communication devices needed to operate efficiently and effectively (Englebardt and Nelson 2002). Much of the infrastructure for the EHR is the same as any information system, such as computers, monitors, network, printers, operating system, and application software. The EHR infrastructure may also include a clinical data repository to centralize the data from the source systems. Another component of the EHR infrastructure is a rules engine that controls alerts, reminders, order sets, and protocols (Amatayakul 2007). The EHR should have access to knowledge-based resources such as MEDLINE, electronic drug references, and research databases. A data warehouse is necessary to provide data mining of the data contained in the EHR. Refer back to Chapter 6 for further information regarding data storage and retrieval.

In the future, the EHR is expected to include a **continuity of care record (CCR)** and a personal health record (PHR) (Hamilton 2009). The CCR is a snapshot of data from the EHR and includes basic information such as diagnoses, allergies, medications, and future treatment. The CCR should be available to all healthcare providers so as to improve the continuity of patient care as well as reduce medical errors. A core data set has been established as the minimum requirements for the CCR (see figure 10.1). In addition to these minimum requirements, the CCR code data set has some optional data elements. The CCR may or may not contain or be used by the healthcare facility. Data contained in the CCR (shown in figure 10.1) can be provided to care providers in electronic format using XML or Health Level 7 (HL7) formats as well as traditional paper format. Unlike the EHR, the purpose of the CCR is not to provide a legal health record, but rather information for the continuity of care (Quinsey 2005).

The **personal health record** (PHR) is a tool for collecting, tracking, and sharing important, up-to-date information on the patient's medical history. A PHR's information is controlled by the patient and includes a wide range of data including allergies, diagnoses, medications, and social and family history. For a full discussion of PHRs, please see Chapter 14.

Figure 10.1.   Core data set for CCR

1. CCR identifying information
   a. Referring ("from") practitioner
   b. Referral ("to") practitioner
   c. Date
   d. Purpose or reason for CCR
2. Patient identifying information—required information to uniquely identify the subject patient; not a centralized system or national patient identifier but a federated or distributed system identifier
3. Patient insurance or financial information—basic information from which eligibility for insurance benefits may be determined for the patient
4. Advance directives—indicators that resuscitation efforts are to be either unrestricted or limited in some way; includes what is commonly known as the Do Not Resuscitate status of the patient as addressed in such documents as living wills, healthcare proxies, and powers of attorney
5. Patient health status
   a. Conditions, diagnoses, problems
   b. Family history
   c. Adverse reactions, allergies, clinical warnings, and alerts
   d. Social history and health risk factors
   e. Medications
   f. Immunizations
   g. Vital signs and physiologic measurements
   h. Laboratory results and observations
   i. Procedures and imaging (this section may be expanded in extensions for clinical specialty-specific information regarding the patient.)
6. Care documentation—detail of the patient-practitioner encounter history, such as:
   a. Dates and purposes of recent pertinent visits
   b. Names of practitioners seen (this section may be significantly expanded in future extensions)
7. Care plan recommendation—includes planned or scheduled tests, procedures, or regimens of care for the patient
8. Practitioners—information about those healthcare practitioners who are participants in the patient's care; links as appropriate to 5a (conditions, diagnoses, problems) and 6 (care documentation) encounters

Source: Quinsey 2005

Why should anyone have an EHR? Healthcare is facing many changes with reductions in reimbursement, the focus on reducing medical errors, increased use of technology, escalating healthcare costs, and a need to coordinate care of the patient. The traditional paper medical record is not meeting the needs of patients or healthcare professionals because of the fragmentation of the record, difficulty in analyzing data in a paper environment, and frequent accessibility issues because of missing information or lost medical records. EHRs can help to improve efficiency and quality of care throughout a facility. For example, alerts built into the EHR can prevent a medication error before the prescription is executed and the EHR can eliminate issues encountered with handwriting and illegibility. Also, medical record accessibility will not be lost or delayed, thus preventing treatment errors such as removing the wrong kidney. **Reminders** can notify physicians of screenings that should be performed based on the patient's age and gender. For example, the physician would be reminded that the patient needs an annual mammogram or a colonoscopy.

Healthcare today can be complicated depending on care and treatment needed. It may require patients to go to multiple physicians and possibly multiple hospitals. The fragmentation of the medical record that results from these patient visits results in a lack of consistency and completeness of the health information (Amatayakul 2007). For example, a patient may be placed on medications that his or her primary care physician is not aware of. The primary care physician may also be unaware of past serious medical or surgical conditions, restricting the thoroughness and accurateness of the patient care rendered. The EHR allows for patient information to be complete and accurate because the system can be programmed to require key data elements be entered before a user can proceed on to the next screen, ultimately improving the quality of the documentation captured. Patients can also receive individually designed and detailed patient instructions (Hamilton 2009).

The United States spends about two trillion dollars, which is approximately 15% of its gross national product, on healthcare (Sanderson 2009). This percentage continues to escalate. A large percentage of these expenses are a result of performing administrative tasks and the EHR is designed to help reduce these tasks to save time and money (Hamilton 2009). For example, HIM staff will no longer have to search for medical records, and the infrastructure to transport the paper medical record from one point to another is no longer needed. Benefits of the EHR are numerous and will be discussed later in the chapter.

Check Your Understanding 10.1

1. A subset of the EHR that is used for subsequent patient care is called:

   A. PHR
   B. CCR
   C. core data set
   D. mini-EHR

2. A reason to implement an EHR is to:

   A. determine the cost of care
   B. improve patient care
   C. eliminate medical errors
   D. meet Joint Commission mandate for the EHR

3. The infrastructure required for the EHR includes which of the components not found in most information systems?

   A. Hardware
   B. Network
   C. Software
   D. Rules engine

4. The system that includes patient information from both the patient and the healthcare provider is called the:

   A. CCR
   B. PHR
   C. core data set
   D. mini-EHR

5. The phrase "womb to tomb" refers to:

   A. completeness of health information
   B. PHR
   C. CCR
   D. longitudinal record

Status

The EHR has not been widely implemented for reasons such as financial constraints, concerns about the technology, privacy and security, a lack of standards, and conflicting standards. Many of these issues are being addressed by Congress, federal agencies, and independent organizations. Many of these initiatives will be addressed either later in this chapter or in Chapter 14. A number of organizations are leading the way, such as the **Office of the National Coordinator for Health Information Technology (ONC)**.

Adoption

A number of studies have been conducted to determine the adoption level of the EHR, especially for physician practices. The Commonwealth Fund reports that the United States trails other countries in EHR adoption. Although the United States is seeing growth in the diffusion of EHR to physicians, in 2006 the adoption rate was still only 28%. In the Netherlands, 98% of the physicians utilize an EHR and in New Zealand the rate is 92%, a rate much higher than that of the United States (Davis et al. 2009). A study conducted by the Institute for Health Policy in late 2007 and early 2008 found that only 4% of physicians had a fully functioning EHR, with 13% having a basic EHR (AHIMA 2008b).

Research shows that EHRs are used more by:

- younger physicians

- primary care physicians

- physicians in the western United States

- physician in large physician practices (50 physicians or more) (RWJF 2009)

Ash and Bates (2004) studied EHR adoption for the inpatient and ambulatory settings, and found that the adoption rate is low. They also found that barriers to the EHR include costs and patient safety issues. Other studies also show concerns over return on investment and fear that the system will become obsolete quickly due to ongoing changes in technology and developing standards. The American Hospital Association reported in 2006 that 68% of hospitals had partial or full EHRs. Only 11% of these hospitals, which were generally large, urban hospitals or teaching hospitals, had fully functional EHRs (AHA 2007).

There are many initiatives across the country taking steps to develop the infrastructure needed to implement and support the EHR. Many of these initiatives are being developed or supported by ONC, which was established by President George W. Bush to prepare the way for a **national health information network (NHIN)**. The NHIN will be a network of networks sharing patient information to provide immediate access across the nation. For more on ONC, please see Chapter 14.

Other ongoing initiatives include the:

- development and implementation of universal standards for data content

- development and implementation of messaging standards

- development and implementation of vocabulary standards

Many laws, both federal and state, that hinder the EHR are being changed and new laws to support the EHR such as the Health Information Portability and Accountability Act (HIPAA) and the American Recovery and Reinvestment Act (AARA) of 2009 have been passed.

One of the newest initiatives is the certification of EHRs. The Certification Commission on Health Information Technology (CCHIT) is the sole certifier of the EHR. This process is discussed in detail in Chapter 14. The healthcare system is not the only one preparing for the EHR. Because of the Internet and other resources, patients are becoming savvier regarding their care. This knowledge makes them active participants in their care and as such, patients are demanding access to their provider and their health information (Howrey 2008).

Another player in the EHR initiatives has been the **American Health Information Community (AHIC)**. AHIC was an advisory committee to the U.S. Department of Health and Human Services. It was developed in 2005 (HHS 2009a). Seven workgroups were created: chronic care; confidentiality, privacy, and security; consumer empowerment; electronic health records; personalized healthcare; population health and clinical care connections; and quality (HHS 2009b). The ultimate goal was interoperability. AHIC was formally disbanded in 2008 (HHS 2009a). The successor of AHIC is the **National eHealth Collaborative (NeHC)**. NeHC is working with other stakeholders to address "issues and effecting the change needed to enable the secure and reliable exchange of electronic health information nationwide" (NeHC 2009).

Stark Law Exception

The Stark Law is frequently called the anti-kickback law. The Stark Law prohibits physicians or their family members from owning businesses to whom the physician refers patients for health services. It prevents physicians from receiving a fee for referring patients for any healthcare services whose care is paid for by a federally funded program such as Medicare and Medicaid. Violation of this law is a felony and can lead to penalties up to $100,000.

Because of the desire for adoption of e-prescribing and the EHR, the **Centers for Medicare and Medicaid Services (CMS)** granted an exception to the Stark Law. This exception took effect in October 2006. There are limitations regarding what the systems have to be able to do, that hardware cannot be included, and that donations cannot exceed 85% of the costs for the systems.

Components of EHR

The EHR is a complex system comprised of a number of components. These components provide the mechanism to collect, store, analyze, and access health information. The components include:

- Order communication/results retrieval

- Electronic document/content management

- Clinical messaging

- Patient care charting

- Computerized physician/provider order entry system

- Electronic medication administration reporting

- Clinical decision support system

- Patient provider portal

- Personal health record

- Population health (Amatayakul 2007)

The consolidation of these functions/systems into one allows health information to be used in ways that were impossible with the paper record. The time and staff required to go through a paper record to analyze data is much more costly compared to the readily available information contained within the EHR. It is for this reason that EHRs can be a significant source of information for identifying trends and ensuring protocols are followed. For example, a facility can analyze data to determine compliance practices are being followed, such as whether or not physicians performed a routine foot exam for patients with diabetes. A brief overview of each of these components follows.

Order Communication/Results Retrieval

The order communication system notifies clinical departments, such as the laboratory, radiology, physical therapy, and dietary departments, of orders made by the physician. These orders are not entered by the physician, but rather by the nurse, unit secretary, or other authorized user (Amatayakul 2007). Because the orders are generally written down and then transcribed into the order communication system, the facility does not receive the benefits of a **clinical provider order entry** (CPOE) system. The CPOE contains preprogrammed clinical decision support designed to assist the user through making an entry appropriately. Although the CPOE is a more robust system, the basic need to enter orders and access results is critical for the implementation of an EHR (Amatayakul 2007). Once tests are performed, results of the diagnostic studies are compiled from their respective clinical information systems (that is, laboratory information system or radiology information system) and transferred into the EHR. The results are then available for viewing, which in turn speeds access to the information because the report does not have to be printed, filed in the medical record, and transported to the provider before it is available for use.

Electronic Document/Content Management

Electronic document/content management may also be called **electronic document management system (EDMS)**. The EDMS may utilize scanning to capture patient information from the paper record. Data may be captured through the use of enterprise report management (ERM) or computer output to laser disk (COLD), voice, e-mail, and e-fax systems. The EDMS may utilize workflow technology to direct specific documents or patient records to coders, risk management, analysts, and other users. For a full discussion of EDMS, please see Chapter 6.

Clinical Messaging

Clinical messaging connects the medical staff and hospital by providing access to systems such as **order entry/results reporting** and EDMS systems. Web-based technology often is utilized to access information in an internal system such as an intranet, or it can use the Internet. Amatayakul (2007, 422) defines clinical messaging as "the secure transmission of clinical information from one entity to another, including providers to providers, patients to providers, payers to providers, and among members of a healthcare community, such as within a regional health information organization." Clinical messages can use e-mail, portals, virtual private networks, and other means to provide the secure means of communication needed for patient information. These messages are shared in such a way as to protect the privacy of the patient (Amatayakul 2007). Standards have been established to control clinical messaging. These standards are discussed later in this chapter.

Patient Care Charting

Patient care charting may utilize many different systems to accommodate all of the different healthcare professionals who document in the medical record. There may be separate systems for physicians, nurses, physical therapists, respiratory therapists, and others. These systems may use bedside terminals, personal digital assistants, and other wireless devices to enable the care provider to document in the medical record as the information is obtained from the patient (LaTour and Eichenald Maki 2006). These systems generally allow entry of both structured and unstructured data. **Structured data** are generally found in checkboxes, drop-down boxes, and other data entry means whereby the user chooses from options already built into the system. **Unstructured data,** also called narrative data, can be entered in a free text format by the user, usually by typing (Amatayakul 2007). Structured and unstructured data will be discussed later in the chapter.

Computerized Physician/Provider Order Entry System

As previously discussed, the computerized physician/provider order entry system (CPOE) is designed for orders to be entered by the healthcare providers. The use of a CPOE can lead to significant improvements in patient safety because of the reminders and alerts built into the system. These alerts and reminders are provided to the physician or other healthcare provider as data are entered, thus identifying problems and key information at the point of capture rather than after review by nurses, pharmacists, or others. These alerts and reminders are controlled by clinical decision support built into the system that are able to help prevent medication errors and improve the quality of care through its validation mechanisms (Amatayakul 2007). Alerts may notify the physician of medication contraindications or that a prescription is about to expire. Reminders usually notify the physician of laboratory test results and preventive measures such as a patient is due for a mammogram.

Although alerts and reminders are useful, too many become frustrating to the physician because they have to constantly stop their data entry to address the alerts and reminders (Amatayakul 2007). CPOE can be used to avoid duplicate testing and ordering of medications not covered by the patient's insurance. This would be accomplished by reminding the physician that there is a recent test or by letting the physician know that the test is not covered or requires preapproval from the insurer.

Using CPOE can be time consuming for physicians; many are reluctant to adopt the systems or try to pass the responsibility of entering the orders to the nurses or other support staff. The benefits of CPOE are realized when the physicians are the users of the system. Because of the importance of physician users and the decision support such as recommending alternative medications, catching inappropriate dosages, and other edits, the providers must be involved in developing it.

Electronic Medication Administration Record

The **electronic medication administration record (EMAR)** automates many of the medication administration processes in a healthcare facility. The level of sophistication varies by system and can be as simple as printing out a list of medications to be administered to the patient and documenting the medications given to the patient. It can be much more sophisticated by using barcodes or **radiofrequency identification devices (RFID)** to properly identify the patient. RFID is the implantation of a microchip to an item to allow tracking of that item (Abdelhak 2007, 245). The EMAR can also provide alerts to assist in medication timing and provide the nurse with reference material on the medication itself (Amatayakul 2007). The more sophisticated EMAR can automate the entire medication administration process. This process includes identifying the drug to administer, identifying the patient, and documenting the administration of the medication or the exception. An example of an exception would be to record that medication was administered late. Some EMAR systems are designed to store commonly used medications on the nursing unit for dispensing through the use of kiosks.

Clinical Decision Support System

The **clinical decision support system** (CDSS) is "the help provided in association with data entry into an EHR system performed directly by the caregiver at the point of care" (Amatayakul 2007, 13). The CDSS may be active, which means that it has alerts or reminders the user must address, or passive, which means the user may choose to utilize or ignore the alerts. Alerts may notify the care provider of patient allergies or contraindications for the medication or other treatment. It may notify the user that the drug being ordered is off-formulary (Amatayakul 2007). The CDSS may also have the clinical practice guidelines advice installed and provide access to knowledge-based systems. Clinical guidelines advice provides recommendations to the physician on how to care for the patient given the patient's circumstances. Rules engines are used to control the reminders and alerts as well as the clinical practice and benchmarking (Amatayakul 2007). Benchmarking compares internal data to external data. In a CDSS, benchmarking is used to standardize practice patterns and reduce the usage of high-cost drugs and other treatments. For more on CDSS, please see Chapter 8.

Patient Provider Portal

The **patient provider portal** is a secure method of communication between the healthcare provider and the patient, just the providers, or the provider and the payer. The patient provider portal may include secure e-mail or remote access to test results, and provide patient monitoring. Monitoring may include monitoring of pacemaker activity, blood sugar, and breath sounds. Patients could also have access to patient education materials to help them manage their own care. This would be especially valuable for chronic conditions such as diabetes mellitus and chronic obstructive pulmonary disease (Amatayakul 2007).

Personal Health Record

The personal health record (PHR) is an application designed for the patient to manage his/her own health information for personal maintenance purposes and to provide to healthcare providers for complete and accurate histories. The PHR may be linked to the EHR and accessibility through a patient-provider portal. For more information on the PHR, see Chapter 14.

Population Health

Population health is the capture and reporting of healthcare data that are used for public health purposes. It allows the healthcare provider to report infectious diseases, immunizations, cancer, and other reportable conditions to public health officials. This reporting is required at the local, state, and national levels and includes infectious diseases. A population health system also can connect with public health officials to receive alerts regarding health issues (Amatayakul 2007). The traditional methods are cumbersome because of the manual processes and disparate systems. The use of technology can speed up the reporting process, thus speeding up the management of disease outbreaks.

Check Your Understanding 10.2

1. The component of the EHR that reports infectious diseases is:

   A. population health
   B. PHR
   C. patient provider portal
   D. clinical decision support system

2. Clinical decision support to enhance physician orders is found in which component of the EHR?

   A. Order communication/results reporting
   B. PHR
   C. CPOE
   D. Patient-provider portal

3. The ability of a healthcare facility to provide EHR software to physicians is allowed through:

   A. the Stark Law
   B. an exception to the Stark Law
   C. health information exchange
   D. Patient-provider portal

4. CCHIT's role in the EHR is

   A. standard development
   B. certification
   C. health information exchange
   D. Stark Law

5. Which statement is true about the state of adoption of the EHR?

   A. EHRs are widely used throughout the United States
   B. The United States is ahead of other countries in EHR adoption
   C. Most EHRs are found in small physician practices
   D. Most EHRs are found in larger facilities and physician practices

Benefits of the EHR

The many benefits to the EHR are both economic and clinical in value. Economic benefits include cost savings and cost avoidance as well as productivity improvement. Cost savings may include reduction in staff, reductions in liability insurance, and reduction in cost of forms, microfilming, and storage of the paper record. Reduced transcription also saves money and provides faster access to health information. Cost avoidance may include not having to expand the file area to accommodate the paper records, not hiring additional staff, and not repeating tests. Overall, the EHR improves productivity; however, it may be difficult to quantify and prove because some tasks take longer. For example, it takes physicians longer to enter data into the EHR than it does to handwrite it.

One of the clinical benefits of the EHR is easier access to clinical information. The EHR provides immediate access, which in turn, speeds diagnosis and treatment to improve the quality of care provided. The EHR provides current information on tests, medications, allergies, and past diagnoses and treatments (among many more) required for decision making and disease management. As previously discussed, the use of tools such as reminders and alerts can remind a physician to schedule mammograms and colonoscopies and to avoid adverse drug events and allergies. The EHR can also enhance the documentation captured because the traditional paper medical record is frequently illegible, incomplete, inaccurate, and redundant. These problems can be avoided with the use of required fields, uniform data entry practices, and trained personnel.

Patient education is important for the continued improvement of a patient's condition. The EHR strongly supports patient education materials such as discharge instructions and medication information can be personalized for the individual patient. The EHR allows healthcare providers to spend more time with patients because of the benefits in workflow and administrative tasks since most documentation can occur at the bedside (Amatayakul 2007).

The EHR improves the level of communication between providers. With the use of bedside terminals, care providers have the latest information at all times from any location (Hamilton 2009). The edits and required fields in the EHR also reduce or eliminate incomplete information. With paper records, the medical record is not updated immediately following the care but, rather, periodically through the nurse's shift.

The EHR can improve the efficiency of the healthcare system in many ways. The use of bedside terminals means that when the patient leaves the facility the medical record documentation can be completed, thus enabling the immediate coding and billing of the encounter. Test results can also be available immediately upon completion. If time spent looking for lost or misplaced medical records was quantified, administration would be horrified at the waste of time and money. Time savings can be realized by nursing and other care providers through the elimination of duplicate data collection and improved availability. Other time savings can be realized through e-prescribing, dual access to the patient's medical record, and reduction in the dependence on medical transcription.

Barriers to the EHR

The EHR is a powerful tool that can completely revolutionize healthcare. As discussed previously, the EHR provides a multitude of benefits, but there are many issues and barriers that must be addressed in order to encourage adoption and interoperability.

One of the primary barriers to EHR implementation is cost. It is expensive, and many are hesitant to invest in one without a guarantee of a return on their investment. Accurate and flexible budget planning must be completed for a successful implementation. The facility must be sure to account for every cost, no matter how large or small, in planning the budget. Costs will include items such as hardware, software, construction or reconstruction of space, training, and maintenance to name a few. Additional technical staff may be required to address technical issues that arise, such as the system crashing or virus infection.

Another main issue is the lack of uniform standards to support the functions and purpose of the EHR (Hamilton 2009). Standards needed include content, clinical protocols, data integrity, and decision support. The lack of standards prevents interoperability of the various systems that make up the EHR. Although standards are being developed, there is not always consensus on which should be followed. The lack of consistent standards makes it difficult for systems to talk to one another, setting up the system to fail in meeting those standards required in the future. Please see the standards section of this chapter for further details.

The third barrier mentioned here will be training. A learning curve is associated with all training associated with the EHR. With new software and policies, physicians, healthcare professionals, and support staff will initially lose efficiency in performing their everyday job duties, which will create backlogs. As users become more confident, productivity will increase.

The final barrier to be discussed is fear. Not only do documentation practices change, but workflow and other processes in the healthcare facility change as well. Many potential users of the EHR fear the system will crash and that security of the system will be breached. Some people fear losing their jobs and some fear change altogether. Change management issues should be addressed prior to and during implementation. EHRs change the dynamic and environment of the facility. It is a considerable change for staff to undertake and many will be apprehensive. One employee may discontinue tasks that have been a key part of his or her job duties (such as filing and pulling charts) and are now assumed by the EHR. A situation like this will be intimidating to an employee and should be dealt with immediately. Communication is critical.

Functionality

Functionality and performance of an EHR will vary by setting (Amatayakul 2007). In other words, an EHR for the ambulatory setting will be different than one for an acute care hospital. However, regardless of setting, there are universal functions that all EHRs must have. Many of these functions have been described throughout this chapter and include clinical decision support, CPOE, results reporting, and charting. EHRs must also have the necessary infrastructure in place to support it. An infrastructure is made up of many different components such as the hardware, network, database, server, personnel, and processes necessary, among many others, to operate the EHR (Amatayakul 2007).

The core function of the EHR is storing patient information. The patient information collected and stored includes but is not limited to the problem list, diagnosis/procedures, test results, advance directives, discharge summary, history and physical, documentation of treatment provided, operative reports, and medication lists.

To support the users in the documentation and retrieval of health information, users should be able to control their view of the data (Abdelhak et al. 2007). For example, a nurse would need to immediately see new orders and any significant changes in the patient's condition. A cardiologist would need to see significant changes in the patient's condition and cardiac test results such as electrocardiograms or catheterization report. A pulmonologist would rather see the arterial blood gas, chest x-rays, and other pulmonary tests before the cardiac test results.

The EHR can also link to medical devices, allowing for automatic capture of monitoring and testing (LaTour and Eichenwald Maki 2006). For example, fetal monitoring, electrocardiograms, electroencephalograms, blood pressure, and pulse oximetry results can be automatically captured and thus monitored from a remote location by the physician or other authorized user in real time.

With the paper medical record, reporting is limited to a copy of the individual forms filed in the medical record. Documentation is recorded in chronological order and broken up by encounter. The data cannot be manipulated into different views within each encounter, much less across encounters. With the EHR, test results can be viewed longitudinally so blood pressure, blood sugar, and other results can be viewed over time. Other manipulations of data can be performed with just a few keystrokes or clicks. Reports can also be designed to meet the needs of the users or requester. An example of a report would be to help monitor compliance of the HIPAA minimum necessary rule.

The ambulatory EHR frequently is combined with the practice management system that performs the billing scheduling and other administrative tasks. The ambulatory EHR generally has a scheduling or in-basket function allowing the user to retrieve the patient's medical record quickly and easily. There is typically a summary screen that quickly accesses parts of the medical record. There are generally templates for documenting patient care and entering orders as well as pop-up boxes providing alerts. E-prescribing allows prescriptions to be sent to the retail pharmacy. A report writer allows the facility to develop ad-hoc reports as well as routine ones (Amatayakul 2007).

The acute care EHR is still very departmental in its design. The acute care EHR is made up of many components that evolve over time. These components are designed for a specific function, such as nursing documentation or clinical provider order entry, rather than overall value of the EHR (Amatayakul 2007).

Check Your Understanding 10.3

1. The time taken to enter data is considered to be a _____ to the EHR.

   A. barrier
   B. benefit
   C. component
   D. asset

2. What function is typically found in the ambulatory EHR but not the inpatient EHR?

   A. Decision support
   B. Practice management
   C. Security
   D. CPOE

3. Which of the following is a benefit of the EHR?

   A. Improved efficiency
   B. Costs
   C. Fear of technology
   D. Security concerns

4. Which statement regarding patient education is true?

   A. The EHR allows for patient education whereas the paper record did not
   B. The patient education is only provided online with an EHR
   C. The patient creates the patient education curriculum
   D. Patient education can be customized for each individual patient

5. Which statement is true about the EHR?

   A. The EHR is the same regardless of the setting in which it operates
   B. The EHR is different based on the setting in which it operates
   C. The EHR does not utilize reminders
   D. The EHR does not allow for the use of CPOE

Signatures

Signatures are an important part of the EHR because the authentication of medical record entries is a requirement of state licensing, accreditation, and other standards. The purpose of signatures, in both the paper and electronic environment, is to record the identity of the individual who performed the entry.

One of the benefits of the electronic signature is that it automatically stamps medical record entries with the date and time of the entry. It also records user identification so that the identity of the individual who created the entry into the system is automatically recorded. There are three levels of signatures found in the EHR. The **digitized signature** is a scanned image of an individual's actual signature. This method is very insecure because anyone who has access to the image can use the signature. The next level is the **electronic signature**, which requires a password or even a two-tiered authentication method to be entered before the signature is executed. The **digital signature** is similar to the electronic signature except that it uses encryption and nonrepudiation to prove the authenticator's identity (Kohn 2009).

Classification Systems

Classification systems are used for secondary data. The purpose of a classification system is to group similar items together. According to Giannangelo, "a classification is a system that is clinically descriptive and arranges or organizes like or related entities" (Giannangelo

2006, 2). An example of a classification system is *International Classification of Diseases, Ninth Edition, Clinical Modification (ICD-9-CM)*. Classifications provide outputs such as the reporting of diagnoses and procedures on patient accounts, but it does not act as an input device by performing tasks such as documenting the discharge summary or other patient information (Giannangelo 2006). This information is part of the EHR.

Common classification systems such as ICD-9-CM and CPT are used to organize diagnoses and procedures. Although an important part of the common medical language necessary for the EHR, they are not detailed enough to provide adequate information to describe the patient's encounter. Classifications are used for reimbursement, quality of care, planning, statistics, and public health reporting. One of the problems with classification systems is that there is not a central oversight organization over them such as those used for coding (Campbell and Giannangelo 2007). For example, ICD-9-CM diagnosis codes are controlled by the National Center for Health Statistics while the ICD-9-CM procedure codes are under the auspices of the Centers for Medicare and Medicaid Services, and CPT, a proprietary system, is maintained by the American Medical Association. The American Procedural Association's **Current Procedural Terminology** (CPT) are the terms used in professional billing. The ICD-9-CM and CPT coding updates are published at different times of the year, thus complicating the management of the systems (Campbell and Giannangelo 2007). Because of the EHR and tools such as natural language processing, code assignment can be performed automatically. Please see Chapter 14 for details.

The United States of America currently uses ICD-9-CM for reimbursement and *International Classification of Diseases*, 10th Edition (ICD-10) for mortality statistics. The United States is converting to *International Classification of Diseases*, Clinical Modification (ICD-10-CM) and *International Classification of Diseases*, 10th Edition Procedural Coding System (ICD-10-PCS) effective October 1, 2013. Codes can be used in several ways. They can represent words in a language, terms in a terminology or vocabularies, and even groups in a classification system.

Standards

Standards are important to the EHR because they streamline the communication method that allows systems to speak to each other and for data to be stored using the same formats, language, and terms to describe and execute functions. There are a multitude of standards that exist, yet no universal one is required to be followed. **Health Information Technology Standards Panel (HITSP)** is making attempts to overcome this issue.

HITSP works collaboratively with public and private sectors to achieve what they call "widespread interoperability among healthcare software applications." HITSP membership is available to anyone interested in participating, which includes standards development organizations. HITSP publishes their work products prior to approval in order to obtain public feedback. HITSP meetings are open for the participation of all members. HITSP was established in 2005. Rather than developing standards, HITSP works to obtain widespread consensus on existing standards (HITSP 2008).

In the following sections, standards development organizations and the various standards required by the EHR will be discussed. These standards include:

- vocabulary standards

- messaging standards

- data content standards

Standards Development Organizations

Standards development organizations (SDOs) are organizations that create standards. **American National Standards Institute (ANSI)** is responsible for accrediting SDOs in the United States. To be accredited, the standard must be open, voluntary, and have input from stakeholders. Anyone can join an SDO and participate in the development of standards.

American National Standards Institute

ANSI does not develop standards but, rather, provides a neutral environment for others to work together to settle on a common agreement. Before a standard can be approved, it must meet the rules of ANSI and the following requirements:

- Made from consensus

- Due process

- Openness

- Balance (ANSI 2009)

Through ANSI, diverse stakeholders work together to develop standards. The stakeholders must be willing to compromise in order to develop consensus-based standards. Due process comes from the fact that standard development must occur in an open manner that is responsive to the needs of the stakeholders, and the development should be equitable, thus balancing the needs of all of the stakeholders during the development process. The openness of standards development allows any interested party to participate in the development process (ANSI 2009).

Data Content Standards

Data content standards facilitate interoperability through the standardization of the structure and content of data elements (Rollins 2007). Data content standards identify the structure and content of data elements to be collected by the EHR. Data content standards allow organizations to collect data once and use it many times in many ways. It also assists in data storage and mining as well as sharing data with external organizations for use in benchmarking and other purposes. The use of data content standards also assists in the health information exchange process, which is discussed in Chapter 14. There are a number of standards that have been developed, but many of these overlap or replicate each other (AHIMA 2008a).

Vocabulary Standards

Vocabulary standards address the problem of multiple ways to define, classify, and represent language. Amatayakul (2007) states that "language generally refers to a system of communication using an arbitrary set of vocal sounds, written symbols, signs, or gestures in conventional ways with conventional meanings" (Amatayakul 2007, 200). Medicine has its own language. The problem is there are many terms used in medicine that have multiple synonyms. The use of synonyms makes it difficult to identify all patients with a specific disease or condition. There are a number of terms that fall into the concept of vocabulary standards including language, vocabulary, terminology, and nomenclature:

- Language is a system of communication used by a group of people

- Vocabulary is all the terms that can be used for communication within the area of specialization

- Terminology is the terms used for a specific purpose

- Nomenclature is a system used to assign names (Amatayakul 2007)

Vocabularies require terms to be evaluated for inclusion. Each term included in the vocabulary should have a unique meaning; however, it should be noted that synonyms are allowed. Terminologies, along with classification systems, are necessary to support the

EHR, PHR, safety, clinical trials, and population health reporting as well as quality reporting, biosurveillance, and reimbursement (Campbell and Giannangelo 2007). Because of the proprietary nature of terminologies as well as uncoordinated life cycles and a lack of standardization, they are currently unable to meet the current and future healthcare needs (Campbell and Giannangelo 2007). As a result, national and international initiatives are underway to overcome some of these obstacles.

Systematized Nomenclature of Medicine (SNOMED)

As stated previously, nomenclature refers to systems that identify the names used. The nomenclature system uses established rules to assign names. The most widely recognized nomenclature in healthcare is the **Systematized Nomenclature of Medicine (SNOMED)**. It was developed and maintained by the College of American Pathologists until recently when the responsibility was transitioned to the International Health Terminology Standards Development Organization. The current version is SNOMED Clinical Terms (SNOMED CT). The use of a nomenclature allows for comparison and aggregation of data (Giannangelo 2006).

SNOMED CT is a terminology that is designed to capture detailed clinical information, which then makes it possible to share and aggregate data. SNOMED is used for the EHR and for research, and clinical decisions. The information that SNOMED captures includes items such as diagnoses, procedures, signs, symptoms, and cause of injury. SNOMED CT has a concepts table that consists of 344,000 concepts, each of which has a unique meaning and format definitions. It also contains descriptions tables with more than 900,000 language descriptions or synonyms (LaTour and Eichenwald Maki 2006). This allows for flexibility in expressing clinical concepts. A relationships table contains over a million semantic relationships (Giannangelo 2006). These relationships are important to data retrieval. Figure 10.2 provides a short example of how clinical information is coded in SNOMED CT.

Logical Observation Identifiers Names and Codes (LOINC)

Logical Observation Identifiers Names and Codes (LOINC) is a laboratory vocabulary that is used to order and report laboratory tests and record clinical observations for use in patient care, outcomes management, and research (LOINC 2008). It is controlled by the Regenstrief Institute for Health Care, an international research organization. LOINC was created in 1994 to assist in the electronic transmission of laboratory data between laboratories, care providers, and third-party payers. LOINC was not intended to share all data collected about a laboratory test, but instead to identify test results. The standardization allows

Figure 10.2.   SNOMED CT working behind the scenes in an EHR

In the following excerpt from an electronic health record (EHR), a few of the applicable SNOMED CT codes are noted in parentheses to illustrate what SNOMED CT is doing behind the scenes. It is automatically identifying standard terms and tagging them for future references.

This 85-year- (258707000) old (70753007) female (248152002) was admitted via the emergency department (50849002 ED admission) from the nursing home (42665001) with shortness of breath (267036007), confusion (22544008 onset of confusion), and congestion (85804007). There was no history of (14792006) fever (386661006) or cough (49727002) noted. Patient also has a history of (392521001) senile dementia (15662003) and COPD (13645005)…

Prior to admission, the patient was on the following medications:

Prednisone (116602009), Lasix, Holdol (349874003), and Colace. Patient also has been on lorazepam 0.5 mg tablet (377147002) 2x a day as needed for anxiety (48694002). Patient is noted to have a vitamin C deficiency (76169001)…

Source: Giannangelo 2006

the results from multiple laboratories to be easily understood. The laboratory terms found in LOINC include blood chemistry, hematology, serology, and other specialized areas of clinical laboratories (Giannangelo 2006).

RxNorm

RxNorm is a vocabulary for medications developed by the National Library of Medicine (NLM), Veterans Administration, the Food and Drug Administration, and input from HL-7. It is nonproprietary and provides the standards for drug ingredients and strength as well as dose formats and relationships to other drugs. RxNorm is not used independently and is only available through the UMLS Metathesaurus (Giannangelo 2006).

Unified Medical Language System (UMLS)

Developed by the National Library of Medicine (NLM), the **Unified Medical Language System** (UMLS) is a database that catalogues bibliographic citations for biomedics (Giannangelo 2006). The UMLS catalogues more than 4,500 references into Index Medicus and MEDLINE and was developed to help improve search capabilities. The improvement in search capabilities improves with semantics that are organized in a hierarchical structure. Amatayakul (2007, 207) describes semantics as a "branch of linguistics dealing with the study of meaning, including the ways meaning is structured in language and how changes in meanings and form occur over time." Syntax is described by Amatayakul as "the study of the patterns of formation of sentences and phrase from words and of the rules for the formation of grammatical sentences in a language" (2007, 207). In other words, how words are sequenced can change the meaning of the phrase. For example, "appendicitis, ruled" out has a very different meaning than "rule out appendicitis." In the former, ruled out means that the condition was considered and eliminated as a possibility. In the latter, the condition is still under consideration. UMLS is a thesaurus of medical terms. It groups various terms according to concept, thus improving retrieval of information across multiple resources. Knowledge sources are used to help retrieve data across many databases. Knowledge sources are UMLS Metathesaurus, SPECIALIST Lexicon, and UMLS Semantic (Giannangelo 2006). UMLS Metathesaurus is used to convert the terms supplied by the user into the terms used by UMLS, thus improving search results. The UMLS Metathesaurus includes more than 60 vocabularies and standards. It retains the meanings, relationships, and other attributes of the original vocabulary system while adding information and identifying relationships not contained in its original vocabulary. This is used by information systems staff predominantly, but may also be used by librarians and other information management specialists. The UMLS SPECIALIST Lexicon contains biomedical terms. Each of these terms has information about how the word is formed, the sound of the term, and other information that describes the term. UMLS Semantic Network contains information on all UMLS Metathesaurus concepts and the relationships between them (Giannangelo 2006).

National Drug Codes

National drug codes (NDC) were developed by the Food and Drug Administration to act as a universal unique identifier for human drugs. The NDC identifies the labeler/vendor, product, and trade package size, as shown in table 10.1. This is one of the codes mandated for use by HIPAA. Each code is 10 digits and is divided into three sections. The first section of the NDC code identifies the company that manufactures, packages, and distributes the drug. The second section of the code identifies important information about the drug itself such as drug name, strength, form, and formulation for a particular firm. The third and final section identifies the package size (Giannangelo 2006).

MEDCIN

MEDCIN is a nomenclature and knowledge-based system. It was developed by Peter S. Goltra. It is now controlled by Medicomp Systems, Inc. It was designed to provide "an

Table 10.1.   Examples of NDC codes

Drug	NDC Code
Fluoxetine 100 mg Caps	00172-4363-70
Prenatal Plus Tab	0093-9111-01
Hydrocodone/APAP 7.5/500 mg Tab	00591-0385-05
Glycolax 3350 NF POW	62175-442-31
Flonase 0.05% Nasal Spray	00173-0453-01
Progesterone 600 mg Supp	51927-1046-00
Seraquel 100 mg Tab	00310-0271-10
Axert 12.5 mg Tab	00603-2213-32
Amitriptyline 25 mg TAB	00603-2213-32
Amoxicillin 400 mg/5 Susp	63304-0907-04

Source: LaTour and Eichenwald Maki 2006

intelligent clinical database for documentation by the clinician at the time of care" (Giannangelo 2006, 127), which allows it to be used for documentation in the EHR. MEDCIN includes 250,000 concepts that fall into the following categories: symptoms, history, physical examination, tests, diagnoses, and therapy. MEDCIN is unique in that it contains 68 million links between clinically related findings.

Mapping

To allow for interoperability, a crosswalk between the various terminologies must be created. This crosswalk is called **mapping** (Wilson 2007). An example of a map is to link the code for acne in ICD-9-CM to the code for acne in ICD-10-CM. Before the map can be created, there must be an understanding of how the data will be used, because the map must be consistent. LaTour and Eichenwald Maki state that mapping is frequently done through the use of categories. Examples of the categories are as follows:

- One-to-one: An exact match is made between the systems
- Narrow-to-broad: A more granular term in the starting system maps to a more general term in the receiving system
- Broad-to-narrow: A more general term in the starting system maps to a more granular term in the receiving system
- Unmappable: There is no matching into the receiving system (LaTour and Eichenwald Maki 2006, 337)

In order for this mapping to be performed correctly, individuals performing the mapping must have a complete understanding of how the data will be used. The HIM professional has this knowledge as well as an understanding of classification systems (Wilson 2007). This makes the HIM professional a qualified candidate for this job. Table 10.2 is an example of mapping between ICD-9-CM and ICD-10-CM.

Use cases are frequently used to create maps. According to Washington (2008, 60), **use cases** are "an extension of workflow analysis, an early and essential step in selecting or designing new health information technology." The use case is part of the information system design process. It describes how the user will interact with the system and what the system will do. Use cases are tools that provide very detailed information for programmers to use when developing the system. Use cases will be required for each of the processes in the EHR (Washington 2008).

Table 10.2.   Example: ICD-9-CM → ICD-10-CM

ICD-9-CM	Description	≈ =	ICD-10-CM	Description
			M25.141	Fistula, right hand
			M25.142	Fistula, left hand
719.84	Other specified disorders of joint, hand –calcification of joint –fistula of joint	≈ =	M25.149	Fistula, unspecified hand
			M25.841	Other specified joint disorders, right hand
			M25.842	Other specified joint disorders, left hand
			M25.849	Other specified joint disorders, unspecified hand

Source: Butler and Wilson 2006

Check Your Understanding 10.4

1. The most secure type of signature used in the EHR is:

   A. there is no difference in security between the types of signatures
   B. electronic signature
   C. digital signature
   D. digitized signature

2. ICD-9-CM is an example of a:

   A. nomenclature
   B. classification system
   C. vocabulary
   D. language

3. The nomenclature used in the EHR to capture detailed clinical information is called:

   A. DICOM
   B. UMLS
   C. LOINC
   D. SNOMED CT

4. Which of the following organizations is an SDO?

   A. ANSI
   B. HITSP
   C. CCHIT
   D. National Library of Medicine

5. The concept of a crosswalk between two terminologies is called

   A. interoperability
   B. granularity
   C. use cases
   D. mapping

Messaging Standards

Messaging standards may also be called interoperability standards or data exchange standards. The purpose of messaging standards is to support communications between information systems. With messaging standards, proprietary systems are able to talk to one another, allowing the exchange of data. Standards do this by mapping proprietary forms to other formats. Existing standards have allowed for flexibility, which has caused problems with the interoperability between systems (Amatayakul 2007). Figure 10.3 shows the various types of messaging standards used today.

The ANSI-Accredited Standards Committee X12-Insurance Subcommittee develops messaging standards for electronic data interchange (Amatayakul 2007). ANSI-ASCX12N was adopted by the HIPAA Transactions and Code Sets. This standard is the messaging standard for many of the transactions covered by HIPAA such as claims eligibility inquiry and response, claims status inquiry and response, and payment and remittance advice (Giannangelo 2006). ASTM International develops standards for security, record content, the continuity care record, and for the exchange of laboratory data (Abdelhak et al. 2007).

A number of messaging standards have been approved by the National Committee on Vital and Health Statistics (NCVHS). These standards include (Amatayakul 2007):

- Health Level 7 (HL7)
- Digital Imaging and Communications in Medicine (DICOM)
- National Council for Prescription Drug Programs

HL7 is the standard used in most applications; however, other standards have been developed for special purposes (Amatayakul 2007). For example, DICOM is used for medical imaging.

Health Level 7 (HL7)

HL7 is an SDO that is accredited by ANSI and specializes in standards for clinical and administrative data for the healthcare environment (Giannangelo 2006). According to the HL7 Web site, its mission is to provide "standards for interoperability that improve care delivery, optimize workflow, reduce ambiguity and enhance knowledge transfer among all of our stakeholders, including healthcare providers, government agencies, the vendor community, fellow SDOs and patients. In all of our processes we exhibit timeliness, scientific rigor and technical expertise without compromising transparency, accountability, practicality, or our willingness to put the needs of our stakeholders first" (HL7 2009). HL7 is the most common healthcare application level standards that assists in communication across information systems (Giannangelo 2006). HL7 transfers demographic data, orders, test results, history, and physical results (LaTour and Eichenwald Maki, 2006).

Figure 10.3.   Messaging standards

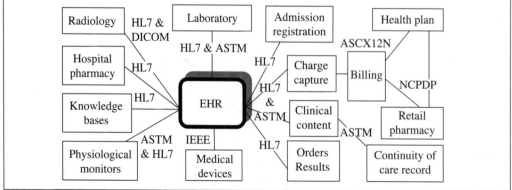

Copyright © 2008, Margret\A Consulting, LLC. Reprinted with permission.

The use of HL7 standards allows patient care information to be shared across computers while not changing the meaning of the information in the process. HL7 utilizes industry experts to advise and participate in the development of the standards. In addition to the messaging standards, HL7 creates other specific standards such as (Edwards 2008):

- Electronic Health Record System (EHR-S) functional model: EHR-S lists the functions that may be present in an EHR and supplies a common language for these functions. This functional model has hundreds of criteria and serves as the basis for CCHIT's EHR criteria.

- Clinical Context Object Workgroup (CCOW) Standard: This standard is for a single interface that allows the user to interact with one system even when accessing multiple systems.

HL7 is also working on standards on the PHR, clinical document requirements, and record management (Edwards 2008).

Digital Imaging and Communications in Medicine

Digital Imaging and Communications in Medicine (DICOM) standard retrieves images and other information from imaging equipment of a variety of different vendors. Areas covered by the standard include message exchange, data dictionary, data structure, and encoding. Although DICOM started out in diagnostic medical imaging, it has broadened to include specialties such as cardiology, dentistry, and radiology. The use of DICOM standards allows images to be transferred between systems from different vendors, ultimately allowing imaging in the picture archival and communication systems to share information with clinical information systems and the EHR (Giannangelo 2006).

National Council for Prescription Drug Programs

The **National Council for Prescription Drug Programs (NCPDP)** is a standard developed for and used by pharmacies and payers. These standards control data to be shared for new prescriptions, refills, and other communications between physicians and pharmacies. NCPDP is mandated by HIPAA for pharmacy reimbursement and insurance transactions (Giannangelo 2006).

Data Structures

Data structures refers to the data stored in the EHR and the way it is managed. Data structures include data sets, databases, data repositories, and data warehouses. Data structures control individual data elements such as formats and its valid characters, how data is stored, and how it can be manipulated.

Data Sets

Data sets are a group of data elements that are the minimum accepted level of information to be collected for a specific purpose along with uniform definitions (LaTour and Eichenwald Maki, 2006). The reason for the data set is to collect and report data in a standardized manner. Standardized data collection allows for comparisons and aggregate data. There are many data sets used in healthcare. Some of these are (Amatayakul 2007):

- Uniform Hospital Discharge Data Set (UHDDS)

- Uniform Ambulatory Care Data Set (UACDS)

- Minimum Data Set (MDS)

- Data Elements for Emergency Department Systems (DEEDS)

- Health Plan Employer Data and Information Set (HEDIS)
- Outcomes and Assessment Information Set (OASIS)
- ORYX

UHDDS is the data set for hospital discharge data in 34 states. UACDS is used for ambulatory care patient records. The MDS is used in long-term care for care and resident assessment protocols. It must be completed for each patient within 14 days of admission. DEEDS was developed for emergency departments and has been incorporated into LOINC and HL7. OASIS was developed by the Department of Health and Human Services for home health data collection. HEDIS was developed by the National Committee for Quality Assurance (NCQA) for managed care accreditation data collection. ORYX was developed by Joint Commission to study outcomes and healthcare performance. The purpose of data sets is to allow comparisons across healthcare facilities (Giannangelo 2006). For a full discussion of datasets, please see Chapter 3.

Database

A **database** is defined as "a collection of data carefully organized to be of value to the user" (Austin and Boxerman 2003, 127). Databases are an important part of the EHR. The EHR is partially a collection of databases because the EHR is made up of many information systems. This collection of databases frequently results in duplication of data and because of a lack of interoperability; they may be unable to communicate with each other. These issues can be overcome with a data repository or data warehouse. For a full discussion of databases, refer to Chapter 4.

Data Repository

A **data repository** is a database that is developed in an open format, thus allowing the facility to use it for multiple systems (Amatayakul 2007). This allows the facility to access data stored in various systems to be retrieved from one source. The data repository is updated by the various systems in real time, thus providing access to the most current information available. For a full discussion of the data repository, refer to Chapter 4.

Data Warehouse

A **data warehouse** is a database containing data from other source systems in the healthcare facility such as laboratory information system, hospital information system, or radiology information system. The data warehouse is not updated in real time, but is better formatted to allow for querying and data analysis. These secondary data are then used for executive decision support purposes. Analyses may include research and health-related management additional to the executive queries. A data mart is a subset of the data warehouse. It can be used for specialized purposes such as research. The data contained within the data warehouse may be used for revenue management, outcomes management, operations management, research, patient care, and other purposes. For a full discussion of data warehouse, refer to Chapter 4.

EHR Tools

The EHR utilizes a multitude of tools in its presentation layer. The **presentation layer** controls screen layout, data entry, and data retrieval. The flexibility of the presentation layer is what allows the various healthcare providers to manipulate it (Amatayakul 2007). This flexibility allows users to control the screens to meet their needs. The EHR also makes it possible for users to graph information to identify trends over time. Other tools in the EHR ease process and function in areas such as data retrieval, alerts, and data entry.

Data Retrieval

When developing the EHR, the healthcare facility should understand how the data is to be used to ensure that it will be present and in the desired format for retrieval. Data retrieval should also take into account printing format. Because of privacy issues, the EHR should also allow for identifying information to be removed automatically. This process is called deidentification. For further discussion of data retrieval, please see Chapter 6.

Graphical User Interface

GUI technology is used to navigate through an information system. Tools such as icons, colors, buttons, menus, and other tools are used to help make the system user friendly. For example, an icon containing an image of a printer would notify the user that clicking it will trigger printing the document. A poorly developed GUI can confuse and hinder use of the system, leading to frustration for the user (Williams 2006).

Alerts and Reminders

Alerts are one of the key benefits to the EHR that can help reduce errors and improve the quality of care rendered. This topic was discussed in detail earlier in the chapter.

Data Entry

Data entry is important to the EHR. Data entry can take a lot of time, and errors can cause mistakes that could be detrimental to the patient. Because of this, a lot of care should be taken to improve data quality and speed data entry. A full discussion of data quality is presented in Chapter 3. Typing, voice recognition, transcription, and other means of data entry can be used to get data into the system. When entering data, unstructured and structured data—or a combination of these—may be used.

Unstructured Data Entry

Unstructured data is also called narrative or free text data. It is usually entered using a keyboard, but other methods such as dictation or voice recognition may also be used (Amatayakul 2007). Unstructured data allows the data entered to be more specific and detailed for each patient than structured data. In these fields, the provider could enter a patient's history of present illness, level of compliance with medical regimen, or anything else not captured in the structured data. The level of detail is much greater with unstructured data because the choices designed in the system are not limited. The user can use his or her own words. A disadvantage of unstructured data is that it is not beneficial for reporting purposes. Because unstructured data does not have a data model, it will be difficult for the system to identify and gather desired information provided in a report.

Structured Data Entry

Drop-down lists, check boxes, radio buttons, and other forms of controlled data entry are used in structured data entry. The choices must be clearly defined, comprehensive, and applicable. Use of structured data entry allows quickness, but there is a learning curve in the beginning while users get familiar with the choices and the GUI (Amatayakul 2007). For example, when entering a patient's gender, the options would be male, female, and unknown; or, if the data being entered were the number of dilation centimeters for an obstetric patient, the choices would range from 0 to 10.

Structured data entry is frequently used for physician EHRs, with the menus developed specifically for the physicians' medical or surgical specialty. Because it is easy for the user to overlook entry, defaults should not populate an entry but rather should be left blank, forcing the user to address the field. The EHR should be able to convert structured data into a narrative format (Amatayakul 2007). An example would be structured data of "no tobacco use" and "no alcohol use" converts to "Patient denies the use of tobacco and alcohol". One of the advantages of structured data is that it can easily be used for reporting purposes. Data can also be graphed, allowing for trending. An example of the use of graphing is the ability to trend blood sugar or blood pressure levels over time. Figure 10.4 shows an example of a structured data entry template.

Figure 10.4.   Example of a structured data entry template

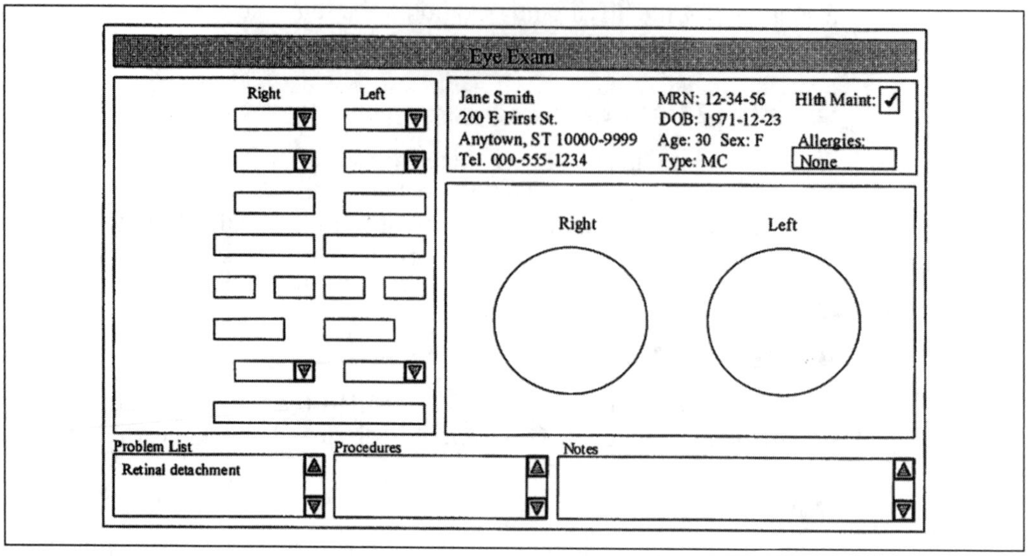

Copyright © 2006, Margret\A Consulting, LLC. Reprinted with permission.

Template-Based Entry

Template-based entry is a cross between free text and structured data entry. The user is able to pick and choose data that are entered frequently, thus requiring the entry of data that change from patient to patient (Amatayakul 2007). Templates can be customized to meet the needs of the organization as data needs change by physician specialty, patient type (surgical/medical/newborn), disease, and other classifications of patients. Templates may be used to cut and paste words from one note and place into another note, thus saving time. This option should be used judiciously, however, because the wrong data could be copied and/or pasted into the wrong patient's record. All templates have predefined parameters that are checked as data are entered. They can check for logic, but not accuracy (Amatayakul 2007). For example, templates can prevent a data entry that shows a patient has a temperature of 200°F, but would not catch entering 100.4°F instead of 100.8°F. Also, too many checks can slow down the system, so templates should be used judiciously.

Natural Language Processing

Natural language processing (NLP) converts unstructured text into a structured format. This requires sophisticated computer software to separate the narrative into little packets. These packets can be used for storage, analysis, and retrieval. This is not a required function of the EHR, but will be valuable for research. The technology is still being developed. Please see Chapter 14 for additional information (Amatayakul 2007).

Legal Issues

There are a number of legal issues facing the EHR. Some of these issues are being addressed as laws and regulations catch up with technology. The EHR must be designed so that it is admissible in court. State laws vary as to what is and is not acceptable in a court of law regarding EHRs. Healthcare providers frequently receive subpoenas requesting the production of the medical record. Data in the EHR will be used to meet the requirements contained in the subpoena. The documentation provided to the court must be in a useable format, not just screen prints or other unformatted data. The subpoena may require the production of audit trails, decision support rules, clinical guidelines, and other information that was never an issue with the paper medical record. A number of other legal issues that must be addressed are retention, storage, security, privacy, signatures, and data quality. These topics are discussed throughout this book.

EHR Data

Data in the EHR are similar to the paper medical record; because the chief complaint, review of systems, patient demographics, and other data elements are present, it would still be subject to UHDDS and other data sets. The EHR, however, allows these data to be viewed in multiple formats. For example, the patient's temperature can be viewed as individual elements, a line graph, or other format. Data collected are controlled by data standards discussed earlier in this chapter and data sets discussed in Chapter 4.

Interoperability

The NCVHS (2000, 8) defines **interoperability** as "the ability of one computer system to exchange data with another computer system." Interoperability is divided into three levels: basic, functional, and semantic. With basic interoperability, a computer can send data to another computer but the receiving computer is unable to interpret the data. Functional interoperability defines the structure of messages so that the receiving computer can interpret the data. The most advanced level, semantic interoperability, allows the information to be used in a meaningful way. Interoperability will require uniform standards for data capture, storage, and transmission. Data cannot be shared and stored without ensuring data integrity, privacy, and security (Heubusch 2006).

Transition Period—Hybrid Record

The conversion to an EHR does not happen overnight. Throughout the system and implementation life cycle, the healthcare organization will have to manage paper records, microfilms, scanned images, and the EHR. Because the health information is fragmented, there may be some risk to the quality of patient care. The fragmentation comes from the information being on several different sources such as paper, microfilm, and the EHR. The facility must have a means of pulling all information together when it is needed.

In order to make paper medical records available, facilities have provided many different options. Some facilities back scan paper records into the EHR while others manually enter in basic information so that it is quickly available for patient care. Some even keep the paper records as is and maintain the same system and processes until the EHR is fully functional. The AHIMA e-HIM Workgroup on Hybrid Records defines the **hybrid record** as a system with functional components that include both paper and electronic documents and use both manual and electronic processes (AHIMA e-HIM Work Group on Health Information in a Hybrid Environment 2003b, 1). Hospitals need policies and procedures to define the sources of where the components of the patient's health information are and will be for easy and accurate access, use, and disclosure. Some facilities do this by recording the presence of additional information in the EHR (AHIMA e-HIM Work Group on Health Information in a Hybrid Environment 2003a).

Some facilities print out documents from the electronic sources to compile the contents of the legal health record. This practice prevents the facility from realizing the benefits of the electronic system. Unnecessary printing is not only costly, but complicates operational issues in managing the hybrid records; facilities frequently establish policies that discourage superfluous printing of documents.

Impact on HIM

The EHR will not eliminate the HIM department; however, the functions performed by the HIM department will undergo significant changes. Issues facing the HIM department in a hybrid environment include authoring and printing issues, and access and disclosure issues, for example. Table 10.3 illustrates differences in HIM functions in the paper, hybrid, and EHR environments.

Table 10.3.   Differences in HIM functions in the paper, hybrid, and EHR environments

Function	Paper Health Record	Hybrid Paper-Electronic Health Record	Electronic Health Record
Abstracting data elements	Manual or data entered into computerized system	Function could be minimized due to initiation of structured data collection through online forms and data entry templates for documentation at the point of care. HIM involvement needed for the process of designing and revising forms to meet data collection, regulatory, and bylaw needs.	Function could be completely eliminated if automated data capture implemented (except for free-form documentation, such as narrative notes, dictations, and natural language processing). HIM staff may be qualified to perform data analysis and data administration or verification and reporting. Documentation templates may be developed to conform with state, federal, tribal, and local laws.
Admission and discharge processing and reconciliation	Accounting for records to ensure 100-percent retrieval of cases for filing and coding; function performed by clerks.	Accounting for paper records to ensure 100-percent retrieval of cases for filing portions of paper record, scanning, and coding; function performed by clerks or scanning staff.	Accounting for paper records received from external sources for scanning; function performed by scanning staff. Online reconciliation of cases for revenue stream; function performed by coders.
Adoption record change	Minimal	Minimal	Minimal
Analysis (or deficiency analysis)	Manual assessment for compliance with regulatory and internal medical staff bylaw requirements.	Assessment rules and rules to force completion will begin to be developed, with some analyst work reduction. Opportunity to reallocate staff to preadmission analysis via work queues (e.g., ensuring H&P is adequate prior to surgery or MD orders complete for nursing home or rehabilitation facilities). Physicians will receive electronic notification of incomplete items in the health record.	Function should be minimal because of automated rules. In the absence of rules, HIM staff will need to check documents (e.g., handwritten documents, voice recognition, dictations). Physicians will receive electronic notification of incomplete items in the health record.
Assembly of paper record	Manual	Manual for remaining paper documents	Staff may be redeployed for document preparation, indexing, imaging, and quality control.
Backup, downtime, and recovery processes	Paper-based charts used	Organizations must develop a plan for worst-case scenarios when the EHR is unavailable; HIM staff should coordinate daily system disaster plan (e.g., printing of key documents, maintenance backup, paper systems, coordination of data entry or scanning of key data elements after unplanned down times). Necessary forms revert to paper processes and must be readily available. Staff must be trained in their use.	Same as hybrid state. The backup system could be a CD with appropriate documents that can be accessed from a local drive rather than the network. Downtime processes could include use of PDAs or tablet PCs with uploading of data when the system has been recovered.

Table 10.3.   **Differences in HIM functions in the paper, hybrid, and EHR environments** *(continued)*

Function	Paper Health Record	Hybrid Paper-Electronic Health Record	Electronic Health Record
Birth and death certificate preparation	Conduct interviews, collect data, type, fill out paper forms or electronic submissions, and obtain signatures required by state law.	Clerical staff may continue to abstract and collect data for vital records. However, state or county laws may mandate use of an electronic data submission process. Electronic data submission processes may not require validation by provider. Birth facility may continue to prepare and provide a signed paper document to parents.	Same as hybrid state
Charge description master (CDM) administration	Function is moving into the realm of HIM department to ensure accurate and timely codes and updates.	HIM staff ensure accurate and timely codes and updates and begin to link codes to online-structured documentation. Staff test and verify mapped codes.	HIM staff ensure accurate codes and maintenance updates are performed on time and continually link codes to online-structured documentation. Staff test and validate mapped codes and application software. CDM will be linked such that there is notification when changes occur.
Charge ticket verification	Some HIM departments manually verify all charges on charge ticket against documentation.	HIM staff validate mapped codes, some manually and some online based on location of documentation. Super bills may be created by physicians or specialty clinics and are maintained and updated on a regular basis.	Computer-assisted coding will continue to require validation of structured documentation against unmapped codes and validation of unstructured documentation against charges. If computerized physician order entry and medication administration record are implemented, this could become completely automated.
Coding and documentation training for all providers (physicians, nurse practitioners, physician assistants)	Provider training for documentation and relationship to coding is rudimentary, generally focused on specific providers or disciplines where reimbursement is a concern. Query process for providers for additional documentation of information is typically done on paper.	Same as paper record	Number of positions will increase as traditional coding positions decrease. Function is critical to ensuring that charge description master and documentation templates correspond to internal and external reporting requirements as well as billing. HIM staff should educate clinicians on changes and develop and maintain templates and charge capture process to ensure accuracy of coding and documentation. Query process for providers requesting additional documentation or information will be automated.
Coding CPT	Manual assignment using books or encoders, often done outside HIM department.	Transition to coder-managed chargemaster would eliminate need for manual code assignment. Auditing function will still be needed to ensure charges are entered for all documented services rendered.	Coding may be automated. Validation of charge capture against documentation still required. Auditing or coder intervention for ad-hoc documentation required. Reduced staffing expected.
Coding: E/M and physicians at teaching hospitals	Manual	Manual	Function will change focus from coding all procedures to validation and comparison of document and computer-suggested codes.

(continued on next page)

Table 10.3.   Differences in HIM functions in the paper, hybrid, and EHR environments *(continued)*

Function	Paper Health Record	Hybrid Paper-Electronic Health Record	Electronic Health Record
Coding ICD-9-CM, ICD-10-CM, ICD-10-PCS	Use of books or encoders. Paper documents are the source of information.	Function moves toward automated encoding as online medical record systems support functions that are computerized.	Computer-assisted coding could change coding to become more of an auditing function to ensure full capture of all codes, especially from free-form sources such as natural language processing; SNOMED-CT use adopted for data reporting and research. As clinical care is documented by providers in an EHR, SNOMED-CT codes are automatically applied, and mapping tables are used to identify related codes in another terminology. As rules-based maps are developed for multiple-use cases and become increasingly sophisticated, the level of human review at the individual code level will diminish and human roles will primarily be focused on the development and maintenance (including quality control) of maps for a variety of use cases and the development of algorithmic translation and concept representation. Availability of computer-aided coding applications would relieve the shortage of expert coders and enable them to perform other critical data management roles in the electronic HIM environment. ICD-10 coding will be important as a global tool.
Data quality, integrity, and reconciliation processes (including EHR and other specialized application work queue management)	Verification of computer reports and statistics against paper record and reports.	HIM staff begin online reconciliation of autogenerated reports and monitor parts of the EHR such as inboxes and failed interface report transfers (e.g., documents from transcription or laboratory systems that fail to post in the EHR).	Function will fully transition from paper verification to computer-based reconciliation of EHR functions and work queues. Patient-entered data will include entering results of self-monitored clinical data (such as daily blood pressure), registration data verification, and registration for appointments and tests. Insurance verification will be completed automatically during the preregistration process. Patients without coverage will automatically be directed to a financial counselor.

Table 10.3.   Differences in HIM functions in the paper, hybrid, and EHR environments *(continued)*

Function	Paper Health Record	Hybrid Paper-Electronic Health Record	Electronic Health Record
Data reporting and interpretation	Ad-hoc and routine reporting	Function will begin transition to ad-hoc reports and data mining. Methods will be required for tracking inception, revisions, and deletions of specific online-structured data fields that are a component of the EHR.	Data interpretation and data mining skills will be new focus. Healthcare organizations will need staff that understand coded data and classification systems for efficient data mining, accurate reporting, and interpretation as well as development of metadata definitions. Relational database management skills will be needed. The healthcare world will move toward disease management, where the patient is managed across the healthcare continuum and health problems are identified more quickly. Healthcare data will be used as the basis for developing treatment protocols and critical pathways for disease management.
Denial management	Manual	May include both manual and electronic follow-up	Activity could be minimized if improvements are made in health plan and benefits validation programs or claims processing programs and charge description master software become more sophisticated. Audits may be done virtually. With electronic provision of required documents, turnaround time should decrease.
Document and records management	Primary focus is paper medical record and some required logs and registers.	As focus moves away from paper medical record management, time shifted to assume organization-wide document management functions, including processes to eliminate shadow medical records, radiographic images, photographs, patient videotapes, business document imaging, image reproduction, retention, storage, access planning, record organization, and data collection.	Same as hybrid record
Document identification	Often manual; a key component of filing paper.	Function will transform to barcoding, indexing methods, or optical character recognition as appropriate for the electronic systems implemented (such as document imaging). The process must ensure correct posting including date of service, correct patient, or document type.	Process expands from the hybrid state to all documents in the EHR. There should be monitoring to ensure correct posting of electronic documents.

(continued on next page)

Table 10.3. **Differences in HIM functions in the paper, hybrid, and EHR environments** (*continued*)

Function	Paper Health Record	Hybrid Paper-Electronic Health Record	Electronic Health Record
Document preparation, indexing, and scanning	Document repair only; performed as part of record assembly.	Function requires manual preparation of documents, except those that are COLD fed (come directly into the EHR electronically). Decisions must be translated into policy and procedure for which documents are to be scanned.	Generally this function includes only paper documents received from external sources. This will continue as long as paper documents need to be part of the EHR. It should decrease as interoperability allows more document exchange electronically.
Documentation improvement training	Minimal except for coding training. It has increased with programs such as DRG Assurance or through correct E&M coding initiatives	Same as paper record	Function will decrease as structured forms or data fields are designed to capture regulatory and billing needs. HIM staff should ensure rules and structured data fields meet regulatory needs. Automated tools will allow online queries of and by providers. Online tools should provide training 24 hours a day, seven days a week through real-time feedback.
DRG or documentation auditing program	Manual	Function consists of a combination of manual review of paper records and review of electronic documentation.	Daily concurrent follow-up should be minimized as templates and rules are implemented. Initial review will be necessary if the primary document is the unstructured H&P. This could be performed remotely.
Filing records	Manual	Some manual filing may remain through the transition state.	Function eliminated as move to EHR is completed.
Filing reports, concurrent (charting)	Manual	If printed record is maintained, some printing and filing will be necessary. But activity will be reduced as documents become available electronically.	Function eliminated. Staff can be redeployed to prepare documents for scanning, indexing, and other activities in that process.
Filing reports, retrospective	Manual	Manual for paper record, but potentially only key documents during transition to fully electronic health record.	New function will be resolution of electronic documents and reports that cannot be matched to a record. The frequency of this activity is dependent on system activity and mismatches.
Form and template design	Function includes standardization of data elements, placement (format), logical flow for data capture.	Function includes screen design and data field definition and print formats as well as development of standard online data collection procedures and data dictionary definitions. Processes for requesting and implementing new forms will be standardized to optimize use of existing data.	Same as hybrid record. Data dictionary will encompass all medical documentation.
Imaging	Minimal	Function will significantly increase during transition to hybrid state and then to a fully electronic health record.	With most documents online, imaging will be a function to capture temporary forms and external records only. HIM advisory role will develop for imaging acquisitions and implementation for business records. Imaging may become minimal as external documents become available electronically.

Table 10.3.   Differences in HIM functions in the paper, hybrid, and EHR environments *(continued)*

Function	Paper Health Record	Hybrid Paper-Electronic Health Record	Electronic Health Record
Master patient index (MPI) maintenance	Manual or electronic, including card file and online systems; may be limited to HIM applications.	Function will expand to system-wide database coordination for integrated EHR. For reasons of patient safety, dedicated MPI reconciliation staff may be required to maintain up-to-the-minute patient identifiers. Roles will likely expand to person identity management (guarantors). Number of disparate systems with patient information will increase the number of staff dedicated to this function. Number of staff will also be influenced by enterprise medical record number needs for integrated health systems. Staff will monitor medical record number and correct source documents with accurate number.	Positive patient identification at the point of registration may reduce staff dedicated to this function, but this depends on the size of immigrant and transient populations. Population predictions for the next 25 years forecast that immigrant populations will continue to have larger families, so there will be continued MPI challenges, especially in the pediatric population. Computer algorithmic scripts will need to be implemented that run on a concurrent basis to identify duplicate registrations (or possible duplicates). Pictures of patients may be included in the EHR to ensure identification.
Ongoing record review	Manual	Function will extend to paper and online records.	Function should decrease with use of templates, alerts, and reminders. It will likely be based on exception reports for items designated for review using autogenerated reports for review. Focus will shift to follow-up as reporting becomes routine.
Reconciliation of inboxes and other online files	Does not exist	A concurrent monitoring program of all systems concurrently should be developed, and HIM staff should perform reconciliation to ensure system files are complete and accurate.	Same as hybrid record
Record completion process	Manual	As electronic signatures are implemented, completion could be accomplished remotely.	Rules will be in place for automated monitoring of unsigned reports, monitoring of unreviewed results, and missing reports.
Registries, specialized (cancer, cardiac, PICU, trauma, Alzheimer's)	Manual or computerized	HIM staff should be able to gather data from the EHR if rules are implemented identifying cancer cases requiring physician staging. Staff may continue to submit paper to state registries until they are able to accept data electronically.	HIM staff may continue to submit paper abstracts depending on state registry computerization. Staff could fill out abstracts online and submit electronic data transfer from health facility data repository or warehouse to state system. Data will be coded in SNOMED-CT or ICD-10 so information can be translated in a global environment.
Release of information for continuity of care	Manual	Manual for caregivers without remote access or without privileges.	Protocols will be developed to provide electronic versions of information that can be shared as appropriate. This could be made available as a read-only version or placed in a queue with a specific date by which it is no longer accessible.

(continued on next page)

Table 10.3.   Differences in HIM functions in the paper, hybrid, and EHR environments *(continued)*

Function	Paper Health Record	Hybrid Paper-Electronic Health Record	Electronic Health Record
Release of information, other	Manual	Manual, but will begin process of identifying methods to allow access to both paper and electronic record.	HIM staff will continue to assist external sources needing access to PHI through batching individual or groups of records, setting up and monitoring work queues, and tracking disclosures. Depending on state law, organizations may be able to eliminate paper records for legal purposes (e.g., court) and provide a view that is certified as a legal copy using an electronic signature.
Release of information to patients	Manual	Function may continue to be manual. There may be new responsibilities assisting patients with access to their information through a secure Web site or portal.	HIM staff will continue to assist patients to access records through Web site as well as in paper for those without computer access. New process of assisting patients moving data from the main medical record to the personal health record will emerge. Staff will continue to assist court system and other external requests needing certified copies. Paper copies may continue to be generated but should be reduced as interoperability progresses and patients are able to access EHRs. Electronic signatures may be developed that signify a view as certified for legal purposes.
Retrieving records	Manual	There will be reduced record pulling as records are scanned or online documents become available, but function will be needed for historical files not yet scanned (if there is a decision to scan old files). Physicians may be asked to identify information from paper charts that should be scanned to eliminate the need to pull same paper chart at a future date.	Function eliminated except for historical files maintained in paper or on microform.
Revenue stream management (DNFB, charge entry, provider completion of documentation; organization of follow-up efforts)	Manual	Function will include more online management through computer-generated reports using logic rules.	The revenue cycle should be managed completely online.

Table 10.3.   Differences in HIM functions in the paper, hybrid, and EHR environments *(continued)*

Function	Paper Health Record	Hybrid Paper-Electronic Health Record	Electronic Health Record
Security, clinical access by users to the health record	Manual	Function will be performed manually and online through the use of role-based, context or individual access rights to clinical information. There will be increased emphasis on auditing access history to ensure adherence to policies.	Routine auditing and monitoring of access history will be in place.
Statistics	Manual	Function will be performed manually, though some statistics will be produced through automated reporting tools.	Function will include increased use of dashboard and other types of automatically generated statistical reports.
Transcription, natural language processing, direct charting by clinicians	Manual	Addition of processes such as natural language processing to support creation of the EHR will begin. HIM roles include training staff, system administration, development of templates, monitoring accuracy, and a new role for transcriptionists as document editors.	There is potential for reduced transcription staff due to use of natural language processing (NLP), direct charting, and point-and-click charting by clinicians. There will be a potential of increasing the number of typed documents and shifting available transcriptionists to NLP editing or other situations in which structured notes may not be appropriate.

Source: Tegan et al. 2005

Transcription is a very labor-intensive process. The EHR decreases the dependence on transcription as providers more often perform data entry into the EHR, and the system can create discharge summaries and other documents automatically from data entered into the system.

Release of information traditionally has been a slow process because the paper medical record had to be retrieved, copied or faxed, and then refiled. With the EHR, a few keystrokes will print or fax the document(s) needed to fulfill requests.

Record processing varies widely by facility, but generally includes assembly, analysis, and chart completion. The assembly process is eliminated completely with the implementation of the EHR because there is no need to organize paper documents. Dependent on organizational policy and quality levels, the analyst may or may not have to verify that all pages belong to the same patient, which will reduce the time needed for analysis. Finally, the system will not allow an entry to be made without a signature, thus reducing the number of deficient charts.

In a hybrid record environment, paper records do not cease to exist immediately with the advent of the EHR but rather the paper records disappear over time. The file room will ultimately be eliminated as the existing paper records are destroyed according to the retention schedule or the records are scanned into the EHR. For a discussion of disposal of electronic data, please see Chapter 12.

These changes do not signal the end of the HIM department or the HIM profession; rather, this is only the beginning. It is the knowledge and skill set of the HIM professional that is needed to maintain and manage data quality, evaluate the system, evaluate standards, perform project management, and more. The HIM profession as we know it will change with some tasks being eliminated, others changed, and still others created (Tegan et al. 2005).

Check Your Understanding 10.5

1. Which of the following standards is the messaging standard used in most information systems?

   A. DICOM
   B. NCPDP
   C. ICD-9-CM
   D. HL7

2. DICOM is an example of a:

   A. data content standard
   B. vocabulary standard
   C. classification system
   D. messaging standard

3. Which of the following is a database that is not updated in real time?

   A. EHR
   B. Data repository
   C. Relational database
   D. Data warehouse

4. Check boxes is a method of data entry used in:

   A. structured data entry
   B. unstructured data entry
   C. narrative data entry
   D. all types of data entry

5. The term used to describe a medical record that is partially online and partially paper-based is:

   A. interoperability
   B. use case
   C. hybrid record
   D. NLP

References

Abdelhak, M., S. Grostick, M.A. Hanken, E. Jacobs. 2007. *Health Information: Management of a Strategic Resource*. St. Louis, MO: Saunders Elsevier.

AHIMA e-HIM Work Group on Health Information in a Hybrid Environment. 2003a. Complete Medical Record in a Hybrid EHR Environment: Part II: Managing Access and Disclosure.

AHIMA e-HIM Work Group on Health Information in a Hybrid Environment. 2003b. Complete Medical Record in a Hybrid EHR Environment: Part III: Authorship and Printing the Health Record.

Amatayakul, M.S. 2007. *Electronic Health Records: A Practical Guide for Professionals and Organizations*. Chicago: AHIMA.

American Health Information Management Association. 2008a. Data Content Standards: Part and Parcel of Data Integrity Management. *AHIMA Advantage* 12(2):1, 3–5.

American Health Information Management Association. 2008b. Survey seeks definitive look at EHR adoption. http://journal.ahima.org/2008/08/04/survey-seeks-definitive-look-at-ehr-adoption/.

American Hospital Association. 2007. Continued progress: Hospital use of information technology. http://www.aha.org/aha/content/2007/pdf/070227-continuedprogress.pdf.

American National Standards Institute. 2009. Standards activities overview. http://www.ansi.org/standards_activities/overview/overview.aspx?menuid=3.

Ash, J.S. and D.W. Bates. 2004. Factors and forces affecting EHR system adoption: Report of a 2004 ACMI discussion. http://www.jamia.org/cgi/content/full/12/1/8.

Austin, C.J. and S.B. Boxerman. 2003. *Information Systems for Healthcare Management.* Chicago: Health Administration Press.

Butler, R. and P. Wilson. 2006. Navigating Uncharted Territory: Mapping ICD-9-CM to ICD-10-CM and ICD-10-PCS. *Proceedings of the American Health Information Management Association's 78th National Convention and Exhibit.*

Campbell, K.E. and K. Giannangelo. 2007. Language barrier: Getting past the classifications and terminologies roadblock. *Journal of AHIMA* 78(2):44–48.

Davis, K, M. M.M, Doty, K. Shea, and K. Stremikis. 2009. Health information technology and physician perceptions of quality of care and satisfaction. *Health Policy.* http://www.sciencedirect.com/science?_ob=ArticleURL&_udi=B6V8X-4V11H9V-1&_user=10&_rdoc=1&_fmt=&_orig=search&_sort=d&view=c&_acct=C000050221&_version=1&_urlVersion=0&_userid=10&md5=73aac9799cae03ba04cbf2f534256b99.

Department of Health and Human Services. 2009a. American Health Information Community. http://healthit.hhs.gov/portal/server.pt?open=512&objID=1199&parentname=CommunityPage&parentid=11&mode=2&in_hi_userid=10882&cached=true.

Department of Health and Human Services. 2009b. American Health Information Community. http://healthit.hhs.gov/portal/server.pt?open=512&objID=1253&&PageID=15692&mode=2&in_hi_userid=10732&cached=true.

Edwards, W. 2008. Standards development and HIM: HL7's IT standards work and its uses in health information management. *Journal of AHIMA* 79(7):58–59.

Englebardt, S. and R. Nelson. 2002. *Health Care Informatics: An Interdisciplinary Approach.* St. Louis, MO: Moseby.

Giannangelo, K., ed. 2006. *Healthcare Code Sets, Clinical Terminologies, and Classification Systems.* Chicago: AHIMA.

Hamilton, B. 2009. *Electronic Health Records.* Boston, MA: McGraw-Hill Higher Education.

Health Information Technology Standards Panel. 2008. Program of work. http://www.hitsp.org/.

Health Level 7. 2009. What is HL7? http://www.hl7.org/about/hl7about.htm.

Heubusch, K. 2006. Interoperability: What it means, why it matters. *Journal of AHIMA* 77(1):26–30.

Howrey, L. 2008. Weighing the Stark Laws exceptions. *Journal of AHIMA* 79(8):30–32.

Kohn, D. 2009. How information technology supports virtual HIM departments. *Journal of AHIMA* 80(3): Web extra.

LaTour, K M. and S. Eichenwald Maki. 2006. *Health Information Management: Concepts, Principles, and Practice.* Chicago: AHIMA.

LOINC. 2008. Logical Observation Identifiers Names and Codes. http://www.loinc.org/.

National Committee on Vital and Health Statistics. 2000. *Report to the Secretary of the U.S. Department of Health and Human Services on Uniform Data Standards for Patient Medical Record Information as required by the Administrative Simplification Provisions of the Health Insurance Portability and Accountability Act of 1996.* http:www.ncvhs.hhs.gov/hipaa000706.pdf.

National eHealth Collaborative. 2009. http://www.nationalehealth.org.

Quinsey, C.A. 2005. CCR—Not an EHR. *Journal of AHIMA* 76(3):58–59, 61. http://library.ahima.org/xpedio/groups/secure/documents/ahima/bok1_026061.hcsp?dDocName=bok1_026061.

Robert Woods Johnson Foundation. 2008. Physician adoption of electronic health records still extremely low, but medicine may be at a tipping point. http://www.rwjf.org/qualityequality/product.jsp?id=31632.

Rollins, G. 2007. Unwrapping data standards. *Journal of AHIMA* 78(1):25–29.

Sanderson, S.M. 2009. *Electronic Health Records for Allied Health Careers.* Boston, MA: McGraw-Hill Higher Education.

Tegan, A., et al. 2005. Practice brief: The EHR's impact on HIM functions. *Journal of AHIMA* 76(5):56C–H.

Washington, L. 2008. Understanding Use Cases. *Journal of AHIMA* 79(2):60–61.

Williams, A. 2006. Design for better data: How software and users interact onscreen matters to data quality. *Journal of AHIMA* 77(2):56–60.

Wilson, P.S. 2007. What mapping and modeling means to the HIM professional. *Perspectives in Health Information Management* 4:2. http://library.ahima.org/xpedio/groups/publicdocuments/ahima/bok1-033815.pdf#page%3D2.

Chapter 11
Speech Recognition

Objectives

- Identify the history of speech recognition technology from its earliest beginnings until now and how this is integrated into the computerized health record.

- Compare and contrast the differences between front-end and back-end speech recognition technology from the health information management (transcription) viewpoint.

- Explain some of the benefits of using speech recognition technology when coupled with the computerized health record for clinical documentation.

- Discuss what problems could arise with dictation and editing with speech recognition if the dictator did not use basic key recommendations according to the *ASTM International's E2344 Standard* Guide.

- Explain the process of dictation by the dictator in front-end speech recognition as well as the back-end process of editing by the transcriptionist.

- Provide an example of a bigram in the language model when building the vocabulary in speech recognition technology software.

Key Terms

Artificial neural networks (ANN)

Back-end speech recognition (BESR)

Bigram

Continuous speech recognition

Discrete speech

Front-end speech recognition (FESR)

Hidden Markov model

Interactive voice response system

Key-word spotting

Macro

Medical transcriptionists (MTs)

Natural language processing technology

Quadgram

Semantics

Speaker dependent

Speech recognition technology (SRT)

Syntax

Template

Trigram

Turnaround time (TAT)

VoiceXML (VXML)

Introduction

The computerized record and the electronic health record may be thought of as wonderful documentation tools. Speech recognition, also referred to as voice recognition, technology allows the replacement of written or data entry text with the human voice entry. Voice recognition is a software package that uses the human voice as the medium for input. Since it was first introduced back in the late 1980s, this technology has made vast technological improvements. Originally viewed as a new "gadget," voice recognition was not well received by physicians. Over the years and many enhancements later, this technology is now one that can be used as a method of input for computerized records with far better results. This chapter will explore the advantages and disadvantages of SRT, starting with the history of the technology and through the capabilities of the technology now as used with the Internet and XML language.

Definition

Voice or **speech recognition technology (SRT)** by definition is the "technology that converts spoken words to machine-readable input" (AHIMA and MTIA Joint Task Force on Standards Development 2008, 18). The software programs used in SRT are "trained" to recognize the user's voice and translate spoken language into typed text. There are basically two types of SRT: the front-end speech recognition (FESR) and the back-end speech recognition (BESR). FESR is "the specific use of SRT in an environment where the recognition process occurs in real time (or near real time) as dictation takes place" (AHIMA and MTIA Joint Task Force on Standards Development 2008, 18). By definition, back-end speech recognition is the "specific use of SRT in an environment where the recognition process occurs after the completion of dictation by sending voice files through a server" (AHIMA and MTIA Joint Task Force on Standards Development 2008, 18). During FESR the physician does the editing after the notes are transcribed. During BESR, the transcriptionist is more of a quality control editor who performs the task of reviewing the dictated report for quality purposes. As this technology is discussed within this chapter, the advantages and disadvantages of both types of SRT as well as the future of speech recognition within the computerized health record will be examined.

History of Speech Recognition

Some of the earliest attempts "to design systems for automatic speech recognition were mostly guided by the theory of acoustic-phonetics, which describes the phonetic elements of speech (the basic sounds of the language) and tries to explain how they are acoustically realized in a spoken utterance" (Juang and Rabiner 2005, 6). Prior to the 1980s, speech recognition was based on **key-word spotting**, in which a command would be triggered when a user would say a simple phrase or key word. This type of speech recognition is used frequently when phoning and getting a call-in line to direct the user to the correct department or area for help. The prompt might ask the user to say a certain word ("If you need car service, say *service,*" "If you need sales, say *sales,*" or "If you need customer billing, say *billing*"). These examples show key words that have been preprogrammed into phrases the speech recognition software uses to direct calls to the appropriate area. Research continued in the mid 1980s to move the technology past key-word spotting so that it could expand as the capabilities of technology were rapidly advancing. One basic research idea was the **hidden Markov model (HMM)**, which was understood early on in a few laboratories (IBM and the Institute for Defense Analysis (IDA)) and became the preferred method for speech recognition (Juang and Rabiner 2005, 6). At the time, many companies were attempting to use this new technology, all while vendors were trying to develop it for the market. Some healthcare facilities and physicians liked the concept but were not impressed overall with the product. Because SRT was a new concept, research at this point was not fully developed to please all customers. According to van Terheyden of Philips Speech Recognition Systems, he recalls when "Philips introduced SpeechMagic in 1993, there was an overwhelming response, but because it was still in early stages, the results were disappointing" (Macios 2007, 25).

Another technology that was introduced in the late 1980s was the idea of **artificial neural networks (ANN)**, which use "neural networks for speech recognition centered on simple tasks like recognizing a few phonemes or a few words" (Juang and Rabiner 2005, 15). As researchers at various universities and companies continued to increase the vocabularies for continuous speech recognition, newer theories and models were developed. Because speech is a continual conversation with pauses, inflections that have meaning, and hidden meanings of words, speech recognition software must be capable of recognizing and interpreting them. As software applications were developed, these were tested against the data or words within the dictation to determine the word error rate. With continuous use, by the user, of the algorithms within the software application, it will be considered "trained" to his or her voice. The more frequently the user dictates, the more the word error rate will decrease and become more accurate and faster. It is a well-accepted target that in order for virtually any large vocabulary speech recognition task to become viable, the word error rate must fall below a 10% level (Juang and Rabiner 2005, 17).

Speech recognition is very similar to natural language processing technology. The **natural language processing technology** is speech recognition but also uses "sentence structure (**syntax**), meaning (**semantics**), and context to accurately process and/or extract free-text data, including speech data for application purposes" (LaTour and Eichenwald Maki 2006, 50). This technology basically teaches the meaning of a word or phrase to a software application after several uses. This is done by a statistical algorithm; as the applications "can then compare and code these similar expressions accurately and quickly" (LaTour and Eichenwald Maki 2006, 50). Speech technology currently integrates with natural language processing technology (there are those who argue that these are different, and those who say these are one and the same); however, the computerized health record is being merged with this type of technology to bring efficiency of data flow and information within the patient record. A timeline of the history of speech recognition is shown in figure 11.1.

Figure 11.1.   Milestones in speech and multimodal technology research

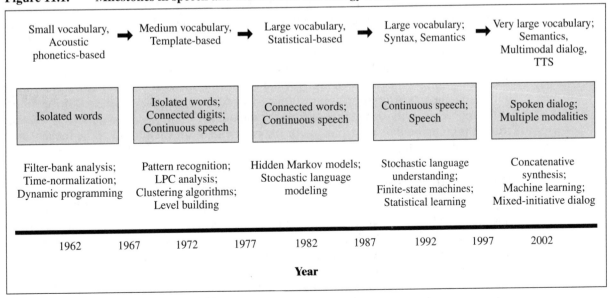

Source: Adapted from Juang and Rabiner 2005, 21

Over the past 50 years, speech recognition began as research examining sound patterns of isolated words and has advanced into the current vocabularies of data. Speech recognition and natural language processing technology is now capable of recognizing the user's voice, meaning, and (in most cases) inflection. This advancement leads to the future of technology, which holds more development into natural language processing and artificial intelligence. Artificial intelligence can be compared to the human brain. By definition, artificial intelligence uses "artificial neural networks (ANN) which seek to provide mathematical models and computer algorithms that operate in a similar manner to the nervous system, in particular, the brain" (LaTour and Eichenwald Maki 2006, 560).

Benefits of Speech Recognition

There are many positive aspects of implementing speech recognition into the HIM arena of the healthcare facility. The primary reason is to speed efficiency with documentation in the health record. The healthcare practitioner can dictate notes directly into the electronic health record, which can then be easily edited by the practitioner or a transcription editor and quickly completed while remaining in the patient's record. This is the ultimate situation in ensuring that history and physical examinations, progress notes, operative reports, and discharge summaries among other medical reports are legible and timely for use in the treatment of the patient. Not only is the clinical documentation typed and legible, it is dictated directly into the system, saving hours of time from the previous method of having to dictate a report, transcribe it, and then physically take the report to the nursing unit to file it into patient record.

The use of electronic health records (EHRs) is on the rise in healthcare facilities and as speech recognition is coupled with this technology, healthcare practitioners are finding that it provides a good combination of feasibility and effectiveness. One facility that uses the EHR and speech recognition, "New York-based Nassau Orthopedic Surgeons and its seven physicians estimate that practice costs are down by $100,000 (annually) and volume is up by approximately 3 percent" (AHIMA e-HIM Work Group on Speech Recognition in the ERH 2003, 2).

Lack of Transcriptionists

One benefit of SRT is that it reduces staffing needs when there is a lack of transcriptionists. There are "not enough experienced **medical transcriptionists (MTs)** to meet current and future demands" (AHIMA e-HIM Work Group on Speech Recognition in the ERH 2003, 2). Transcription has been outsourced in the past few decades as the cost of transcription as a business practice continually rises. This rise in cost is due in part to the "needed hardware and software and because there are not enough trained, expert medical transcriptionists available" (Abdelhak et al. 2007, 181). The future of SRT for clinical documentation will signal a change for the transcriptionists and their duties. No longer will the medical transcriptionist be a typist of words; instead, they will become an editor of the report and will remain responsible for the quality of information dictated. Whether editing is completed on the front end or the back end of the dictation will be the decision of the healthcare facility.

Increase in Patient Load

Another benefit of speech recognition is that the physician's patient load increases. As physicians in busy emergency departments, clinics, or other outpatient settings use speech recognition, the speed of this technology can free the physician to see more patients or use their time elsewhere. Speech recognition can be used to "offer clinicians a way to immediately dictate, sign, and produce a report independently" (Abdelhak et al. 2007, 275). SRT has "the capability of enhancing physician productivity, leaving more time for direct patient care" (AHIMA e-HIM Work Group on Speech Recognition in the ERH 2003, 3).

Demand for Turnaround Time

SRT offers healthcare practitioners legible dictated reports in a shorter completion time. **Turnaround time (TAT)** is defined as "the elapsed time from completion of dictation to the delivery of the transcribed document either in printed medium or electronically to a repository" (AHIMA and MTIA Joint Task Force on Standards Development 2008, 18). Although signatures may or may not be present on this documentation, the presence of the note that has been typed and checked for errors and quality and now resides in the patient record is considered to be the completed chart note.

In the transcription field, the TAT measurement is used as a gauge by the HIM department to determine the productivity and success factor of the area. Turnaround time is also used as a measure of quality. The healthcare facility also defines the amount of time for health reports such as the history and physical (H&P), operative report, and the discharge summary to be completed by physicians. The HIM department can then use the TAT in transcription as a way of determining whether their area has any backlogs in dictation that need immediate attention.

Some facilities use outsourcing companies on a full-time basis to resolve backlogs and other transcription needs. Facilities that perform in-house transcription would need to outsource reports to backup transcriptionists until the backlog is resolved or have the current staff work overtime. Backlogs are costly, and transcription duties are an expensive business.

The TAT for the dictation to be completed and for the transcribed reports to be filed in the patient record is a major factor in the transcription area of HIM. Improving TAT has been an ongoing issue with the paper-based record. As SRT grows more popular and reliable within healthcare facilities, the delays once seen will fade. Speech recognition can deliver documentation more efficiently from voice to text or screen for computerized records.

Southern Hills Medical Center, a facility located in Nashville, TN, has the physicians "able to dictate, edit, and sign reports in one complete step within minutes from commencement to electronic signature" (AHIMA e-HIM Work Group on Speech Recognition in the ERH 2003, 2). The speed of getting information to the patient record can only improve the quality of patient care provided. Another study compared speech recognition software to a traditional transcription service for physician charting in an emergency department. After dictation of 47 health records by two physicians, the study concluded that the speech recognition was accurate and economical. The speech recognition software was "nearly as accurate as traditional transcription, it has a much shorter turnaround time and it is less expensive, we recommend its use as a tool for physician charting in the ED" (Zick and Olsen 2001, 298). Within the emergency department and critical care areas, minutes and seconds are vital to the patient's care. The reduction of time that this technology can provide can "improve patient outcomes and reduce patient care days as well" (AHIMA e-HIM Work Group on Speech Recognition in the ERH 2003, 3).

Handwriting and Legibility Issues

Handwriting is the most common data input in the paper-based health record. With computerized health records, "handwriting is becoming less and less acceptable—although it provides an immediate record, the documentation is frequently not as comprehensive as a dictated note, and legibility is an issue" (AHIMA e-HIM Work Group on Speech Recognition in the ERH 2003, 2). Physicians spend much of their time writing in health records when their valuable time could be used more wisely seeing patients or performing other tasks. Handwritten charts are time-consuming and tedious to complete and "are often difficult to defend" (Zick and Olsen 2001, 295). The quality of the patient's care begins with the patient's documentation in the health record and the communication among the healthcare providers. If this communication between providers cannot be read, patient care is jeopardized. Complete and accurate documentation is the focal point of healthcare and decision making for the treatment and the safety of the patient. Joint Commission lists patient safety goals as their focus. The "legibility of handwriting has long been identified as a problem and now with the use of technology, inaudible dictation has fallen into this same category" (Hurley and Sims 2006, 3). SRT is "not only less time-consuming than handwriting, but typewritten records are legible and usually more detailed and complete" (AHIMA e-HIM Work Group on Speech Recognition in the ERH 2003, 3).

Electronic Health Record

SRT in its simplest form is basically a software application (used with hardware) acting as an input device so the spoken word can be transmitted digitally into text using a computer system. "Software for voice recognition can exist on an individual PC or be a shared application across a network" (Abdelhak et al. 2007, 275). Speech recognition also can be set up where the system "is turned on while an individual clinician dictates . . . the transcriptionist receives a draft document and the voice version and is more quickly able to complete the document and present it for signature" (Abdelhak et al. 2007, 275). Speech recognition "is a technology just as a database or keyboard is a technology . . . that when used together make the EMR data valuable (Macios 2007, 26).

SRT systems are set up differently in various healthcare areas; there are different uses for each type of client, but all have the same goals of efficiency and legibility of clinical documentation as well as sharing the communication with other providers in the treatment of the patient. Coupling the SRT with the EHR is a win-win situation. All documentation is in electronic format for all practitioners to communicate instantly; there is a reduction of illegible charting due to electronic records throughout the record, and upon discharge, billing is faster when documentation of the record is complete and legible. Speech is faster than handwriting and currently is the most common type of communication. When speech is used as the means to input data within the health record, all processes of the health record are completed faster for more efficient care for the patient. This aids the patient as well as all the caregivers and allows the physicians to use their time more wisely. Facilities use speech recognition in conjunction with other technology. Thus, "finding technology that works best for an organization can include using a combination of dictation, speech recognition, templates, and revisionists (also known as medical transcriptionists)" (Macios 2007, 25). The "widespread use of speech recognition throughout the healthcare enterprise is just beginning to be taken seriously, and it is likely to give a significant boost to the goal of making 100 percent of all patient health records electronic" (AHIMA e-HIM Work Group on Speech Recognition in the ERH 2003, 1).

Speech Recognition Software

There are several types of speech recognition software used to convert the human voice to an electronic file. The electronic file can then be imported into the electronic health record. Speech recognition includes voice dialing, call routing, discrete speech recognition, and continuous speech recognition, all of which will be discussed in further detail in this section.

Interactive Voice Response Systems

The **interactive voice response system** is one of the earliest speech recognition systems, taking its root from the key-word spotting systems from the early 20th century. Some "applications, such as voice dialing and call routing, usually involved only short utterances of limited vocabulary and consisted of only a few words" and "there was an emphasis of the research at Bell Laboratories on what is generally called the *acoustic model* (the spectral representation of sounds or words) over the language model (the representation of the grammar or syntax of the task)" (Juang and Rabiner 2005, 11). The key-word spotting is used in call routing systems by a client who when prompted by the system will speak a name or key word and the system will route the caller to the appropriate area or department for phone assistance. This is currently used in many companies with large client bases for directory assistance.

Types of Speech Recognition Software

As software applications, the SRT applications can be simple to reside "on an individual PC or be a shared application across a network" (Abdelhak et al. 2007, 275). Speech recognition as hardware in and of itself can be an input device because the spoken word can be electronically digitized and input as data into the computerized health record through the hardware (Abdelhak et al. 2007, 274).

Older voice recognition applications require each word to be dictated slowly and distinctly by the user. This allows "the software to determine where one word begins and the next stops" (ATRC 2009, 2). This is known as **discrete speech**. As SRT advanced through the years, newer software applications developed. **Continuous speech recognition** "means that the user can use the system naturally and does not have to speak as slowly and distinctly as with previous systems" (Abdelhak et al. 2007, 275). The continuous speech recognition application can recognize speech at up to 160 words per minute (ATRC 2009, 2). Speech recognition systems use a neural net to "learn" to recognize the speaker's voice and remember the way the user says each word, regardless of varying accents and inflection (ATRC 2009, 2).

SRT uses algorithms within the software applications to predict the next word before it is said. Most applications "require an initial training session in which the software is taught to recognize the user's voice and dialect" (Abdelhak et al. 2007, 275). The technology also uses grammatical context and frequency of use to predict the word the user wishes to input (ATRC 2009, 2). Speech recognition has made significant progress since its introduction into the industry. The future of this technology coupled with natural language processing has unlimited possibilities.

Front-End Speech Recognition (FESR)

When a person dictates using **front-end speech recognition (FESR),** "the words appear on the screen and are corrected if they are not displayed correctly" (LaTour and Eichenwald Maki 2006, 189). Thus, the physician or the dictator is the editor of the document that is dictated and it is considered complete when dictating and editing is complete. The distribution process may still be controlled by the system and how the facility has determined setup. However, if there are parties external to the facility who need to receive the document, someone at the originating facility will still need to perform this service.

FESR offers "clinicians a way to immediately dictate, sign and produce a report independently" (Abdelhak et al. 2007, 275). "Front-end speech recognition is also the most effective use of SRT with an EHR, enabling the dictator to respond to prompts from the EHR for more complete and accurate documentation" (AHIMA e-HIM Work Group on Speech Recognition in the EHR 2003, 5). One drawback to this type of speech recognition is the time it takes to train the physician or dictator to use the system. This "is a time-consuming process that takes time away from patient care" (AHIMA e-HIM Work Group on Speech Recognition in the EHR 2003, 5). And "in the amount of time it takes to make the corrections, a clinician can see three additional patients" (AHIMA e-HIM Work Group on Speech Recognition in the EHR 2003, 5). Healthcare facilities must weigh the advantages and disadvantages to the tasks of FESR and BESR to their particular facility and the computerized health record. Each facility must assess their own needs to make the best decision for their patients.

Back-End Speech Recognition (BESR)

The other type of speech recognition is known as **back-end speech recognition (BESR)** and is also referred to as "server-based speech recognition" (AHIMA e-HIM Work Group on Speech Recognition in the EHR 2003, 5). With BESR, "the physician dictates in the usual manner, the audio is sent as a draft text along with the speech file to the transcriptionist who serves as an editor to listen to the audio in comparison with the displayed text and to make changes to the text document" (LaTour and Eichenwald Maki 2006, 189). In other words, the transcriptionist is an editor and the document is sent to the dictator for approval following the editing process. There is no change in the way physicians dictate with back-end speech recognition from how it has been traditionally done (LaTour and Eichenwald Maki 2006, 275). Physicians are more attracted to this type of SRT because the dictation process does not change for them and they do not have to perform the time-consuming task of editing (AHIMA e-HIM Work Group on Speech Recognition in the EHR 2003, 5). However, even with the use of BESR, physicians dictate sentences such as:

> "take out that third sentence and move it to the top of the page and insert my usual drug regimen at that place"

These physicians will find that SRT does not work for them. SRT will type this sentence exactly as it is dictated. Computers are advancing to the natural language processing enabling the "think" process and may one day be capable of performing such actions as the above, but they currently do not act as human transcriptionists do and thus cannot think or perform as such.

Check Your Understanding 11.1

1. The first efforts in SRT was based on what?

    A. key-word spotting
    B. hidden Markov model (HMM)
    C. artificial neural networks (ANN)
    D. semantics

2. The physician acts as the editor within which type of speech recognition technology method?

    A. Back-end speech recognition
    B. Front-end speech recognition
    C. Hidden Markov model
    D. Artificial neural networks

3. Key-word spotting was an early effort in SRT that was used mainly with _____.

    A. medical dictation
    B. emergency departments
    C. call routing
    D. radiology departments

4. Older voice recognition systems use this method where slower talkers must pause between each word that is said, which is called _____.

    A. continuous speech
    B. discrete speech
    C. front-end speech
    D. back-end speech

Templates and Macros

The facility may also choose to use a macro or a **template** that is a preapproved document outline designed so that the practitioner only dictates to fill in the blanks within the template. Figure 11.2 is an example of a template that might be used for dictation.

Some vendors develop their own templates and sell them to their customers; these can vary with a client's needs or can be customizable by the customer. A template "includes fields that enable a user to skip from one field to the next using speech commands" (AHIMA e-HIM Work Group on Speech Recognition in the EHR 2003, 6). A **macro** is similar to a template in the SRT. It basically uses "a series of keystrokes and/or commands that are executed on command;" macros are especially suited to generating "large amounts of text using only a few commands that are easily recognized" (AHIMA e-HIM Work Group on Speech Recognition in the EHR 2003, 7).

Common Speech Recognition Software

There are various types of speech recognition systems available for healthcare facilities, which range from the individual personal computer (PC) station software to the enterprise network-level system. The most popular or common name brand for the individual software application is Dragon NaturallySpeaking, version 10 by (Nuance Communications, Inc. 2009). This company lists two versions for Windows: (1) personal and home version and (2) a business and professional version and the Macintosh editions as: Mac OSX and Simply Dictation (ATRC 2009).

For the commercial speech recognition software, the vendors offering products are Loquendo, ICommunicator, Fonix, and VoiceIn (ATRC 2009).

There are also other vendors, Olympus and iListen, that offer products such as digital voice recorders, which "allow a user to dictate text which can be translated at a later date by a voice recognition system" (ATRC 2009). Microphones are also listed as products by other vendors such as Parrot TalkPro, Andrea, Telex, and Plantronics. These products are compatible with the Dragon NaturallySpeaking systems and the IBM ViaVoice speech recognition systems.

Figure 11.2.   Example of a completed dictation template

<u>**Dictation Template**</u>

<u>PREOPERATIVE DIAGNOSIS:</u> Bilateral otitis media with effusion; adenoidal hypertrophy.

<u>POSTOPERATIVE DIAGNOSIS:</u> Bilateral otitis media with effusion; adenoidal hypertrophy.

<u>PROCEDURE:</u> Bilateral pressure equalizing tubes; adenoidectomy.

<u>OPERATION, IN DETAIL:</u> The patient was brought to the operating room and kept on the gurney. General mask anesthesia was attained. Using an operating microscope, a myringotomy was made through the anterior inferior quadrant of the right tympanic membrane. A Shepard Grommet pressure equalizing tube was then placed through the myringotomy. A similar procedure was performed on the left side.

General endotracheal anesthesia was then attained. A Crowe-Davis mouth gag was then introduced and suspended on a Mayo stand. A red rubber catheter was then placed through the left nares and used to retract the soft palate. Under mirror visualization the adenoidal bed was ablated using coagulation cautery. Care was taken at all times to keep the cautery away from the torus tubarius.

The patient's anesthesia was reversed, and the patient was taken to the recovery room in stable condition.

Speech Pattern Issues

Capturing spoken words and interpreting them into text is the basis of SRT. The success of the software application technology and the editor of this technology must work together to accomplish complete and accurate clinical documentation. There "is no doubt that the complexity of the language of medicine, the dynamics of the healthcare environment, and the sophistication of the dictation systems today present a formidable challenge for dictating authors" (Hurley and Sims 2006, 1). Many times, "the dictator is often frustrated with blanks left in a report; the medical transcriptionist is perplexed when trying to decipher important passages obscured by background noises; the report is delayed in turnaround time as several quality assurance editors try to decipher those same critical passages; the coder needs the report to initiate the reimbursement cycle; and other healthcare professionals look at a report with blanks as risky to important decisions needed for patient care" (Hurley and Sims 2006, 1).

Healthcare facilities must use standards in dictation whether SRT is used or not; however, when SRT is used, standards for dictating and prompts when dictating are a must. A lot of bad habits are picked up throughout the years of practice such as having a conversation or responding to a nurse while in the middle of a dictation. This software is not human and cannot distinguish between a conversation and dictation. Thus, providers who have been dictating for years must be retrained about the rules of dictation. The use of macros and templates (previously discussed) might be a good starting point for practitioners who have trouble with speech recognition software and many "commercial speech recognition engines have programming to eliminate 'um' and 'uh' from the text" and find that commercial software are helpful (AHIMA e-HIM Work Group on Speech Recognition in the EHR 2003, 6).

The Association for Healthcare Documentation Integrity (AHDI) (formerly known as the American Association for Medical Transcription) and the American Society for Testing and Materials (ASTM) International have published materials related to the importance of establishing a system for quality improvement of the dictation process (Hurley and Sims 2006, 1). One of AHDI's publications for established standards of policies and procedures for quality assurance in medical transcription is the Best Practices for Measuring Quality in Medical Transcription (Hurley and Sims 2006, 1; AHDI 2005). Within this document, many key elements are flagged that can pose safety risks to patients, have a negative financial impact to healthcare facilities, have a negative document integrity impact, or promote unprofessional behavior to a healthcare provider's behavior in documentation patterns (Hurley and Sims 2006, 2). The ASTM International has approved "E2344: Standard Guide for Data Capture through the Dictation Process," a guide to improving the quality of healthcare documentation through the dictation process. This guide is a significant effort towards ensuring that standards of professional dictation are followed by providers for error-free, clear, secure, and timely documentation. Some of the key elements of the E2344 standard are shown in figure 11.3.

Rules of Grammar and Punctuation

All healthcare practitioners must review the rules of grammar and punctuation when using SRT. Even though the software applications types exactly what is said, it is best if the user is current on the rules of grammar and punctuation and understands the purposes for commas, semicolons, and other grammatical punctuations. This is also a word of warning for those providers who are in the habit of saying a sentence of dictation and then saying to a transcriptionist "period". Within the speech recognition software, the computer software will of course type the word "period" and not know that the user means that this is a signal to end a sentence.

Voice Inflection and Enunciation

Other thoughts on dictation that should be watched are personal habits such as voice inflection. Some dictators will raise their voice at the end of a sentence, which signals a question. An example of this might be:

"Questionable CAD versus angina?"

Figure 11.3.   ASTM International's E2344 Standard Guide for Data Capture through the Dictation Process

- Use only facility-approved abbreviations within the dictating message and avoid use of other abbreviations, jargon, slang, acronyms, and/or coined terms.
- Maintain a quiet and secure area for the dictation process. Advise dictating authors to use the designated dictation areas to avoid background noise, distractions, interruptions, and confidentiality issues. Advise dictating authors to avoid eating, gum chewing, yawning, smoking, and so on, while dictating. Advise dictating authors to avoid side conversations and background distractions such as voices, telephone ringing, and/or music that may obscure the dictation.
- Advise dictating authors to avoid profanity, and derogatory or other inappropriate comments while dictating.
- Include feedback about the dictation process regarding any mechanical, technical, or other problems that may interfere with a clear, complete, and accurate document.
- Use conversational speed and volume for optimal dictation message.
- Instruct dictating authors on the functions of the dictation system used within their healthcare environment. These include, but are not limited to, the following:
  — Use of the pause mechanism, use of the review mode, use of the insertion mode
  — Use of the types of phones for dictating. Refrain from using speakerphones, portable phones, cell phones, and public phones.
  — Use of microphone settings to avoid clipped words and phrases, proper distance of microphones, and microphone element from mouth.

Source: Hurley and Sims 2006, 2

With a question being dictated, the user's voice inflection rises at the end; however, on the SRT software, this inflection is not recognizable and the punctuation is not added. If the provider says question mark, then of course the word "question mark" gets typed out as "question mark" on the page, rather than the "?" symbol.

Healthcare practitioners must also be careful to enunciate clearly when dictating. This is one of the key factors within the ASTM elements listed in the E2344 standards (Hurley and Sims 2006, 2). Although speech recognition software technology applications are more sophisticated now than over the last 50 years, the user must still be clear in dictation. As long as the practitioner does not mumble, stutter, or slur the words, the software is very capable of producing accurate clinical documentation. If the user keeps this in mind while dictating, this helps all who must use the report , but ultimately it helps the patient with their care.

Acronyms and Spelling

When a healthcare practitioner must dictate an acronym such as an abbreviation, there is a certain method in doing so when using SRT. When Microsoft Vista decided to use the alphabet with its speech recognition component during the testing phase, participants were asked to use the letters of the alphabet, and various words for the letter "A" from what was expected were received (Chambers 2008). According to Chambers, "most products that use speech technology require users to learn the military alphabet (Alpha, Bravo, Charlie, and so on) to spell out words, such as street names that they want to add to the recognized vocabulary" (Chambers 2008). The military alphabet is also called the "NATO alphabet" and is listed in Figure 11.4.

The military alphabet is used when dictation is needed for spelling as well as when the user pauses briefly within the dictation. These pauses do not affect the formatting within speech recognition (Gould 2000). If a user wants to dictate a number, the number must be spelled out. This might be found within a drug dosage or a patient address, and so on.

Examples:

Number: Normal temperature of 98.7° would be said as: "ninety eight point seven degrees"

Time: Time to be reported as 8:30 a.m. would be said as: "eight thirty a.m."

(Source: Gould 2000)

Figure 11.4.   Military alphabet used by many SRT systems

A—Alpha	J—Juliet	S—Sierra
B—Bravo	K—Kilo	T—Tango
C—Charlie	L—Lima	U—Uniform
D—Delta	M—Mike	V—Victor
E—Echo	N—November	W—Whiskey
F—Foxtrot	O—Oscar	X—X-ray
G—Golf	P—Papa	Y—Yankee
H—Hotel	Q—Quebec	Z—Zulu
I—India	R—Romeo	

Source: ATIS 2007

Computer Usage with Speech Recognition

As stated earlier, SRT is an application that can be used simply on an individual PC or across a network. Some of the vendors previously mentioned, such as Dragon Naturally-Speaking and IBM Via Voice, can be installed for a reasonable amount (less than $100 on average) for an individual PC. The PC would need the minimum requirements, which is still 1 GHz, and for RAM, 512 MB on Windows 2000 and XP and 1 GB on Windows Vista (Nuance Communications, Inc. 2009). Wireless microphones or Bluetooth devices may be used for dictation with speech recognition. The Nuance Web site suggests several "plug and play" types that offer the technology device with no training needed and a listing of vendors offering this service (Nuance Communications, Inc. 2009).

Issues with Speech Recognition

Quality of Product—End Result

The outcome of speech recognition is the overall goal for clinical documentation to be efficient, economical, and of quality. Documentation within the record must be complete, accurate, and timely, and yet be clear and economical for the healthcare providers to perform their duties in caring for the patient. The goal of speech recognition must equal or exceed that of the traditional method of dictation and transcription in order for this technology to be successful. The future of natural language processing technology is bright, with even more advancement of this computerization of speech technology in healthcare. As the electronic health record and speech recognition are merged in more and more facilities across the country, more evidence of clinicians and transcription editors partnering for quality documentation will be seen in the patient record. Already discussed within this section has been "decreasing reimbursement, rising costs, growing labor shortages, and increasing demands for more complete documentation provided in a more timely manner" (AHIMA e-HIM Work Group on Speech Recognition in the EHR 2003, 2). SRT must be seen as an answer as the electronic health record age is entered.

Training with the Software

Whether FESR or BESR is used by a facility, the amount of time needed for transcription will continue. If the facility chooses to use FESR, the physician plays the role of dictator and editor. Thus, the amount of time needed for a physician training on the use of the software application will be significant, taking into account the time it will take for the physician to "train" the software to learn his or her voice. Keep in mind that training time also varies by user. If the facility uses BESR, there is no training time needed on the front end. However, the amount of time needed is for the transcriptionist to edit and use the editor function for every report that is dictated. Either way, the amount of time is either spent on the front end with the physician or on the back end with the transcriptionist. This will be a decision that each facility and medical staff will need to make in order to weigh the advantages and disadvantages of costs, technology, hardware, software, time, and any other internal factors. As with all decisions, this should be one that is made not only by administration but everyone involved, including physicians, information systems, HIM administration, and other departments to be affected by the dictation system.

Editing of Dictated Reports

The time allotted for editing completed reports is another factor that must be taken into consideration with SRT. Whether this process is performed by the physician on the front end or the transcriptionist on the back end, the process of editing is time-consuming and must be part of the quality process of the clinical documentation review. When the transcriptionist acts as the editor, costs are reduced and productivity increased "based on the expectation that the MT will no longer be required to manually produce the entire dictation; rather, the MT will review the voice file to the text provided and edit for missing or incorrect content, as well as format the document" (AHIMA e-HIM Work Group on Speech Recognition in the EHR 2003, 3). The "productivity gains should be measured against the generally accepted industry standard of four minutes of transcription time to each one minute of dictation, and average edit review time of two to three minutes per one minute of dictation" (AHIMA e-HIM Work Group on Speech Recognition in the EHR 2003, 3). In one instance, Carle Clinic of Illinois had their transcription volume grow from 15 million lines per year to 40 million lines per year, and once speech recognition was implemented, "the average transcriptionists' productivity increased by roughly 90% because the new model automatically produced accurate and fully formatted first draft documents from clinicians' dictations, which the medical transcriptionists review and edit" (Macios 2007, 25). This productivity gain lowered the cost of transcription for this facility in the editing function with the volume (Macios 2007, 26). What has traditionally taken hours of dictation, transcription and physical filing of a paper document is now reduced to a few minutes for document completion through electronic signature, quality check, editing, and distribution of the document electronically. The "use of speech recognition can reduce the amount of time it takes for information to be made available to other healthcare providers" (AHIMA e-HIM Work Group on Speech Recognition in the EHR 2003, 3).

Speech Recognition Principles

In order for speech recognition technology to be successful, there are various principles or factors that must be considered within the system. These include the distinctions between each human voice, the "training" of the user to the particular SRT system, dialects, accents, voice inflection, and the method of correcting errors. Each of these will be explored within this section.

Decoding Human Voice

Speech recognition works on sound probabilities after the recorder is "trained" to a particular voice. Because every "person's voice is different, the program cannot possibly contain a template for each potential user, so the program must first be 'trained' with a new user's voice input before that user's voice can be recognized by the program" (Baumann 2008). The user must train with a word or phrase several times into a microphone with the speech recognition system. The "program computes a statistical average of the multiple samples of the same word and stores the averaged sample as a template in a program data structure" (Baumann 2008). This is what has been referenced earlier as an algorithm. Some applications such as Dragon NaturallySpeaking have a built-in training wizard that walks a new user through reading different types of passages as part of learning a new user's voice. Speech recognition systems can have large vocabularies, and the more a user trains on these systems the better accuracy of recognition the system. Speech recognition systems can be either discrete or continuous (previously discussed). Discrete systems are the easiest to implement whereas the continuous speech systems are the most difficult to implement (Baumann 2008). A speech recognition system that is "**speaker dependent**" means that it has been "trained" to a particular user and already has an established vocabulary for that user.

Sound Probabilities

Every person's voice is different and because of this, a user must train the speech recognition system to "learn" one's voice. There are also dialects and accents that must be taken into account. SRT has no problem with dialects or accents, but the system must learn these words just as it learns all other words. To the speech recognition system, any word that has a dialect or accent is no different than one without. Regardless of country or region, it still must learn each and every word individually. Once learned, the system then uses probability to determine when the word would be used and in what context.

In addition to the vocabulary within the speech recognition system, language models are used in which bigrams, trigrams, and quadgrams may be found. In the language model, an example of a **bigram** might be the "word pair 'world affairs' over 'whirled affairs' because 'world' occurs more frequently than 'whirled', giving it a higher unigram probability; and because 'world affairs' occurs more frequently than 'whirled affairs' in the speech and writing of target users, resulting in a higher bigram probability" (Voice Perfect Systems 2008). Here, these "two-word sequences sound exactly alike, so the acoustic model can do nothing to differentiate them; the language model calculation is the only information that can help make the right choice" (Voice Perfect Systems 2008). Other word phrases that have three words would be a **trigram** and word sequences with four words are **quadgrams**. These are all within the speech recognition algorithm and are calculated within the language model software.

Correcting Errors

As the user trains the speech recognition software, the vocabulary is developed for that particular user. The "word list adds words in the Dragon NaturallySpeaking active vocabulary (which is loaded into RAM and allows instant recognition) and backup dictionary (which has an expanded number of words for correction purposes) to improve the language model and recognition accuracy when the vocabulary is compiled" (Voice Perfect Systems 2008). Thus, as the user corrects errors within a document, the personal dictionary is continuously being expanded and developed to increase accuracy and reduce errors upfront. If the dictator is also the editor (front end), error correction is completed by using the system according to the facility's approved methods. Approved methods might include amendment to the document (of the error) by the user or by use of system functions such as pause mode, review mode, and/or insertion mode of the word(s) in error (Hurley and Sims 2006, 6).

Using the Speech Recognition System

There are various speech recognition systems on the market, and choosing the right system is a crucial decision and one that should be made using a team approach. The computerized health record or electronic health record and the SRT combination should be a primary consideration in this decision. Speech recognition working in conjunction with the electronic health record is an excellent clinical documentation tool. A well-designed speech recognition program, an EHR system, and a "tightly integrated workflow will ensure that speech recognition is an aid, not a hindrance" (Gater 2008, 20). Speech recognition provides immediate feedback as opposed to having to wait for the transcriptionist, then review the note and possibly make changes to its original format, and have the document retyped once again (Gater 2008, 20).

For the transcriptionist who functions as the editor, it is best that a quality headset be worn for optimal noise reduction for editing to achieve significant recognition accuracy (Gater 2008, 20). If the transcriptionist wishes to use speech recognition to redictate as opposed to typing, separate vocabularies for each physician are recommended. A transcriptionist can type for several types of physician specialties and will need to purchase the medical version of each for SRT. The medical transcriptionist will wear an earpiece connected to the recorder and also wear a headset to hear the redictation. The transcriptionist "will need to use a separate vocabulary when redictating for the cardiologist and switch vocabularies when redictating for the neurologist" (Gater 2008, 20). The recognition accuracy improves when separate vocabularies are used for each specialty rather than trying to redictate from the same vocabulary. Using separate vocabularies increases productivity for the transcriptionist as well as produces a completed report faster.

The physician uses a microphone on a PC or connected to a server within a network for the dictation. The quality of the dictation is extremely important to ensure that background noise is nonexistent and that the words are clearly enunciated and spoken loud enough into the microphone. The spoken words are captured as an audio file and these appear on the computer screen as text. The physician may correct these if there are any errors, as the dictator controls the process (LaTour and Eichenwald Maki 2006, 189). This is the front-end method. In the back-end method, the audio file is captured and is then stored digitally and sent to the transcriptionist for editing. After the editing process, the dictator reviews the document for any changes and approves the document if there are no changes, and the process is completed.

Voice Extensible Markup Language—VoiceXML (VXML)

The Voice Extensible Markup Language or **VoiceXML** is the standard "with which voice applications are developed" (ATRC 2009, 5). The XML standard currently exists and many more languages are being created for SRT by combining several markup languages based on the XML standard (ATRC 2009, 5). Some of the VoiceXML platforms include:

- Java Speech Markup Language by SUN Microsystems
- Accessibility features of Synchronized Multimedia Language (SMIL) and Checkpoints for SMIL
- VoXML at Oasis
- Audiomining by Nuance

These platforms create XML speech recognition on the Internet and index data for audio files that enable searches and location of key words and phrases in audio files (ATRC 2009, 6).

Summary

Speech recognition is proving to be more than a call routing system for phone users. This technology, when combined with the computerized health record, promises an optimistic future with rapid advancements. Speech recognition offers a variety of methods from front end to back end for healthcare facilities to choose from, as well as software types from simple PC versions to high-end network versions. Hardware consists of a microphone, headset, and computer setup. The software consists of the application itself. Training for the user and editor requires time for learning the system and for the editing process that must be taken into account with this technology. However, with any technology, there are advantages and disadvantages; it is the healthcare facility that must decide what is ultimately best for the patient.

Check Your Understanding 11.2

1. How does the speech recognition software handle dialects and accents?

    A. No differently than other words
    B. It must train extra time on the vocabulary builder
    C. The editor corrects these types of words
    D. The dictator must spell these words using the military alphabet

2. For what purpose is the VoiceXML?

    A. To handle speech recognition audio files on the Internet
    B. To create audio and video files
    C. This is a bigram model language
    D. This is a hidden Markov model language

3. The most difficult SRT system to implement is the:

    A. front-end speech
    B. back-end speech
    C. discrete speech
    D. continuous speech

4. True or False: Speaker dependent means that the software has been trained to only one user.

References

Abdelhak, M., S. Grostick, M.A. Hanken, and E. Jacobs. 2007. *Health Information: Management of a Strategic Resource*, 3rd ed. St. Louis, MO: Saunders/Elsevier.

Adaptive Technology Resource Centre. 2009. Technical glossary: Voice Recognition. http://atrc.utoronto.ca/index.php?option=com_content&task=view&id=50&Itemid=9.

AHIMA e-HIM Work Group on Speech Recognition in the EHR. 2003. Practice brief: Speech recognition in the electronic health record. http://library.ahima.org/xpedio/groups/public/documents/ahima/bok1_022107.hcsp?dDocName=bok1_022107.

American Health Information Management Association and Medical Transcription Industry Association Joint Task Force on Standards Development. 2008. (Summer). Transcription turnaround time for common document types. *Perspectives in Health Information Management*.

Alliance for Telecommunications Industry Solutions 2007. ATIS Telecom Glossary. http://www.atis.org/glossary/definition.aspx?id=2568.

Association for Healthcare Documentation Integrity. 2005. Best practices for measuring quality in medical transcription. http://www.ahdionline.org/Portals/0/Downloads/QualityMT.pdf.

Baumann, J. 2008. University of Washington Human Interface Technology Laboratory. Voice Recognition. http://www.hitl.washington.edu/scivw/EVE/I.D.2.d.VoiceRecognition.html.

Chambers, R. 2008. Listening to users is the key to speech recognition at Microsoft. http://www.microsoft.com/enable/microsoft/chambers.aspx.

Gater, L. 2008. Speech Recognition in the ED—and beyond. *For the Record.* 20(3):20. http://www.fortherecordmag.com/archives/ftr_02042008p20.shtml.

Gould, J. 2000. The insider's guide to Dragon NaturallySpeaking. http://www.synapseadaptive.com/joel/NumberFormatting.html.

Hurley, B. and L. Sims. 2006. Dictation best practices for quality documentation. *Proceedings from the American Health Information Management Associations 78th National Convention and Exhibit.* October, 2006: 1–10.

Juang, B.H. and L.R. Rabiner. 2005. Automatic speech recognition—A brief history of the technology development. *Elsevier Encyclopedia of Language and Linguistics*, 2nd ed. http://www.ece.ucsb.edu/Faculty/Rabiner/ece259/Reprints/354_LALI-ASRHistory-final-10-8.pdf.

LaTour, K.M. and S. Eichenwald Maki. 2006. *Health Information Management: Concepts, Principles, and Practice*, 2nd ed. Chicago: AHIMA.

Macios, A. 2007. Finding its voice. *For the Record.* 19(17):24–28.

Nuance Communications, Inc. 2009. Dragon NaturallySpeaking solutions. http://www.nuance.com/naturallyspeaking/resources/faqs.asp.

Voice Perfect Systems. 2008. How NaturallySpeaking works. http://www.voiceperfect.com/naturallyspeaking/howitworks.

Zick, R.G. and J. Olsen. 2001. Voice recognition software versus a traditional transcription service for physician charting in the ED. *American Journal of Emergency Medicine.* 19(4):295–298.

Chapter 12
Privacy and Security

Objectives

- Conduct audit for security violation.
- Develop policies and procedures on security practices.
- Educate staff on security issues.
- Develop policies and procedures related to privacy.
- Control access to protected health information.
- Participate in risk analysis.
- Assist in the development of a security plan.
- Monitor compliance with security plan.
- Develop password management plan.

Key Terms

Access controls
Administrative safeguard
Administrative simplification
ASC X12 standard
Audit controls
Audit reduction tool
Audit trail
Biometrics
Business associate
Certified in Healthcare Privacy and Security (CPHS)
Certified Information Systems Security Professional (CISSP)
Code sets

Contingency plan
Covered entity
Data recovery
Degaussing
Denial of service
Designated standard maintenance organizations
Electronic data interchange
Electronic protected health information (ePHI)
Encryption
Facility access controls
Firewall
Forensics

Health Insurance Portability and Accountability Act of 1996 (HIPAA)
Information system activity review
Integrity
Intrusion detection and response
Malicious software
Mitigation
Network security
One-factor authentication
Passwords
Person or entity authentication
Phishing

Physical safeguards	Security event	Token
Privacy	Security incident	Transactions and Code Sets rule
Privacy rule	Security management plan	Transmission security
Protected health information (PHI)	Security official	Trigger
	Security rule	Two-factor authentication
Redundancy	Spoliation	Username
Risk analysis	Spyware	Virus
Risk assessment	Technical safeguard	Workforce clearance procedure
Security	Telephone callback procedures	Worm
Security awareness training	Termination process	

Health Insurance Portability and Accountability Act of 1996 (HIPAA)

The **Health Insurance Portability and Accountability Act of 1996 (HIPAA)** impacts many areas of healthcare such as insurance portability, code sets, privacy, security, and national identifier standards. HIPAA is divided into five titles or sections. The title that this chapter addresses is Title II: Fraud and Abuse/Administrative Simplification. The purpose of the **Administrative Simplification** title is to improve the efficiency and effectiveness of the business processes of healthcare by standardizing the electronic data interchange of administrative and financial transactions. This title was also designed to protect the privacy and security of **protected health information (PHI)** that is transmitted from one point to another. PHI is individually identifiable health information that covered entities or their business associates transmit or maintain in any form or format. A third purpose was to reduce the cost of doing business in healthcare because of antiquated paper systems, nonstandard formats, and lack of accessibility of medical records due to loss (45 CFR 160, 162, and 164 2003). Many of the issues addressed in the Administrative Simplification title of HIPAA impact the health information management (HIM) profession. These areas are the privacy rule, security rule, and transactions and code sets.

It is important to define privacy and security. **Privacy** is the "right of a patient to control disclosure of personal information" (Johns 2007, 988). **Security** has two definitions according to Johns. They are:

1. The means to control access and protect information from accidental or intentional disclosure to unauthorized persons and from unauthorized alteration, destruction, or loss.

2. The physical protection of facilities and equipment from theft, damage, or unauthorized access; collectively, the policies, procedures, and safeguards designed to protect confidentiality of information, maintain the integrity and availability of information systems, and control access to the content of these systems. (Johns 2007, 992)

To be subject to HIPAA, a healthcare facility must meet the definition of a **covered entity**. Covered entities are one of the following: a health plan, a healthcare clearinghouse, or a healthcare provider that transmits any health information in electronic form for one of the covered transactions. A health plan pays for the healthcare provided to the individuals covered under their plan. These plans include medical, dental, vision, and other forms of health plans. Healthcare providers are hospitals, physician offices, long-term care facilities, ambulatory surgery centers, pharmacies, and other patient care providers. A healthcare clearinghouse collects billing data and processes it for the healthcare provider. The healthcare clearinghouse then submits the claim to the health plan for payment. As stated previously, the health plan, healthcare clearinghouse, or healthcare provider must submit patient information in electronic format for one of the covered transactions. The covered transactions that HIPAA addresses are:

- Health plan premium payments
- Enrollment or disenrollment in a health plan
- Eligibility
- Referral certification and authorization
- Claims
- Payment and remittance advice
- Claim status
- Coordination of benefits
- Health claims attachment
- First report of injury (Davis 2003)

Health plans, healthcare clearinghouses, and healthcare providers that do not share patient information for one of these transactions would not be a covered entity and therefore not subject to HIPAA. Because of the current digital nature of the world, this would be rare. There are a few exceptions to the covered entity rule, such as small providers who bill the Medicare fiscal intermediary but have less than 25 full-time employees.

HIPAA has greatly impacted healthcare and the HIM profession due to changes in processes, emphasis on privacy and security, and patient rights. In this chapter, the **Transactions and Code Sets rule** and the privacy rule will be described briefly. The security rule will be covered in depth. The American Recovery and Reinvestment Act was passed in February, 2009. The act created greater privacy and security restrictions. At the time of publication, specific standards were not available for inclusion.

Transaction and Code Sets

The **Transaction and Code Sets rule** was designed to standardize transactions performed by healthcare organizations. These standards apply to electronic transactions only; however, paper submissions are similar. The Department of Health and Human Services has assigned the responsibility of developing and maintaining standards to seven organizations. These organizations are called **Designated standard maintenance organizations (DSMOs)**. The organizations with this designation are (Scichilone 2002, 74):

- Accredited Standards Committee X12
- Dental Contact Committee of the American Dental Association
- Health Level 7
- National Council for Prescription Drug Programs
- National Uniform Billing Committee
- National Uniform Claim Committee

Many of the standards used to perform the covered transactions were developed by the Accredited Standards Committee (ASC); however, they do work with healthcare providers and users of the standards to develop a consensus. These standards cover the individual data elements and the format of the data. The standards enable the use of **electronic data interchange (EDI)**, the transfer of data from one point to another without human intervention, which can significantly improve the efficiency of healthcare. The HIPAA transactions and code sets requirements adopted ASC X12 standards. The specific **ASC X12 standard** and the transaction for which it is used are (Giannangelo 2006):

Transaction	Standard
Claims, encounters, and coordination of benefits	837
Remittance advice	835
Eligibility inquiry and response	270/271
Precertification and referral authorization	278
Enrollment in a health plan	834
Premium payment	820

Covered entities may follow the transaction requirements themselves and send formatted data to the clearinghouse for submission to the third-party payers. The covered entity also may send unformatted data to a clearinghouse or health plan and have the data converted into the appropriate transaction format.

Code Sets and Standards

Designated **code sets** are also a part of the HIPAA Transactions and Code Set rule. HIPAA defines a code set as a set of codes used to encode data elements (45 CFR 160 and 162 2000). These codes record medical diagnoses, procedures, drugs, dental procedures, and other data elements. A code replaces larger pieces of data. For example, the ICD-9-CM code 250.00 means diabetes mellitus without complication, type II or unspecified type, not stated as uncontrolled. HIPAA mandates the use of certain coding systems in the reporting of diagnoses, procedures, drugs, and more on medical and dental claims. These standards are (45 CFR 160 and 162 2000):

- *International Classification of Diseases, Ninth Edition, Clinical Modification* (ICD-9-CM)

- Current Procedural Terminology, Fourth Edition (CPT-4)

- Healthcare Financing Administration Common Procedure Coding System (HCPCS)

- Code on Dental Procedures and Nomenclature, Second Edition (CDT-2)

- National Drug Codes (NDC)

There are also nonmedical codes that can define medical specialties, claim adjustment reasons, reject reason codes, state abbreviations, remittance remarks, and more.

Privacy Rule

The HIPAA **privacy rule** controls how covered entities may use PHI. As stated earlier in this chapter, PHI is individually identifiable health information that covered entities or their business associates transmit or maintain in any form or format. **Business associates** are individuals or organizations who perform work on behalf of the covered entity that requires access to PHI (Hartley and Jones 2004). Examples are coding, release of information, and billing. The format of the information does not matter because PHI can be on paper or transmitted electronically or with other media. HIPAA lists the specific data elements that determine whether or not information is PHI. If the information includes any of the data elements in table 12.1, it is considered PHI and is therefore subject to the HIPAA privacy rule.

The privacy rule also provides rights to the patient related to their PHI. These patient rights are (LaTour and Eichenwald Maki 2006):

- Patients must be provided a notice of privacy practices that defines how PHI is used in the organization

- Patient has the right to inspect, copy, and receive a copy of the medical record

- Patient has the right to request an amendment to the health information

- Patient has the right to request that communications from the covered entity through alternative means such as a post office box rather than the home address

- Patient has the right to report violations of the HIPAA privacy rule

- Patient has the right to request restrictions on how his or her PHI is utilized by the covered entity

The covered entities must have policies in place to allow a patient to claim these rights. Policies and procedures are important to the privacy rule compliance program because the privacy rule focuses on processes and the people who develop and/or follow them rather than on technology.

The HIPAA privacy rule defines when disclosure of PHI is permitted with and without authorizations. In general, covered entities can use PHI for treatment of patients, payment, and healthcare operations without patient authorization. Although there are other uses of PHI for which patient authorization is not required (such as release to the patient and for the public's interest), most other uses require patient authorization. The privacy rule defines penalties for privacy violations including civil and criminal penalties. Enforcement of the rule has been given to the Department of Health and Human Services Office of Civil Rights (45 CFR 160, 162, and 164 2006).

Table 12.1.   PHI identifiers

1. Name
2. Postal address information, other than town or city, state, and zip code
3. Telephone numbers
4. Fax numbers
5. Electronic mail addresses
6. Social security numbers
7. Medical record numbers
8. Health plan beneficiary numbers
9. Account numbers
10. Certificate/license numbers
11. Vehicle identifiers and serial numbers, including license plate numbers
12. Device identifiers and serial numbers
13. Web Universal Resource Locators (URLs)
14. Internet Protocol (IP) address numbers
15. Biometric identifiers, including finger and voice prints
16. Full-face photographic images and any comparable images

Source: 45 CFR 160, 162, and 164 2006, 66

Check Your Understanding 12.1

1. To be subject to HIPAA, an organization must meet the definition of a:

   A. covered entity
   B. PHI
   C. administrative simplification
   D. designated standard organization

2. One of the purposes of the administrative simplification title is to:

   A. prevent security incidents from ever occurring
   B. create socialized medicine
   C. improve efficiency and effectiveness of healthcare business processes
   D. establish a prospective payment system

3. Which of the following is an example of the designated code set?

   A. ASC X12 837
   B. Health Level 7
   C. ASC X12 820
   D. ICD-9-CM

4. Which of the following would make patient information PHI?

   A. Blood type
   B. Account number
   C. Diagnosis
   D. DNA

5. The document that tells patients how PHI is used is called:

   A. notice of privacy practices
   B. amendment
   C. authorization
   D. code set

Security Rule

The security rule defines the minimum that a covered entity must do to protect **electronic protected health information (ePHI)** which is PHI that is "created, received, or transmitted by covered entities" (45 CFR Parts 160, 162, and 164 37). The security rule does not apply to PHI in other media such as paper and microfilm. Voicemail, fax, and copy machines are also not considered to be in electronic form.

The goals of the HIPAA security rule are to ensure the confidentiality, integrity, and availability of the ePHI. Confidentiality is providing access to ePHI to only those who need it. **Integrity** is ensuring that data are not altered either during transmission across a network or during storage. ePHI must be available when needed for patient care and other uses; availability is ensuring that the ePHI is available to the authorized users whenever it is needed (CMS 2007a).

The security rule was developed to be technology neutral and scalable. Technology changes so fast that the standard would need constant revision if specific technologies were mandated; therefore, the rule mandates not how but what needs to be done. For example, the HIPAA security rule mandates that physical access to electronic information systems is limited to authorized staff. The rule does not tell the covered entity how that limitation is implemented, so they may use card keys, personal identification numbers, keys, biometrics, or other means to control access. Scalable means that the Department of Health and Human Services allows covered entities to take into consideration the size, complexity, and capabilities of the organization when developing the compliance strategy. The covered entity also can consider the infrastructure of the organization regarding technology, software, and hardware as well as the costs of the security measures and the risks to the ePHI (CMS 2004). Because of scalability, the Department of Health and Human Services would expect more from a 1,000-bed hospital than from a 60-bed hospital or a two-physician practice.

Security

Security threats come from three sources: human, environmental, and natural disasters (CMS 2007f). Human error is not intentional and comes from mistakes or misunderstandings. Examples of human threats are cutting electricity to a building when digging, destroying the wrong disk, and entering the wrong configuration setting. There are five types of threats to data security that can result from individuals. These are:

- Threats from employees who make honest mistakes
- Threats from employees who exploit their access to data
- Threats from employees who use their access to data for malice or financial gain
- Threats from external individuals who attempt to access data or steal hardware or other equipment
- Threats from angry employees or others who attack the information systems of the organization (Johns 2007)

Intentional activity is done by current employees, former employees, and hackers who intentionally damage or destroy data or the information systems. Examples of intentional damage are intentional deletion or alteration of data, infecting the information system with viruses, and using data to steal a patient's identity. Natural disasters may cause damage to the facility that destroys the system, or it may temporarily deny access to the system. Examples of natural disasters are floods, tornados, and hurricanes (Johns 2007).

Safeguards

The security rule is designed to ensure that ePHI remains confidential and is protected from unauthorized disclosure, alteration, or destruction. The security rule utilizes administrative as well as technical safeguards in order to protect the ePHI. The security rule has standards related to (CMS 2007a):

- Administrative safeguards
- Physical safeguards
- Technical safeguards

Administrative safeguards are people-focused and include requirements such as training and assignment of an individual responsible for security. Physical safeguards are mechanisms in place to protect hardware, software, and data. The physical safeguards should protect ePHI from fire, flooding, unauthorized access, theft, and other hazards. Technical safeguards use technology to protect data and to control access to the data.

Administrative, physical, and technical safeguards are broken down into implementation specifications and standards. The standards tell the covered entity what must be done, whereas implementation specifications provide direction to the covered entity to help them comply with the standard (Newby 2009). Each standard is identified as required or addressable. Required standards must be implemented by all covered entities to protect the ePHI. Addressable standards must be evaluated by the entity to determine whether or not the standard is reasonable and appropriate. If it is reasonable and appropriate, then the covered entity must implement the standard. If it is not, then the covered entity has the flexibility to identify another equivalent method of accomplishing the same objective (Rada 2003). The covered entity cannot simply document that the standard is expensive and therefore not reasonable and appropriate. If the standard is determined to not be reasonable, the covered entity must document the rationale and what is being done to implement the equivalent method.

Check Your Understanding 12.2

1. The portion of the security rule that provides direction to the covered entity in compliance is called:

   A. standard
   B. implementation specification
   C. safeguard
   D. scalable

2. A healthcare organization can consider size and complexity of the organization when developing the security plan. This is called:

   A. technology neutral
   B. administrative safeguard
   C. scalable
   D. ePHI

3. What type of safeguard is more people-focused in nature?

   A. Technical
   B. Administrative
   C. Physical
   D. Addressable

4. There are some standards where a covered entity can determine whether or not those standards are reasonable and appropriate. This concept is called:

   A. required
   B. addressable
   C. pending
   D. optional

5. Construction workers accidently cut the power to the data center. This is an example of:

   A. human error
   B. intentional activity
   C. misunderstanding
   D. intentional deletion

Administrative Safeguards

Administrative safeguards are standards designed to manage the security of ePHI through a comprehensive security program and to direct the actions of the facilities workforce. Administrative safeguards include (Hartley and Jones 2004):

- Security management

- Assigned security responsibility

- Workforce security

- Information access management
- Security awareness and training
- Security incident procedures
- Contingency plan
- Evaluation
- Business associate contract and other arrangements

The security rule defines **administrative safeguards** as: "administrative actions, and policies and procedures, to manage the selection, development, implementation, and maintenance of security measure to protect electronic protected health information and to manage the conduct of the covered entity's workforce in relation to the protection of that information." (45 CFR 160, 162, and 164 2003, 8376)

A listing of the administrative safeguards required by the HIPAA Security rule can be found in table 12.2.

Security Management Process

The security rule defines a **security incident** as an "attempted or successful unauthorized access, use, disclosure, modification, or destruction of information or interface with system operations in an information system" (45 CFR 160, 162, and 164 2003, 8376). Security incidents cannot be eliminated, but steps can be taken to reduce the risk of the incidents. This is the goal of the security management plan. In the security management process, the covered entity must manage security policies. The policies covered under this **security management plan** must include the policies required to prevent, identify, control, and resolve security incidents (45 CFR 160, 162, and 164 2003, 8346). This process begins with a risk analysis.

Table 12.2.   Administrative safeguards

Standards	Implementation Specifications
Security management	Risk analysis Risk management Sanction policy Information system activity review
Assigned security responsibility	
Workforce security	Authorization and/or supervision Workforce clearance procedures Termination procedures
Information access management	Isolating healthcare clearinghouse functions Access authorization Access establishment and modification
Security awareness and training	Security reminders Protection from malicious software Log-in monitoring Password management
Security incident procedures	Response and reporting
Contingency plan	Data backup plan Disaster recovery plan Emergency mode operation plan Testing and revision procedures Applications and data criticality analysis
Evaluation	
Business associate contract and other arrangements	Written contract or other arrangement

Adapted from 45 CFR 160, 162, and 164 2003, 8380

Risk analysis is the analysis and documentation of potential threats to data security. (Newby 2009) This requires bringing people from across the organization together to identify the data that must be protected. The risk analysis includes estimating the potential costs associated with security breaches and how much it would cost to develop safeguards to prevent these incidents from happening. This analysis must include risks to data confidentiality and integrity, and the availability of the ePHI under its control. To accomplish this, the team has to identify the threats to and vulnerabilities of the facility. Threats are the potential for a vulnerability to be exploited. Examples of threats are disgruntled employees, hackers, and computer viruses. Vulnerabilities are weaknesses that could be exploited thus creating a breach of security. Vulnerabilities may be technical or nontechnical. A technical vulnerability would be configuration in the system that allowed inappropriate access. An example of a nontechnical vulnerability is the lack of policies to guide staff (CMS 2007f). Another example of vulnerabilities would be connection to ePHI through the Internet and lack of detailed security policies and procedures. The organization also must identify existing security controls such as firewalls, employee termination procedures, and virus protection software. In addition, the team must determine the impact of losing one or more systems due to malware, sabotage, hardware failure, breach of privacy, or other failure of the organization. The risk analysis must also look for threats such as floods, fire, errors in data entry, viruses, and unauthorized access to ePHI. The security rule does not define the steps to be taken. It is left to each covered entity to develop and maintain its own plan for compliance.

The seriousness of the failure of an information system will be variable. For example, failure of the patient satisfaction database will not be as critical as the failure of the EHR. If the patient satisfaction system is not working for a week, the data entry will be backlogged and the reports may be delayed, but patient care goes on unimpeded. With the EHR, the patient's test results, allergies, past medical history, and other information may not be available. Not all risks are created equal. Each risk must be evaluated for the likelihood of the event happening. For example, if the healthcare facility is located in Alabama, the risk of an earthquake is low, but the risk of a tornado or hurricane will be high. The covered entity could categorize risks into high, medium, and low based on the impact that the threat would have on the organization.

If a vulnerability is activated, the outcome resulting from the vulnerability could take a number of forms. According to the Centers for Medicare and Medicaid Services (CMS), potential impacts include:

- Unauthorized access to or disclosure of ePHI

- Permanent destruction or corruption of ePHI

- Temporary destruction or unavailability of ePHI

- Loss of cash flow

- Loss of physical assets (CMS 2007f, 11)

Based on the likelihood of risk, the impact on the organization, and other findings, the team must recommend controls to reduce the risk to the organization. Examples of controls are sanction policies, firewalls, encryption, and biometrics. These proposals must be in compliance with the HIPAA security rule and be designed to reduce the risk and vulnerabilities to ePHI. The process, findings, and recommendations of the **risk assessment** process must be documented and retained.

According to Davis, "risk management is the process of assessing risk, taking steps to reduce risk to an acceptable level and maintaining that level of risk." (Davis 2003, 54). The first step in risk management is the development of a risk management plan. This plan sets the priority for the implementation of the security measure identified in the security assessment. The plan should include a description of the risks, the security measures to be established, and an implementation plan for the security measures including dates, resources needed (staff and monetary), and ongoing maintenance required (CMS 2007f). Risk assessment and risk management are not one-time events but rather ongoing processes. Although HIPAA does not mandate the frequency of reviews or updates, it does mandate that it must occur as necessary. This time period could be from 1 to 3 years based on the needs of the organization.

Each covered entity must develop for itself a sanction policy that should address how workforce members will be penalized for failing to follow security policies and procedures. HIPAA does not require specific employee penalties but rather requires the covered entity to determine how breaches and other violations should be handled. Employees should be notified of the policies and procedures and the penalties that come with violations. Members of the workforce should sign an acknowledgment of the security requirements and that they understand that violations may result in disciplinary actions that could include termination of employment. Sanctions should be based on the severity of the failure to comply with the policies and procedures (Burrington-Brown 2003b). For example, an employee who fails to log off of a computer during a medical emergency should not be penalized in the same way as an employee who accesses celebrity ePHI inappropriately and sells that information to the tabloids.

Covered entities are required to conduct an **information system activity review**—the periodic review of the security controls (Rada 2003). HIPAA does not mandate the frequency of this review nor how this review is to be conducted. These reviews should include logs, access, and incident reporting. The covered entity should monitor audit logs and other tracking mechanisms to identify any successful and unsuccessful attempts to access ePHI. This review should include review of audit logs, the incident log, and other internal and external documentation. If risks have increased or technology changes, the security program would need to be updated (Amatayakul 2003).

Assigned Security Responsibility

The security rule mandates an individual to be in charge of the security program for the covered entity. HIPAA calls this individual a **security official**; however, this position is frequently called chief security officer (CSO) by the covered entities. The CSO is responsible for (McWay 2008):

- Developing the security goals and objectives for the covered entity

- Determining how the goals and objectives will be met

- Advising administration regarding information security

- Determining reporting procedures

- Conducting adequate risk assessment and determining the appropriate level of risk acceptance

The CSO does not work alone, but with others who assist in managing the security program of the organization. This individual must have a strong understanding of both technology and the business practices of the organization. HIPAA gives little direction as to the role of the CSO, just that the responsibility should be given to a specific individual. The CSO role may be a full-time or part-time role and may be the same or different individual from the privacy official.

Workforce Security

Policies and procedures should be in place to ensure that members of the workforce have the appropriate access to ePHI for their job. Each workforce member must be authorized to perform various activities such as accessing an information system or viewing data (CMS 2007b). The **workforce clearance procedure** ensures that each member of the workforce's level of access is appropriate (Newby 2009). This access determination should be based on risk analysis and each employee's job description. There must be termination procedures to eliminate access to the information systems by a member of the workforce when their employment with the covered entity ends. This termination should include both voluntary and involuntary separation from the covered entity (CMS 2007b). The **termination process** should also include changes to the access level as the individual's role changes in the organization. The new role may require the employee to have access to more or less ePHI, so a review of the employee's level of access must be conducted to ensure that it is appropriate for his or her job.

Information Access Management

Covered entities are required to limit access to ePHI to individuals with a need for that information. Under this standard, covered entities are required to isolate healthcare clearinghouse functions and control access authorization, access establishment and modification. To isolate healthcare clearinghouse functions, the ePHI must be stored in such a way to prevent employees in a separate component of the parent organization from accessing the information inappropriately (CMS 2007b). There must be policies and procedures defining who has access to ePHI, how those decisions are made, and the process followed. Not everyone with access to ePHI needs the ability to create and modify data. For example, a coder in the HIM department will need to review the ePHI to properly code the admission; however, the coder would not need to add clinical information to the chart. There must be policies and procedures in place to control the specific authorization that a user has such as view, add, delete, and modify. As the individual's role in the organization changes, there must be a mechanism in place to amend the workforce member's rights.

Check Your Understanding 12.3

1. The document that includes policies and procedures to prevent, identify, control, and resolve security incidents is called:

   A. Risk assessment
   B. Workforce security
   C. Security management plan
   D. Business associate contract

2. Employees who violate HIPAA are subject to what policy?

   A. Risk assessment
   B. Sanction
   C. Violation
   D. Vulnerability

3. Security controls should be monitored periodically for effectiveness. This review is called:

   A. Security management process
   B. Trigger
   C. Audit
   D. Information system activity review

4. The process that determines whether or not an employee's access to ePHI is appropriate is called:

   A. Information system activity review
   B. Workforce security
   C. Termination process
   D. Workforce clearance procedure

5. The individual assigned the responsibility of managing the security process is called:

   A. Security official
   B. Privacy official
   C. Chief executive officer
   D. Chief information officer

Security Awareness and Training

All workforce members must receive **security awareness training**. This training provides employees of the covered entities with information and a basic knowledge of the security policies and procedures of the organization (Newby 2009). This training must be provided to all members of the workforce including administration, board of directors, custodial staff, students, volunteers, and all other employees. Security training is not a one size fits all, but everyone should receive basic security training that will cover issues such as general security policies, physical and workstation security, password management, and other issues (Amatayakul and Johns 2002). This security awareness training could be presented as part of the new employee orientation. Many workforce members will require additional security training based on the needs of their job (Hjort 2003a). For example, the management staff will need training on monitoring procedures and security system assessment. Training should be ongoing and provided whenever there are changes to policies and procedures or areas related to security. HIPAA does not mandate the format that the training takes. The face-to-face training classes should be supported with periodic security reminders, which could take many formats, including:

- screen savers with security reminders

- periodic e-mails with security reminders

- articles or statements in an employee newsletter

- notices posted in public areas such as the cafeteria

Documentation of the training must be retained for 6 years as required by HIPAA. Examples of documentation include (Hjort 2003a):

- sign-in sheets

- handouts

- e-mail messages

- training database identifying training and actions taken

Security Incident Procedures

No matter how hard a covered entity strives to eliminate security incidents, they will happen. HIPAA requires covered entities to actively identify and report security incidents. As stated earlier, the security rule defines a security incident as "the attempted or successful unauthorized access, use, disclosure, modification, or destruction of information or interference with system operations in an information system" (45 CFR 160, 162, and 164 2003, 8376). Because this definition is broad, the covered entity should define a security incident for the facility. The security incident policies and procedures should identify how the incidents will be identified and to whom it should be reported. Security incidents from throughout the organization should be reported to a centralized location. The security incidents should include information technology incidents, such as hacking, as well as physical security incidents, such as computer theft. Security incidents must be addressed quickly because inaction could allow the incident to worsen, such as in the case of a virus (Amatayakul 2005b).

Policies and procedures should define how the covered entity will respond to a security incident. These responses should vary by the seriousness of the incident. If the incident suggests criminal activity or compromises the safety of an individual, the local law enforcement agency should be contacted.

The CSO should monitor trends in the types of security incidents that occur. The identification of patterns that this trending can provide yields valuable information regarding threats and vulnerabilities of the organization.

Figure 12.1 provides an example of an incident response report form.

Figure 12.1.   Sample security incident response report form

Sample Security Incident Response Report Form

Privileged and Confidential Attorney-Client Communication/Work Product

INCIDENT IDENTIFICATION INFORMATION

Date and Time of Notification:

Incident Detector's Information:

Name:	Date and Time Detected:
Title:	Location:
Phone/Contact Info:	System or Application:

INCIDENT SUMMARY

Type of Incident Detected:

☐ Denial of Service   ☐ Malicious Code   ☐ Unauthorized Use
☐ Unauthorized Access   ☐ Unplanned Downtime   ☐ Other

Description of Incident:

_____
_____
_____

Names and Contact Information of Others Involved:

_____
_____
_____

INCIDENT NOTIFICATION – OTHERS

☐ IS Leadership   ☐ System or Application Owner   ☐ System or Application Vendor
☐ Security Incident Response Team   ☐ Public Affairs   ☐ Legal Counsel
☐ Administration   ☐ Human Resources
☐ Other:

ACTIONS

Identification Measures (Incident Verified, Assessed, Options Evaluated):

_____
_____
_____

Containment Measures:

_____
_____
_____

Evidence Collected (Systems Logs, etc.):

_____
_____
_____

Eradication Measures:

_____
_____

Recovery Measures:

_____
_____

Other Mitigation Actions:

_____
_____

This form has been developed as a working tool for assessment and improvement activities; it is intended for internal use only.

Journal of AHIMA/January 2008 - 79/1

Figure 12.1.   Sample security incident response report form *(continued)*

Sample Security Incident Response Report Form

Privileged and Confidential Attorney-Client Communication/Work Product

EVALUATION

How Well Did Work Force Members Respond?

Were the Documented Procedures Followed? Were They Adequate?

What Information Was Needed Sooner?

Were Any Steps or Actions Taken That Might Have Inhibited the Recovery?

What Could Work Force Members Do Differently the Next Time an Incident Occurs?

What Corrective Actions Can Prevent Similar Incidents in the Future?

What Additional Resources Are Needed to Detect, Analyze, and Mitigate Future Incidents?

Other Conclusions or Recommendations:

FOLLOW-UP

Reviewed By:
☐ Security Officer   ☐ IS Department/Team
☐ Privacy Officer   ☐ Other

Recommended Actions Carried Out:

Initial Report Completed By:

Follow-Up Completed By:

This form has been developed as a working tool for assessment and improvement activities; it is intended for internal use only.

Journal of AHIMA/January 2008 - 79/1

Source: AHIMA 2007 Privacy and Security Practice Council 2008

Forensics "is the process used to gather intact and validated evidence" (Derhak 2003, 2) and is the process that should be used to gather evidence of the security incident. The steps in forensics include:

- documentation of the investigation conducted

- protection and preservation of any evidence found, the logs reviewed, and reports

- documentation of the chain of custody (who had access)

- the use of an exact copy of the media in the investigation (Derhak 2003)

The investigation may require hardware to be confiscated and stored in a secured location, network logs to be printed, backing up of data, and other investigative steps. Failure to protect data properly may result in the destruction of evidence. This destruction may be intentional or unintentional. Unintentional destruction or alteration of evidence is called **spoliation** (Tomes 2005). During the course of the investigation a number of steps may be taken such as:

- recovering deleted files

- recovering passwords

- analyzing file access, creation, and modification times

- analyzing system and application logs

- determining user and application activity on a system (Derhak 2003, 2)

Once a security incident is identified, the covered entity must mitigate the harmful effects of security incidents and document the incident and the outcomes. **Mitigation** is the process of attempting to reduce or eliminate harmful effects of the breach (45 CFR 160, 162, and 164 2003). It may not be possible to completely mitigate the effects, but the covered entity must do everything that it can to protect the patient. For example, if a patient's social security number is inappropriately disclosed, the covered entity may pay for the patient to monitor his or her credit report for a specified period of time.

An example of the steps to take in the case of a security incident is found in figure 12.2.

Security events are poor security practices that have not led to harm, whereas security incidents have resulted in harm or a significant risk of harm (Amatayakul 2005b). Security events may be mistakes by an employee that occurred, but no disclosure of ePHI resulted in the error. Many of these errors may result from noncompliance with the organization's policies and procedures, such as not logging off the computer system.

Examples of security events include:

- shared logon

- password reminder visible at workstation

- monitor left logged on and unattended

- system access to patient data down with only paper copies of encounter forms

- unencrypted or otherwise unsecured e-mail of protected health information (PHI)

- maintenance personnel fixing equipment with PHI without supervision by your workforce (Amatayakul 2005b)

Examples of security incidents include:

- someone impersonating an IT technician asking for a password

- former employee using old ID and password to access electronic PHI (ePHI)

- virus attack that destroyed current files

Figure 12.2.   Data breach investigation and mitigation checklist

Data Breach Investigation and Mitigation Checklist

Actions to Be Taken Immediately upon Identification of an Incident

1. Notification Process
   - ☐ Notify privacy and security officers
   - ☐ Initiate security incident report form
   - ☐ Record name and contact information of reporter
   - ☐ Gather description of event
   - ☐ Identify location of event

2. Investigation Steps
   - ☐ Establish security incident response team (e.g., security officer, privacy officer, risk manager, administration, and others as needed) and identify team leader (e.g., privacy or security officer)
   - ☐ Identify and take immediate action to stop the source (e.g., hacking) or entity responsible (e.g., work force member, vendor)
   - ☐ Identify system, application, or electronic PHI compromised and then immediately begin identification process of those patients whose information was compromised and what data elements were included (e.g., name, age, date of birth, Social Security number, diagnosis)
   - ☐ Determine need to notify key internal stakeholders not represented on the team:
     - ▫ HIM department (if necessary to sequester records)
     - ▫ Billing and patient accounts department (if necessary to suspend billing process)
     - ▫ Human resources department (if a work force member is suspected)
     - ▫ Vendor relations or purchasing leadership
     - ▫ Others as necessary
   - ☐ Identify the source or suspects involved in event:
     - ▫ If the source is identified as a vendor or business associate, determine if business associate agreement has been established (collect as evidence)
     - ▫ If the source is identified as a work force member, establish existence of criminal background check, privacy and security education and training, etc. Coordinate with human resources to determine appropriate sanctions.
     - ▫ If the source is external, work with law enforcement agency to determine appropriate actions
   - ☐ Carry out IT forensic investigation to gather evidence and determine course of events as well as identify electronic PHI compromised
   - ☐ Identify and sequester pertinent medical records, files, and other documents (paper and electronic)
   - ☐ Determine need for external notification or involvement (see individual sections following):
     - ▫ Legal counsel (identify all communications as "Privileged and Confidential Attorney-Client Communication/Work Product")
     - ▫ IT forensics support
     - ▫ Law enforcement agency (local and federal)
     - ▫ Media
     - ▫ Victims

- ☐ Determine need to contact other additional external stakeholders:
  - ▫ Corporate office
  - ▫ Licensing or accrediting agencies
  - ▫ Centers for Medicare and Medicaid Services, Office for Civil Rights (self-reporting is not required by regulation, it is an organizational decision)
  - ▫ Business associates or partners

Other Actions as Applicable

1. Contact Law Enforcement Officials
   - ☐ Verify event constitutes a crime and is reportable
   - ☐ Determine appropriate law enforcement agency and contact
   - ☐ In cooperation with local law enforcement officials, determine the need to involve other external law enforcement agencies (e.g., FTC, FBI, Social Security Administration, Inspector General)
   - ☐ Obtain name of law enforcement contact to provide upon victim request

2. Collection of Evidence
   - ☐ Security incidence response form
   - ☐ IT forensic evidence (e.g., reports, logs, audits)
   - ☐ Records of communications (e.g., phone logs, e-mail, letters)
   - ☐ Law enforcement agency and police reports
   - ☐ Legal counsel guidance

3. Notification of Victims
   - ☐ Determine need to notify victims. Consider:
     - ▫ Likelihood of harm (e.g., stolen laptop protected by password or encryption, PHI limited to first names and dates only)
     - ▫ Recipient of information, if known (e.g., if recipient is known covered entity, there is less risk than if PHI was disclosed to other individuals)
     - ▫ Regulatory reporting and disclosure requirements (review state regulations)
     - ▫ Type of incident (e.g., targeted theft of data or incidental as part of crime of opportunity such as laptop left unaccompanied in airport waiting area)
     - ▫ Actions of other organizations if involved in event (e.g., information system of vendor hacked containing multiple healthcare clients)
     - ▫ Historical responses by others involved in similar events
   - ☐ Prepare a communication plan to cover oral and written communications to victims as well as information to assist them with personal needs (FTC guidance) and organizational contact person for questions and concerns (privacy officer)
   - ☐ Provide information regarding law enforcement contacts
   - ☐ Consider provision of credit monitoring services (e.g., fees paid by organization? If so, how long?)

Journal of AHIMA/January 2008 - 79/1

(continued on next page)

Figure 12.2.   Data breach investigation and mitigation checklist *(continued)*

Data Breach Investigation and Mitigation Checklist

Actions to Be Taken Immediately upon Identification of an Incident

4. Communication with Media
   - ☐ Determine need to proactively contact media or prepare press release in response to inquiries. Consider:
     - ▫ Likelihood of media awareness or investigation
     - ▫ Scope of event (e.g., number of individuals impacted, type of information disclosed, threat of harm to victims)
     - ▫ Potential for harm to individuals (e.g., patients, business associates, clients, others)
     - ▫ Organizational preventive safeguards and practices
     - ▫ Mitigation efforts
     - ▫ Preparation of talking points for public affairs department outlining organizations privacy and security safeguards
     - ▫ Limitations of disclosure as advised by legal counsel or law enforcement

5. Other Organizational Processes to Be Considered
   - ☐ Determine how best to account for disclosures of PHI (HIPAA requirement):
     - ▫ Update each health record (paper or electronic) with disclosure information
     - ▫ Provide list of patients to privacy officer in response to accounting of disclosure requests (may be preferred for large numbers of disclosures)
   - ☐ If event is result of a business associate's failure to safeguard PHI, consider need to terminate relationship (refer to business associate agreement)

Follow-Up Activities, Identifying Opportunities for Improvement

1. Evaluation of Security Incident Response (Document on Form)
   - ☐ Identify actions:
     - ▫ Identification measures (incident verified, assessed, options evaluated)
     - ▫ Evidence collected
     - ▫ Eradication measures
     - ▫ Recovery measures

- ☐ Determine:
  - ▫ How well did the work force members respond to event?
  - ▫ Were documented procedures followed? Were they adequate?
  - ▫ What information was needed sooner?
  - ▫ Were there any steps or actions that might have inhibited recovery?
  - ▫ What could work force members do differently the next time an incident occurs?
  - ▫ What corrective actions can prevent similar events in the future?
  - ▫ What additional resources are needed to detect, analyze, and mitigate future incidents?
  - ▫ Can missing electronic PHI be recreated to provide continuity of care?
  - ▫ What external resources and contacts proved helpful?
  - ▫ Other conclusions or recommendations

2. Follow-Up
   - ☐ Security incident response form completed and supporting documentation made part of form or filed as attachments (consider restricting access to the form)
   - ☐ Policy and process review completed and all necessary changes made based on shortcomings identified through managing event
   - ☐ Training, education, and awareness activities carried out (balancing need for awareness with disclosure of event)
   - ☐ Event documented as educational case study (de-identified) for internal use

3. Other
   - ☐ Consider the offer of a reward for return of lost or stolen equipment ❖

Source: AHIMA 2007 Privacy and Security Practice Council 2008

- audit trail with evidence that someone misused someone else's password
- corrupt backup tapes with no ability to restore archived data
- physical break-in with ePHI copied or stolen
- PHI posted on the Internet from a Web portal
- misdirected e-mail with ePHI
- terminated employee keeping copies of records with PHI
- CDs containing ePHI found discarded without physical destruction (Amatayakul 2005b)

Contingency Plan

A **contingency plan** is made up of policies and procedures that identify how a healthcare facility will react in the event of an information system emergency such as power failure, natural disaster or a system failure (Newby 2009). A healthcare facility can have redundancy built into the system to reduce the risk of the EHR or other critical patient care systems from being down but it cannot eliminate the possibility. **Redundancy** is duplication of data, hardware, cables, or other components of the system. This is useful in case a cable is cut or a computer fails. With the redundancy, the system is operational with little to no downtime.

There will be times when the system is down for routine maintenance or failure. To prepare for these times when the system crashes or is experiencing downtime for hardware maintenance, loading of updated software, and other reasons, a contingency plan must be developed. The contingency plan should include a data backup plan. The data backup plan should include all critical sources of information such as the EHR and clinical information systems.

There may be a time when disaster strikes and the organization loses data because of flood, fire, tornado, hardware failure, or other failure. The facility must have plans in place to get the system working again and then to update it with all activities that occurred during the downtime. The emergency mode operation plan encompasses procedures necessary to keep the critical business processes of the covered entity in place during system downtime (Davis 2003). Manual processes such as paper laboratory slips, microfilm of the master patient index, and medical record forms must be available in the event that the system is down. The contingency plan must be tested periodically and revised as areas needing improvement are identified. Not all information systems are equivalent. Some information systems such as the EHR cause turmoil in an organization if they are offline. Other systems such as a strategic decision support system have less impact on the organization because there is no direct impact on patient care. Each system should be evaluated to determine how critical it is and a plan of action in place in the event of a system outage. The result should be a prioritized list of applications and data used to determine which system should be addressed first if multiple systems are down simultaneously (LaTour and Eichenwald Maki 2006). The EHR and other patient care systems would have top billing on the priority list, with nonpatient, nonfinancial systems at the bottom.

Data Recovery

System maintenance, hardware failures, and other problems can result in the loss of data and unavailable systems. Contingency and disaster planning prepare the facility to operate in a manual process and to get the information systems up and operational again. When the systems are again functional, data recovery must occur. **Data recovery** is the process of recouping lost data or reconciling conflicting data after the system fails (Microsoft Corporation). These data may be from events that occurred while the system was down or they may be from backed up data. Data captured during the downtime must be entered into the system in order to bring the system up-to-date. Data lost out of the database should be recoverable from backup tapes or other media. Depending on the time since the last backup, little or no data may be lost. The facility must have current backups of the database to be able to re-create the data. Information systems should have a utility to restore data from tape or other media onto the database. This process should be tested periodically to ensure that the utility is working appropriately.

Evaluation

Implementation of the security safeguards is not enough. Covered entities must also critique their security program through ongoing monitoring and evaluation to identify areas for improvement. The evaluation must include both technical and nontechnical processes. Technical processes would include encryption, access controls, and other technical tools. Nontechnical processes would include policies and procedures, training, and other administrative responsibilities (Rada 2003). The evaluation should address whether or not the organization is meeting the HIPAA security rules and whether or not the program is still appropriate for the current status of the organization. Organizations change over time because of growth, changes in policies, changes in technologies used, and changes in laws and regulations. The security program must keep up with these changes.

Business Associate Contracts and Other Arrangements

Business associates are organizations that conduct business on behalf of the covered entity, and as a part of that role they require access to PHI (45 CFR 160, 162, and 164 2006). Business associates are subject to the security rule and are expected to follow the tenets of the rule. In order for the business associate to gain access to the ePHI, they must ensure the covered entity that they will protect the ePHI and will notify the covered entity of any failures. There must be a business associate agreement between the covered entity and the business associate that meets the requirements established in HIPAA (Hartley and Jones 2004). Examples of business associates are contract coders, application service providers, transcription servers, and billing services.

Check Your Understanding 12.4

1. Poor security practices that do not lead to disclosure of ePHI are called:

    A. security incidents
    B. mitigation
    C. security events
    D. noncompliance

2. A security breach has been reported. What concept describes the process used to gather evidence?

    A. Forensics
    B. Risk assessment
    C. Security incident
    D. Security event

3. If the EHR crashes, what plan should be implemented?

    A. Contingency
    B. Workforce clearance
    C. Forensics
    D. Security safeguards

4. Security awareness training must be provided to:
   A. all management employees
   B. all nonmanagement employees
   C. all members of the workforce
   D. all members of the workforce excluding the board of directors

5. HIPAA calls an organization that conducts business on behalf of the covered entity and requires access to PHI to perform this work a(n):
   A. consultant
   B. business associate
   C. contractor
   D. outsource vendor

Physical Safeguards

Physical safeguards are an important part of security. The security rule defines **physical safeguards** as "physical measures, policies, and procedures to protect a covered entity's electronic information systems and related buildings and equipment, from natural and environmental hazards, and unauthorized intrusion" (45 CFR 160, 162, and 164 2003, 8376).

Physical safeguards protect the hardware and software related to the ePHI. The physical plant and equipment must be protected from intentional and unintentional tampering or destruction.

The hardware must be protected from natural disasters such as tornadoes and floods. It must also be protected from fire, theft, and intentional tampering. The policies and procedures should also document how the organization is protecting the equipment from unauthorized access, tampering, and theft. Physical safeguards should include not only the computers and other hardware but also backup tapes. The required physical safeguards are (Newby 2009, 73):

- facility access controls

- workstation location and access

- workstation security

- device and media controls

A summary of the physical standards can be found in table 12.3

Table 12.3.   Physical standards

Standards	Implementation Standards
Facility access controls	Contingency operations Facility security plan Access control and validation procedures Maintenance records
Workstation location and use	
Workstation security	
Device and media controls	Disposal Media reuse Accountability Data backup and storage

Adapted from 45 CFR 160, 162, and 164 2003, 8380

Facility Access Controls

The covered entity must implement **facility access controls** which limit physical access to authorized information system staff to the data centers where the hardware and software for the electronic information systems are held. Visitors to the area frequently are required to sign in and be escorted while in the data center. This type of control must be documented in the policies and procedures. There must also be policies and procedures regarding the handling of contractors and service technicians. In the event of a system outage, the appropriate staff and contractors must be able to access the system so that the system can be operational as quickly as possible. Individuals with authorized access should wear a picture identification tag at all times.

Access to the data center can be controlled by card keys, access codes, or other control methods. The fact that an individual is a member of the workforce does not authorize him or her to be in the data center. Access to the data center should be limited to individuals with a business need. Identification badges are also often required for entry. Cameras may be used to record individuals going into the data center and other areas where hardware is located. The video can be used to determine who had access to the data center or other critical areas in the event of a security incident.

Some of the safeguards are as simple as locking doors, using an alarm system, bolting the equipment to a desk, and using surge suppressors. Other safeguards include monitoring the temperature of the room so that the computers do not become too hot or too cold, because extreme temperatures can damage the computer. Some computers are very sensitive to temperature and may become damaged in temperature extremes. There should also be a system in place to extinguish fires.

These safeguards will need to be maintained and updated as appropriate to ensure that they protect the ePHI. There must be documentation of the repairs performed (CMS, 2007c). This can be as simple as a log book or as complicated as a specialized database, based on the size and complexity of the organization. Workstations, which include computers, personal digital assistants (PDAs), and laptops that access ePHI, should be used appropriately by the workforce members. It is up to the organization to define what is appropriate.

Workstation Use

Workstations include not only a desktop computer but handheld devices, laptops, and other pieces of equipment that manage ePHI (Hartley and Jones 2004). Workstations must be protected from unauthorized access (CMS, 2007c). Policies and procedures should be in place to protect the workstation from viruses, breaches of privacy, and other risky behaviors. For example, employees should log off if they step away from their workstation. Another example would be for the computer to be programmed to automatically log off after a predetermined period of time.

It is easy for thieves to pick up computers or other pieces of hardware. To protect hardware, security measures can include bolting hardware to desks and locking doors. As discussed in more detail in the next section, laptops, PDAs, and other portable devices are especially easy to steal because of their portability. Every item should have a property control tag to track the hardware as it moves throughout the facility (Dinh 2009). The facility may also want to investigate security options for portable devices such as those that monitor the location of devices. When an inventory is performed, the facility knows exactly where pieces of hardware should be located and what has been moved.

Physical security also includes the need for a **contingency plan**. A contingency plan outlines how the facility will operate if the EHR or other information system is inoperable. The plan should include how data will be restored and how they will be updated during the time that the system is down. An emergency mode operation plan is part of the contingency plan where the organization plans for how they will function while the system is down. Paper forms and manual processes must be in place to document patient care, dictate reports, order tests, and report test results and other functions performed by healthcare information systems.

Both the hardware and software should be protected. Members of the workforce who are responsible for accessing the test system and making changes to the software must be controlled so as to reduce errors that occur when many people are involved.

When maintenance is performed to the physical security measures, these actions must be documented. Examples of this maintenance include: installing new security cameras, changing locks, or knocking down walls to expand the size of the data center. This documentation should be retained for future reference.

Physical security goes beyond protecting the hardware, and also includes protecting the data accessed on the computer. For example, computers should be positioned so that unauthorized users cannot view the data on the screen. Another method of controlling access to ePHI is for the workstation to log off automatically after a specified time period of inactivity. This prevents visitors or other employees from sitting down at the workstation and accessing protected health information and attributing the access to the individual logged in. Prior to this logoff, a screen saver that blanks out the screen after a period of inactivity should be activated so that passing individuals would not see protected health information. Besides the technical controls, policies and procedures should specify the need for employees to log out of the system when stepping away from the workstation. Privacy screens may also be used to prohibit authorized viewing of the data on the workstation. Privacy screens require the user to sit directly in front of the workstation to be able to see the data on the screen.

Device and Media Controls

Workstations, hardware, software, and other devices are not the only items that should be protected from loss and destruction. Media, which includes computer hard drives and removable digital storage must also be protected. Examples of removable digital storage are external hard drive, thumb drives, CDs, and optical disks. Media that stores ePHI must have policies and procedures that control its movement and storage. Because media is small and easily portable, it is easy for employees to move the media and for it to get lost. It is also easily stolen. The covered entity could create a log to track receipt or removal of the media so that an individual is responsible for the media. This tracking of devices and media is called accountability (Hartley and Jones 2004).

With the advent of portable devices such as the PDA, tracking media is becoming more and more difficult to do because the devices are moved around for use in patient care. The actions and not the location of the workstation matter, so the policies should apply to computers at employee's workstations and other locations. It is very easy to lose CDs, tapes, and other media that store ePHI, so covered entities must have a policy in place to protect them from loss or destruction. The media must be tracked throughout the organization. Once the computer media is no longer required, it must be disposed of in the appropriate manner.

Once the media is no longer needed there should be a formal process for its disposal. Workstations and other media just cannot be thrown away. There have been numerous stories in the news over the years in which computers were purchased at garage sales and thrift shops and confidential information was found by the new owner. Deletion of the ePHI stored on the media does not render it inaccessible; there are utilities, or software programs, that can undelete files. Because of this capability, the media itself needs to be destroyed or the media should be degaussed. **Degaussing** is application of a magnetic field to the media to render the data on it useless. Degaussing renders data impossible to recover and is not reversible (Hughes 2002). Another method for sanitizing the hard drive of a computer is overwriting the data stored on the hard drive (Keating 2006). The data may have to be overwritten multiple times in order to prevent recovery (Hughes 2002). CDs, floppy disks, and other media may also be pulverized.

There may be times that the facility wishes to reuse media on which ePHI is stored. For example, workstations frequently may be moved from one location to another to make way for more powerful workstations. The security rule does allow this if the ePHI is removed according to policy. Electronic media, computers, and other hardware may be moved within the organization, but there must be a record of the movements and who is responsible for the equipment. When a computer has ePHI stored on it, the data should be backed up before the computer is moved. Another method of protecting ePHI when computers are moved is to store the data on a network so that the ePHI is not at risk. If ePHI is stored on the workstation, that data must be removed before the computer is transferred from one location to another. The movement of workstations and media must be tracked so the facility knows where all of the workstations and media are at any given time. (CMS, 2007c)

Media can become damaged and files can become corrupted. Media also can be destroyed by natural disaster or fire. To protect the facility against loss of ePHI, there should be an exact backup file of the data stored in the EHR, financial information system, and all other systems. One facility that implemented an imaging system properly created a backup file of all of the optical disks. The problem was that this facility stored the backup file 15 feet from the original disk. The HIM department, where the optical disks were stored, was located in the basement so if there had been a flood or other disaster both copies would have been lost. Backup files should be stored at an off-site location that would not be at risk for the same disaster. For example, a healthcare facility in New Orleans could have their data backed up on an information system in Montana. This eliminates the possibility of the same event damaging both the original and the backup databases.

Check Your Understanding 12.5

1. Using a magnet to destroy data on a magnetic disk is called:

    A. degaussing
    B. deleting
    C. disposal
    D. destruction

2. An example of a facility access control is:

    A. contingency planning
    B. locking a computer to a desk
    C. escorting visitors in the data center
    D. tracking PDAs through the organization

3. Which statement is true?

    A. Physical safeguards address only the physical hardware
    B. Physical safeguards address only fire protection
    C. Physical safeguards include not only hardware but data as well
    D. Physical safeguards include protecting the data center only

4. Backup disks should be stored:

    A. in a convenient area
    B. in another area in the facility
    C. in an area that would not be subjected to the same natural disasters as the original data
    D. within 20 miles of the healthcare facility to allow for easy access in the event of loss of data

5. Physical safeguards include:

    A. hardware and software
    B. hardware, software, and backup tapes
    C. hardware
    D. hardware and software located at the healthcare facility

Technical Safeguards

Technical safeguards are defined by the security rule as "the technology and the policy and procedures for its use that protect electronic protected health information and control access to it." (45 CFR 160, 162, and 164 2003, 8370) Technical safeguards use technology as well as policies and procedures to protect the ePHI from unauthorized access and destruction or alteration. The policies, procedures, and documentation standards set define the requirements for the documentation of the security program. Technical safeguards standards are (45 CFR 160, 162, and 164 2003, 8376):

- access control
- audit controls
- integrity
- person or entity authentication
- transmission security

A summary of the HIPAA technical safeguard standards are found in table 12.4.

Access Controls

Access controls are the technical policies and procedures used to control access to ePHI. Access controls must be used to provide users with rights and limitations on what they can do in a system containing ePHI. The specific technology is not mandated, but each user must have unique user identification. The unique user identifier tracks the actions of each user. Some organizations use employee names, for example, jdoe or jane.doe. Others assign a number or identification to each user (Connecting for Health Policy Subcommittee 2006). Each of these users should have access to only the information required to perform their job. There may be times when a user needs to have access to information not normally allowed by their access controls. This situation usually occurs during a medical emergency. In that case, an **emergency access procedure** must be in place so that the individual can access the ePHI required. This access is frequently called "break the glass." This emergency access procedure may require a second password or a reason for access. The use of the emergency access procedures must be monitored to ensure that the system is not abused (Amatayakul 2005a). The system should require a brief note as to why the data are required. Even in an emergency situation, there must be a way to identify who activated the emergency access and why. This access should be audited to ensure validity.

As stated earlier, if a workstation is inactive for a period of time specified by the organization, it should log itself off automatically. This automatic logoff helps prevent unauthorized users from accessing ePHI when an authorized user walks away from the computer without logging out of the system. The monitor of the workstation should also be faced away from the public to prevent an unintentional privacy or security breach.

Table 12.4.   Technical safeguard standards

Standards	Implementation Specifications
Access control	Unique user identification Emergency access procedure Automatic logoff Encryption and decryption
Audit controls	
Integrity	Mechanism to authenticate ePHI
Person or entity authentication	
Transmission security	Integrity controls Encryption

Adapted from 45 CFR 160, 162, and 164 2003, 8380

Audit Controls

The facility cannot just develop a security program and assume that all is well. The covered entity must monitor the program. **Audit controls** are one component of this monitoring program. Audit controls are "mechanisms that record and examine activity in information systems" (LaTour and Eichenwald Maki 2006, 228). Audit controls serve four purposes (Amatayakul 2004a):

- Hold individual users personally responsible for their actions

- Use an investigation tool to identify cause of problem, how bad the problem is, and how to restore the system back to normal operations

- Use real-time monitoring to identify breaches, technical problems, and other security issues quickly

- Watch for intrusions into the system so that the intrusion can be stopped before a breach occurs

These audits review system activities to identify security incidents. **Audit trails** are the record of these system activities such as login, logout, unsuccessful logins, print, query, and other actions. It also records user identification information and the date and time of the activity. Audits should be scheduled periodically, but can also be performed when a problem is suspected.

A review could also be performed when a patient complains that their PHI has been released, or in response to a newspaper article or other suspected incident. Facilities choose a variety of schedules for audit trails. Some turn the audit controls on randomly so that the user never knows if his or her actions are being recorded (Amatayakul 2004a). Others record everything all the time. Whatever the schedule of capture, the data must be audited. This audit should be designed to include a review of the user's actions at different days, times of day, and locations. The security rule does not mandate a specific number of audits, but the facility should base the volume on the size and complexity of the facility. The findings should be reported all the way up the organizational chart to the board of directors.

Audit controls are not without their problems. One is that the audit controls of the various information systems vary in their level of sophistication. Some are only able to record logins and not the specific records accessed. Also, recording audit trail data consumes resources that may slow down the system and require the upgrade of the file server. To protect the audit log data from alteration or destruction, the data should be stored on a different server than the ePHI. In addition, to prevent alteration or destruction, access to the audit log should be restricted to a limited number of users who have a business need to access the information. Another advantage to the audit trail data being stored on a separate server is that the increase in storage space will allow longer retention of the data as needed (Amatayakul 2004b).

A review of the audit trail is not the only auditing that should be performed. Another means of auditing is touring the facility to ensure that security policies and procedures are being followed. Examples of actions that can be monitored in this way include ensuring that monitors are turned away from public areas and that users log out of the system when stepping away from the computer, and also looking for signs of passwords being written down or shared.

Integrity

Technology has advanced to a point where an unauthorized user can capture data in transit and alter it. Covered entities must confirm the integrity of data passed across a network. Integrity is the security principle that protects data from inappropriate modification or corruption. This includes both intentional and unintentional modifications and destructions. Unintentional modifications and destruction could occur if the wrong data are destroyed, the wrong tape is used to restore data, or an electrical fire destroys the computer. Examples of intentional modification and destruction include intentional deletion of data, induction of virus software, and changing the amount that the employee owes for treatment. An example of a tool that can be used to monitor data integrity is checksum verification (LaTour and Eichenwald Maki 2006). Data integrity is where the message received must be confirmed as the one sent (CMS, 2007d). Integrity can be validated with checksum validation. A checksum validation follows the data sent across the network. The checksum links to the data. If the data is changed, the checksum does not properly match the data being transmitted thus indicating that the data has been altered (Rada 2003).

Person or Entity Authentication

Person or entity authentication is required to prove a person's identity. There are three models of authentication that the covered entity can use. These methods of authentication are based on (Dougherty 2004):

- something the individual knows, such as a password or personal identification number

- something the individual has, such as a smart card or token

- something unique to the individual, such as biometrics

Methods of Authentication

Passwords are commonly used in conjunction with a username or identifier. This is an example of a **one-factor authentication** as it only utilizes something you know (Burrington-Brown 2003a). The **username** is usually based on the individual's name, but it could be some other assigned user identification. Two common methods of assigning a username for John Smith are jsmith and john.smith. Social security numbers should never be used as the user identification because of concerns about identity theft. The organization should establish strict rules for the use of passwords. These rules should control the format of the password, the frequency of change, and privacy of the password.

Strong passwords should not be easily guessed; the user's name, child's name, dog's name, and favorite sports team are passwords that may be easy to determine. Passwords should have seven or more characters. They should contain two or more types of characters such as uppercase letters, lowercase letters, numbers, and/or symbols. Ideal passwords would not contain a word found in any language. These passwords should be changed periodically. Many systems force the user to change the password periodically. The number of days is determined by the facility but could be 30 days, 6 months, 1 year, or other defined time period. Best practices state that the user should choose his or her own password and passwords should not be reused (Amatayakul and Walsh 2001).

Policies related to passwords should state that the password is confidential and cannot be shared with anyone else. In years past, users have written passwords down near their computer so they did not have to remember the password. For example, they taped it on the computer or placed it under their phone or some other convenient location. Users also shared their password with other users. For example, if a user forgot to log out of one computer and tried to log onto another computer, the user would frequently ask another user to share his or her password. This password may have been shouted across the nursing unit or other area. Because audit trails record not only what was done but who did it, making the user responsible for every action under that username, usernames and passwords should never be shared with another user. Employees who violate policies related to passwords should be disciplined according to the policies of the organization.

One problem with passwords is that users have too many of them. The different systems that they use frequently have different passwords, thus making it almost impossible for users to remember all of them. One way to overcome this issue is the use of single sign-on systems, which are designed so the user logs in one time (Abdelhak et al. 2007). The user is able to move from one application to another without entering another password. This single sign-on password should be protected so that the system is not at risk of unauthorized access (Amatayakul and Walsh 2001).

Tokens are used in conjunction with a password to provide **two-factor authentication** because a token and a password are two different types of authentications—something you know and something you have (Burrington-Brown 2003a). Tokens are about the size of a credit card and contain a magnetic strip or chip. This strip identifies the user. An algorithm displays a sequence of numbers in an LCD window. The characters in the LCD window change at specified times; for example, every minute. The user must enter the code on the token in order to access the system. The problem with the use of tokens is that the token may be lost (Abdelhak et al. 2007).

Biometrics use information about the person in order to access the data center, an information system, or other secured area. Retinal scans, fingerprints, facial features, and voice prints may be used. This method is very secure because it is not possible to forge a person's identify using biometric data; however, there are times when these authentications do not work (Abdelhak et al. 2007). For example, latex gloves may alter an individual's fingerprint enough to make it unrecognizable.

Another form of entity authentication is **telephone callback procedures**, which are most commonly used when users access the system remotely such as from their home. The user dials into the system and the system requests the phone number from which the call originates. If the phone number is an authorized number, the user is allowed into the system.

Authorization

Once the system authenticates the user, the system authorizes what data and functions the user is able to access. For example, a user may be permitted to delete a patient, change the medical record number, and access the EHR or only the master patient index. There are three methods to determine what the user can do: role-based, user-based, and context-based authentications. In role-based authentications, the functions available to the user are based on the role of the individual. For example, all floor nurses would have the same functions and the same would be true for all medical coders. In user-based authentication, the functions available to the user would be identified based on the needs of the individual user—not all users with the same job title. For example, some Health Information Management Technicians may have the authority to combine duplicate medical record numbers but others would not. This method is more accurate with the assignment of the functionality required, but is much more difficult to manage because every user must be managed individually. Context-based authentication controls access not only on the role that the employee has in the organization but also the individual data elements and the context in which the user is working (Amatayakul and Walsh 2001). This is helpful when there are employees, such as nurses, who work various units or have different roles at different times.

Transmission Security

Transmission security is mechanisms designed to protect ePHI while the data are being transmitted between two points. Network communication protocols such as those discussed in the introduction to Chapter 1 may be used. Other methods are data or message authentication codes. Encryption is frequently used to prevent the reading of ePHI by anyone with access to data during transmission.

Check Your Understanding 12.6

1. An example of a technical safeguard is:
   A. Locked door
   B. Card key
   C. Policy and procedure
   D. Audit control

2. Verifying that the data sent is the same as the data received is called:

   A. Audit control
   B. Integrity
   C. Encryption
   D. Technical safeguard

3. bob.smith is an example of:

   A. Username
   B. Password
   C. Two-factor authentication
   D. Biometrics

4. A token is an example of:

   A. Something you know
   B. Something you have
   C. Something unique to individual
   D. Forensics

5. The phrase "break the glass" refers to:

   A. Trigger
   B. Event
   C. Audit control
   D. Emergency access procedure

Monitoring

Using passwords and other authentication methods is not enough to ensure the security of the data. Audit controls are required by HIPAA to confirm the security of the data. The audit controls also hold users accountable for their actions. Individuals are more likely to follow the rules when they know monitoring is occurring and that penalties will be assessed when violations are identified. Monitoring may also identify attempted and successful intrusions into the system.

One method of monitoring is the use of audit trails. Audit trails are a recording of activities occurring in an information system. Audit trails can monitor system level controls such as who logs on, when they logged on, and applications accessed. System level controls monitor logon/logoff activity and applications accessed by the user. Application level controls track what systems were used, what the user saw, and what they did. User level controls record what actions the user initiated, such as resources accessed (Amatayakul 2004a). Security experts frequently recommend storing audit trail data on a different file server than the system itself. This separation improves the security of the data and provides the necessary storage capability to store the data for long periods of time. The length of time audit trails are stored must be defined by the facility because there are no retention requirements by HIPAA.

Review of the audit trail can identify potential security incidents. The reviews can be reviewed when a known incident has occurred or is suspected to have occurred. It should also be monitored routinely. Policies and procedures should identify frequency and type of review. The security audit process should include **triggers** that identify the need for a closer inspection. These trigger events cannot be used as the sole basis of the review, but they can significantly reduce the amount of reviews performed. Examples of triggers are (Hjort 2003b):

- user has same last name as patient

- patient is a celebrity, employee, or other public figure

- access to sensitive diagnoses

- care providers accessing a patient in whose care they were not involved

Just because a trigger is activated does not mean that there has been a breach. With common names such as Smith and Jones, it would be easy for an employee named Smith to care for a patient named Smith who was not related.

Audit reduction tools review the audit trail and compare it to facility-specific criteria and eliminate routine entries such as the periodic backups (Amatayakul 2004b) There are also trend and variance detection tools that look for variances from the expected behavior of an user (Halpert 2000). For example, if a nurse works only on the weekend and suddenly logs in on Tuesday, a red flag would be raised. Of course, there may be a legitimate reason such as she changed days with another nurse because of a family event, but it could be that the user was sneaking a peek at a neighbor's ePHI. Finally, there are attack signature-detection tools that look for a specific sequence of events that may indicate a security problem.

Actions flagged by these systems should only be viewed as potential problems that should be investigated, because there are legitimate reasons for variances and failed login attempts. For example, a coder may be coding late at night because he or she may be taking classes during the day.

Network Security

Healthcare facilities rely heavily on networks to share information. These networks frequently allow users across the healthcare facility's campus and beyond to access ePHI. HIPAA mandates the use of network security methods to protect the ePHI as it travels across the network. **Network security** is using technology to protect the data transmitted across the network and includes fire walls, encryption, and data integrity.

Firewalls are designed to control access to a network from the outside or to control access to the outside from the facility (Abdelhak et al. 2007). This gatekeeper is physically located between the routes of a public network like the Internet and a private network like that of a healthcare facility. All data entering and leaving the facility must pass through the firewall, which evaluates everything that passes in or out of the network based on user-defined rules. If the data pass the evaluation, the data are allowed in or out of the network (LaTour and Eichenwald Maki 2006). The term used to describe the data passing through the firewall is packet filtering (Newby 2009). The firewall can attach confidentiality messages to e-mails, it can limit the size or type of file entering the network, and it can limit access to specific Web sites. The firewall may even scan the data to determine if a virus is attached (Newby 2009).

Intrusion detection and response "is the act of monitoring systems or networks for unauthorized users or unauthorized activities and the actions taken for correction to these acts." (Ruano 2003, 5). The firewalls can only contain intrusion detection systems that set off alarms if there have been inappropriate attempts to access the network.

Encryption converts data from a readable form to unintelligible text. Only authorized users are able to convert the data back into a readable format. The science of cryptography (encryption) uses mathematics to convert data into unintelligible data and back again. Encryption uses cryptography to manipulate digital data. Encryption is needed to protect data as it moves across networks. If data are intercepted during transmission, the health information is protected because the individual who intercepted the data cannot view it. Only authorized users would be able to decrypt the data back into a readable format.

There are two categories of encryption: symmetric and asymmetric. Symmetric encryption assigns a secret key to data. The computer sending the data uses the key to turn the message into the unintelligible format. The receiving computer uses the same key to revert the data back into its original format. In asymmetric encryption, also known as public key infrastructure, two keys are used. The sending computer uses a private key to convert the data. The public key is provided to the computer with whom the sender is communicating. This public key converts the data into readable format. A licensing agency called a certification authority confirms the receiver's identity and relationship to the public key. In doing this, the certification authority issues a digital certificate to the receiver. This digital certificate is part of the integrity process because it ensures that plaintext messages are received without any alterations. This encryption and decryption occurs in the background. When conducting business transactions over the Internet, secure socket layer (SSL) public key infrastructure is used to transmit the protected information (LaTour and Eichenwald Maki 2006).

Public key encryption is extremely popular. In public key encryption, the user gives a public key to everyone who should have access to the system. A private key is retained by the sender. The private key and public key must work together to encrypt, send, and decrypt the message.

Check Your Understanding 12.7

1. An activity, based on facility standards, that should be reviewed to determine whether or not it is a security incident is a(n):

   A. Trigger
   B. Event
   C. Audit control
   D. Cryptography

2. What audit control tracks when a user logs in and out of the system?

   A. Firewall
   B. Data recovery
   C. Audit trail
   D. Monitoring

3. Audit trails should be stored:

   A. On a different computer from the data
   B. On the same computer as the data
   C. Forever
   D. For 10 years

4. A type of network security is:

   A. Audit reduction tool
   B. Audit trail
   C. Monitoring
   D. Encryption

5. The network security method of monitoring data entering and leaving the network is called:

   A. Encryption
   B. Audit reduction tool
   C. Monitoring
   D. Firewall

Data Security

Data must be protected against loss, destruction, tampering, or inappropriate alteration. Methods of data security include passwords and other access control mechanisms as well as preventing the loss of data through the use of backups. Data is also protected through the physical and network security measures. These data security measures are discussed elsewhere in this chapter. There are other threats to data such as malicious software, which will be discussed next.

Malicious Software

Malicious software or malware is designed to harm a computer. The specific damage varies by virus or other malware. Some of these viruses or malware are more of a nuisance, whereas others destroy data or other files that may prevent the computer from operating. HIPAA mandates that the covered entity take steps to protect the data and information system from malware.

There are a number of different types of malware. One type of malware is masqueraders. Masqueraders give the appearance of being exactly what the user needs, but when activated actually perform malicious actions. The Trojan horse is a masquerader that appears to be useful, but performs unexpected actions instead. Some files appear to be nonexecutable files that when opened execute a software program that performs unexpected actions. Macros are frequently used in this way, which is why computers provide notification when macros are used and ask if the user still wants to open the file (Joint NEMA/COCIR/JIRA Security and Privacy Committee 2003).

Another type of malware is incapacitation. These programs are designed to disable the computer. Two examples of incapacitation are time bombs and denial of service (DoS). Time bombs are activated when the trigger established by the programmer occurs. This trigger could be a date or performing a specific task or other action. The outcome will vary according to the type of time bomb, but formatting of the hard drive or destruction of the startup files may occur. **Denial of Service** is a type of malware that is designed to overload a Web site or other information system so that the system cannot handle the load and eventually shuts down (Joint NEMA/COCIR/JIRA Security and Privacy Committee 2003).

Viruses and spyware corrupt data. **Viruses** are designed to do a variety of destructive behaviors. For example, they can destroy data or damage the system/boot record. It is the term commonly used to indicate malware, but it is technically a specific type of malware. Viruses are frequently spread through e-mail. They can spread through the e-mail server and even the user's e-mail address book (Abdelhak et al. 2007) **Spyware** may be used to track keystrokes and passwords, monitor Web sites visited, or other actions, and report these actions back to the creator of the spyware. The spyware may slow down the computer system and contribute to identity theft or other breaches of privacy.

Worm is a type of misuse malware. The **worm** installs itself onto a computer attached to a computer network and then moves to all computers on a network. It may harm the system or initiate a DoS. The worm frequently spreads through e-mail attachments as well as files downloaded from the Internet. The worm spreads to the e-mail server and then to all of the users listed in the e-mail mailbox (Abdelhak et al. 2007).

Phishing is an e-mail that appears from a legitimate business that asks for account number or other personal information. The e-mail is actually from a phisher who uses the account number or other information maliciously. Large companies such as eBay or AOL are frequent targets of phishing because so many people have an account with these companies and may not realize a scam is being perpetrated (Joint NEMA/COCIR/JIRA Security and Privacy Committee 2003).

Actions must be taken to protect computers from malicious software. Antivirus and other software packages are designed to identify and stop or clean up malicious software.

Organizational Requirements

As discussed earlier in this chapter, a covered entity must have a contract with each business associate. If the organization discovers that the business associate is in noncompliance with the security rule, the covered entity has a responsibility to work with the business associate to bring them into compliance. If all efforts fail, the covered entity should terminate the contract. The contract should mandate the business associate to notify the covered entity of any security incidents. The contract should also allow for the termination of the contract.

The need for policies and procedures to document security processes is mentioned throughout this chapter. These policies and procedures should be in writing and may be updated at any time. Policies and procedures and other documents must be maintained for a minimum of 6 years from the date of creation or the date it was last in effect (Rada 2003). The time period utilized must be the one that is longer. This documentation must be available to members of the workforce responsible for implementing the procedures referred to in the documentation. The documentation must be available to the employees to whom the policy applies. Documentation should be periodically reviewed and updated as appropriate (Rada 2003).

Penalties

The oversight of the HIPAA security rule has been given to the Centers for Medicare and Medicaid Services. They have the right to award civil and criminal penalties. Civil penalties can be up to $100.00 per violation. The security rule provides a maximum penalty of $25,000.00 per person per year for each requirement violated. Criminal penalties are more severe. These penalties are awarded when the individual knowingly and willfully violates the security rules. There are three tiers of criminal penalties. These penalties are (Rada 2003):

- Up to $50,000.00 and 1 year in prison may be awarded for obtaining and disclosing PHI.

- Up to $100,000.00 and up to 5 years in prison may be awarded if the individual obtains or discloses PHI under false pretenses.

- Up to $250,000.00 and up to 10 years in prison may be awarded for obtaining and disclosing PHI and using it for commercial gain, personal gain, or malicious intent.

Certifications

There are two privacy and/or security certifications: Certified in Healthcare Privacy and Security (CHPS) and Certified Information Systems Security Professional CISSP. The CHPS is designed specifically for healthcare whereas the CISSP is a general security certification.

Certified in Healthcare Privacy and Security

The **Certified in Healthcare Privacy and Security** credential is an area of specialization and is much more advanced than the privacy and security skills of the Registered Health Information Administrator or Registered Health Information Technician examinations. It is sponsored by the American Health Information Management Association (AHIMA).The CHPS examination includes both technical and managerial issues, including a number of topics related to privacy and security (AHIMA 2008).

To be eligible to sit for the examination, the candidate must meet one of the following eligibility requirements.

- Baccalaureate degree and a minimum of four (4) years experience in healthcare management

- Master's or related degree (JD, MD, PhD) and two (2) years experience in healthcare management

- Healthcare information management credential (RHIT, RHIA) with a baccalaureate or higher degree and a minimum of two (2) years experience in healthcare management (AHIMA 2008)

Figure 12.3 shows AHIMA's 2008 CPHS competency statements.

Figure 12.3.   2008 CPHS competency statements

1. **Management and Administration**
   A. Provide guidance regarding applicable standards of accreditation agencies (Joint Commission, AAAHC, AOA, NCQA).
   B. Administer an appropriate organizational infrastructure for privacy and information security.
   C. Create, document, and communicate company privacy and security policies, procedures, and guidelines.
   D. Review relationships to identify business associates.
   E. Ensure appropriate contract development and management procedures comply with business associate requirements.
   F. Ensure the maintenance of the inventory of software, hardware, and all information assets.
   G. Participate in business continuity planning for planned downtime and contingency planning for emergencies and disaster recovery.
   H. Perform data criticality analysis.
   I. Establish and maintain facility security plan to safeguard unauthorized physical access to information and prevent theft or tampering.
   J. Participate in analysis, implementation, and decisions regarding privacy and security solutions.
   K. Develop, deliver, evaluate, and document training and awareness of privacy and security.
   L. Work with appropriate organization officials to ensure information used or disclosed for research complies with applicable privacy regulations.
   M. Facilitate ongoing assessments of organizational policies, procedures, and practices related to privacy and security.

2. **Regulatory Requirements, Investigation, and Compliance 8 16 10 34**
   A. Assess and communicate risks and ramifications of breaches of privacy and security, including those by business associates to leadership.
   B. Establish incident response plan and identify team members (for example, Human Resources, Legal, Risk Management, Physical Security, Legal Law Enforcement, Public Relations).
   C. Coordinate privacy and security compliance documentation required by law.
   D. Ensure and monitor compliance with state and federal laws and regulations related to privacy and security.
   E. Coordinate the organization's response to inquiries and investigations from external entities relating to privacy and security.
   F. Develop system to maintain and retain applicable documentation.
   G. Establish compliance indicators and develop methods to measure compliance to improve organizational performance.
   H. Coordinate incident investigations and response.
   I. Develop, implement, and ensure follow-through on a system to evaluate risk.
   J. Enforce privacy and security policies, procedures, and guidelines to enable compliance with federal, state, and other regulatory or accrediting bodies.
   K. Monitor appropriateness of access to identifiable health information.
   L. Establish a complaint investigation and resolution process.

3. **Information Technology**
   A. Monitor data backup plan.
   B. Develop and manage strategic information security plan.
   C. Assess security risks and identify threats and vulnerabilities.
   D. Establish audit controls (for example, logging guidelines, administrative access).
   E. Ensure technical safeguards such as configuration management, intrusion detection, and preventive countermeasures are adequate for the organization.
   F. Ensure the documentation of the maintenance of software, hardware, and all information assets.
   G. Ensure that preventive measures are in place to prevent attacks (for example, malicious code, hacking).
   H. Establish internal standards to determine compliance to security requirements by system, network, application, and user.
   I. Ensure that the transmission of secure and private information is protected appropriately.
   J. Implement disaster recovery plan as needed after disaster has occurred.
   K. Establish guidelines, procedures, and controls to ensure the integrity, availability, and confidentiality of communication across networks (for example, wireless Internet, secure sockets, VPNs, and PKI).
   L. Ensure the use of event triggering to notify abnormal conditions within a system (for example, intrusion detection, denial of service, and invalid logon attempts).

Figure 12.3.   **2008 CPHS competency statements** *(continued)*

M. Establish and manage process for verifying and controlling access authorizations and privileges including emergency access (for example, context-based access, role-based access, and user-based access).

N. Establish and manage authentication mechanisms (for example, guidelines, unique user ID, password, biometrics, PIN, token, telephone callback).

O. Develop process for the use of cryptography, digital signatures, and public and private key infrastructure technologies.

P. Provide forensic services (for example, data recovery, evidence preservation, and event tracing).

4. **Physical Safeguards**

A. Establish media control practices that govern the receipt, removal, or disposal (internal and external destruction) of any media containing data.

B. Establish physical security mechanisms to limit the access to authorized personnel for approved activities (for example, workstation placement, fax machine control, printer control).

C. Establish reasonable safeguards to reduce incidental disclosure.

D. Ensure use of generally accepted physical and system security principles.

5. **Health Information Management**

A. Recommend appropriate deidentification methodologies.

B. Ensure that recipients of secure and private information are permitted to receive the information (subpoena, court orders, search warrants).

C. Ensure the rights of the individual who is a subject of individually identifiable health information. (amendments, access, restrictions, confidential communications).

D. Define HIPAA-designated record sets for the organization.

E. Identify information and record sets requiring special privacy protections.

F. Identify permitted disclosures (for example, research, marketing, fund development, valid authorizations).

G. Identify permitted uses of health information (for example, treatment, payment, healthcare operations, minimum necessary, need-to-know).

H. Ensure protocols are in place to verify identity of recipients of health information.

Source: AHIMA 2008, 7–10.

Certified Information Systems Security Professional (CISSP)

The **Certified Information Systems Security Professional** (CISSP) certification is sponsored by the International Information Systems Security Certification Consortium [(ISC)^2]. It is a generic security certification and therefore is not healthcare specific. To be eligible, an individual must have 5 years full-time experience in security. This experience must be in 2 or more of the 10 domains. These domains are:

- Access control
- Application security
- Business Continuity and Disaster Recovery Planning
- Cryptography
- Information security and risk management
- Legal, regulations, compliance and investigations
- Operations security
- Physical (environmental) security
- Security architecture and design
- Telecommunications and network security

To maintain the certification, 120 continuing education credits must be reported every 3 years. ((ISC)^2 2008)

Check Your Understanding 12.8

1. An e-mail that looks legitimate but is actually trying to obtain personal information is called:

   A. spyware
   B. denial of service
   C. virus
   D. phishing

2. The term used to describe viruses and spyware is called:

   A. malicious software
   B. spiteful software
   C. masqueraders
   D. macros

3. The security rule is enforced by:

   A. Office of Inspector General
   B. Office for Civil Rights (OCR)
   C. National Center for Health Statistics
   D. National Institutes of Health (NIH)

4. Policies and procedures related to HIPAA must be retained for _____ years.

   A. 3
   B. 5
   C. 6
   D. 10

5. Which type of malware is designed to overload a website or other information system and force it to shut down?

   A. Denial of Service
   B. Phishing
   C. Virus
   D. Worm

References

45 CFR 160 and 162. Health Insurance Reform: Standards for Electronic Transmission: Announcement of Designated Standard Maintenance Organizations; Final Rule and Notice. 2000 (Aug. 17). http://www.cms.hhs.gov/TransactionCodeSetsStands/Downloads/txfinal.pdf.

45 CFR 160, 162, and 164. Healthcare Reform: Security Standards; Final Rule. 2003 (Feb. 20) http://www.cms.hhs.gov/SecurityStandard/Downloads/securityfinalrule.pdf.

45 CFR 160, 162, and 164 HIPAA Administrative Simplification Regulation Tex (Unofficial Version, as amended through February 16, 2006). 2006 (March.). t http://www.hhs.gov/ocr/privacy/hipaa/administrative/privacyrule/adminsimpregtext.pdf.

Abdelhak, M., S. Grostick, M.A. Hanken, and E. Jacobs. 2007. *Health Information: Management of a Strategic Resource*. St. Louis, MO: Saunders Elsevier.

AHIMA 2008. 2008 Candidate Handbook CPHS. 7–10. http://www.ahima.org/certification/documents/CHPS.PDF.

AHIMA 2007 Privacy and Security Practice Council. 2008. How to react to a security incident. *Journal of AHIMA* 79(1):66–70. http://library.ahima.org/xpedio/groups/public/documents/ahima/bok1_036247.hcsp?dDocName=bok1_036247.

Amatayakul, M. 2003. Practice brief: Security risk analysis and management: An overview. *Journal of AHIMA* 74(9):72A-G.

Amatayakul, M. 2004a. Kick starting the security risk analysis. *Journal of AHIMA* 75(7):46–47.

Amatayakul, M. 2004b. The trouble with audit controls. *Journal of AHIMA* 75(9):78–79.

Amatayakul, M. 2005a. Access controls: Striking the right balance. *Journal of AHIMA* 76(1):56–57.

Amatayakul, M. 2005b Reporting security incidents. *Journal of AHIMA* 76((3):60.

Amatayakul, M. and M.L. Johns. 2002. Compliance in the crosshairs: Targeting your training (HIPAA on the job). *Journal of AHIMA* 73(10):16A-F.

Amatayakul, M. and T. Walsh. 2001. Selecting strong passwords (HIPAA on the job). *Journal of AHIMA* 72(9):16A-D.

Burrington-Brown, J. 2003a. On the line—Professional Practice solutions: What is multi-factor authentication? *Journal of AHIMA* 74(5):64.

Burrington-Brown, J. 2003b. Sorting out employee sanctions. *Journal of AHIMA* 74(6):53–54.

Centers for Medicare and Medicaid Services. 2007a. 1 Security 101 for covered entities. (HIPAA security series). http://www.cms.hhs.gov/EducationMaterials/Downloads/Security101forCoveredEntities.pdf.

Centers for Medicare and Medicaid Services. 2007b. 2 Security standards: administrative safeguards (HIPAA security series). http://www.cms.hhs.gov/EducationMaterials/Downloads/SecurityStandardsAdministrativeSafeguards.pdf.

Centers for Medicare and Medicaid Services. 2007c. 3 Security standards: Physical safeguards (HIPAA security series). http://www.cms.hhs.gov/EducationMaterials/Downloads/SecurityStandardsPhysicalSafeguards.pdf.

Centers for Medicare and Medicaid Services. 2007d. 4 Security standards: Technical safeguards (HIPAA security series). http://www.cms.hhs.gov/EducationMaterials/Downloads/SecurityStandardsTechnicalSafeguards.pdf.

Centers for Medicare and Medicaid Services. 2007e. 5 Security standards: Organizational, policies and procedures and documentation requirements (HIPAA security series). http://www.cms.hhs.gov/EducationMaterials/Downloads/SecurityStandardsOrganizationalPolicies.pdf.

Centers for Medicare and Medicaid Services. 2007f. 6 Security standards: Basics of risk analysis and risk management (HIPAA security series). http://www.cms.hhs.gov/EducationMaterials/Downloads/BasicsofRiskAnalysisandRiskManagement.pdf.

Connecting for Health Policy Subcommittee. 2006. Authentication of system users. *The Connecting for Health Common Framework*. http://www.connectingforhealth.org/commonframework/docs/P5_Authentication_SysUsers.pdf.

Davis, J.B. 2003. *HIPAA Compliance Manual: A Comprehensive Guide to the Administrative Simplification Provisions for Health Care Professionals*. Los Angeles: PMIC.

Derhak, M. 2003. Uncovering the enemy within: Utilizing incident response, forensics. *In Confidence* 11(9):1–2.

Dinh, A. 2009. Securing portable devices. *Journal of AHIMA* 80(1):56–57.

Dougherty, M. 2004. The 10 security domains. *Journal of AHIMA* 75(2):56A-D.

Giannanglo, K., ed. 2006. *Healthcare Code Sets, Clinical Terminologies, and Classification Systems*. Chicago: AHIMA.

Halpert, A.M. 2000. Access audit trails: En route to security. *Journal of AHIMA* 71(8):43–46.

Hartley, C.P. and E.D. Jones III. 2004. *HIPAA Plain and Simple: A Compliance Guide for Health Care Professionals*. Chicago: American Medical Association.

Hjort, B. 2003a. Practice brief: HIPAA privacy and security training (Updated). http://library.ahima.org/xpedio/groups/public/documents/ahima/bok1_022114.hcsp?dDocName=bok1_022114.

Hjort, B. 2003b. Practice brief: Security audits (Updated). http://library.ahima.org/xpedio/groups/public/documents/ahima/bok1_022113.hcsp?dDocName=bok1_022113.

Hughes, G. 2002. Practice brief: Destruction of patient health information (Updated). http://library.ahima.org/xpedio/groups/public/documents/ahima/bok1_016468.hcsp?dDocName=bok1_016468.

(ISC)² 2008. CISSP® - Certified Information Systems Security Professional. https://www.isc2.org/cissp/default.aspx.

Johns, M., ed. 2007. *Health Information Management Technology: An Applied Approach*. Chicago: AHIMA.

Joint NEMS/COCIR/JIRA Security and Privacy Committee. 2003. Defending medical information systems against malicious software. http://medicalimaging.org/documents/medical-defending.pdf.

Keating, A. 2006. Hard Drive Sanitation – Best Practices and State of the Industry. *Proceedings from the American Health Information Management Association's 78th National Convention and Exhibit*. (October, 2006).

LaTour, K. M. and S. Eichenwald Maki, eds. 2006. *Health Information Management: Concepts, Principles, and Practice*. Chicago: AHIMA.

McWay, D.C. 2008. *Today's Health Information Management: An Integrated Approach*. Clifton Park, NY: Thomson Delmar Learning.

Microsoft Corporation. 2002. *Microsoft Computer Dictionary*, 2nd ed. Redmond, WA: Microsoft Press.

Newby, C. 2009. *HIPAA for Allied Health Careers*. Boston: McGraw-Hill Higher Education.

Rada, R. 2003. *Health Information Security: HIPAA*. Chicago: HIPAA-IT LLC and Healthcare Information and Management Systems Society.

Ruano, M. 2003. Understanding telecommunications, network security, and HIPAA. *In Confidence* 11(5):5.

Scichilone, R.A. 2002. DSMOs shed light on future coding systems, data sets. *Journal of AHIMA* 73(7):74–77.

Tomes, J.P. 2005. Spoliation of medical evidence.*Journal of AHIMA* 76(9):68–72.

Chapter 13
Role of HIM Professionals in Information Systems

Objectives

- Discuss various technology-driven roles performed by health information management (HIM) professions.

- Discuss information technology tasks performed by HIM professionals in traditional and nontraditional settings.

- Discuss the role of Knowledge Clusters and Domains, Subdomains, and Tasks on the HIM educational process.

- Describe the skills of the HIM professionals.

Key Terms

Clinical vocabulary manager
Commission on Accreditation of Health Information and Informatics Management Education (CAHIIM)
Data analyst
Data miner
Data navigator

Data quality and integrity monitor
Data resource manager
Data security, privacy, and confidentiality manager
Data translator
Domains, subdomains, and tasks
Health information technology

Knowledge clusters
Registered health information administrator
Registered health information technician
Terminology asset manager
Work and data flow analyst

Overview

According to AHIMA's Health Information Careers Web site, HIM is "the study of the principles and practices of acquiring, analyzing, and protecting digital and traditional medical information vital to providing quality patient care" (Health Information Careers 2007). As indicated by this definition, health information managers are becoming more and more involved in information systems as the data they manage are digitized.

HIM professionals have a unique combination of skills that make them a valuable asset to the information systems team. This set of skills frequently places the HIM professional in the role of liaison between the technical information system staff who do not understand healthcare and the clinicians who do not understand technology. For example, computer programmers do not understand documentation and the needs of the nursing staff anymore than the nursing staff, laboratory staff, or other clinical departments understand computer programming, system implementation, and other system issues. The HIM professional is valuable because of his or her understanding of information systems, documentation, the medical record, and other issues.

As the legal health record becomes more electronic, it is important that the HIM professional be a part of the team leading the change to the electronic health record (EHR); otherwise, issues related to retention, data quality, security, release of information and other data management topics may be ignored or incorrectly implemented, thus increasing the risk of HIPAA violations, state licensing problems, and lawsuits.

In the Summary Findings from the HIM Workforce Study, three changes to the HIM environment were identified. These changes were:

- changes in the environment
- impact of evolving technology on HIM and the healthcare field
- EHRs (AHIMA 2005)

The changes in the environment come from changes in the overall healthcare delivery system, increases in the use of technology such as the EHR, and the trend toward consumer-driven healthcare and patient-centered care. HIM professionals must rapidly adapt to the changes that are creating new roles for this profession as well as the need for more HIM professionals. Education is critical in preparing new HIM professionals for these new roles.

The **Commission on Accreditation for Health Informatics and Information Management Education (CAHIIM)** is responsible for establishing the content that accredited bachelor and associate programs must teach their students. **Domains, Subdomains, and Tasks** along with the **Knowledge Clusters**, are updated periodically to remain current. These documents define the content that the accredited programs must cover. Topic areas covered in the **health information technology** curriculum include:

- Biomedical sciences
- Health data structure, content, and standards
- Healthcare information requirements and standards
- Clinical classification systems
- Reimbursement
- Healthcare statistics and research
- Healthcare delivery system

- Healthcare privacy, confidentiality, legal, and ethical issues
- Information and communication technologies
- Data storage and retrieval
- Data security and healthcare information systems
- Organizational resources

The Domains, Subdomains, Tasks and Knowledge Clusters are based on research focused around what HIM professionals are currently doing in the field and what the profession is expected to do in the future. Many of the areas required are technological in nature whereas many others, while not technical themselves, impact the EHR. For example, although reimbursement itself is not an information system topic, computers are valuable to coding, chargemaster, compliance, and other reimbursement-related functions. CAHIIM is currently developing standards for the Master's level as well. Table 13.1 lists the Knowledge Clusters required for the associate degree program. Table 13.2 lists the domains, subdomains, and tasks for the associate degree program.

Table 13.1.   Knowledge cluster content assessment, Associate Degree Program

Knowledge Cluster Content
Biomedical Sciences
• Anatomy
• Physiology
• Medical Terminology
• Pathophysiology
• Pharmacotherapy
I.A. Health Data Structure, Content, and Standards
1. Data vs. information
2. Structure and use of health information (individual, comparative, aggregate)
3. Health information media (such as paper, computer, Web-based)
4. Health record data collection tools (such as forms, screens, and so on)
5. Data sources (primary, secondary)
6. Data definitions, vocabularies, terminologies, and dictionaries
7. Data storage and retrieval
8. Data quality and integrity
9. Healthcare data sets (such as OASIS, HEDIS, DEEDS, UHDDS)
10. Data monitoring and compliance reporting
11. National Healthcare Information Infrastructure (NHII)
I.B. Healthcare Information Requirements and Standards
1. Type and content of health record (paper, electronic, computer-based, e-health-personal, Web-based)
2. Health record documentation requirements (such as accreditation, certification, licensure)
3. Health record monitoring and compliance reporting

(continued on next page)

Table 13.1.   Knowledge cluster content assessment, Associate Degree Program *(continued)*

Knowledge Cluster Content
I.C. Clinical Classification Systems
1. Classifications, taxonomies, nomenclatures, terminologies, and clinical vocabularies
2. Principles and applications of coding systems (such as ICD-9-CM, ICD-10, CPT/HCPCS, DSM-IV)
3. Diagnostic and procedural groupings (such as DRG, APC, RUGs, SNOMED-CT)
4. Case mix analysis and indexes
5. Medicare Severity Diagnosis-Related Groups (MS-DRGs)
6. Coding compliance strategies, auditing, and reporting (such as CCI, plans)
7. Coding quality monitors and reporting
I.D. Reimbursement
1. Commercial, managed care, and federal insurance plans
2. Payment methodologies and systems (such as capitation, prospective payment systems (PPS), RBRVS)
3. Billing processes and procedures (such as claims, EOB, ABN, electronic data interchange)
4. Chargemaster maintenance
5. Regulatory guidelines (such as LMRP, peer review organizations)
6. Reimbursement monitoring and reporting
7. Compliance strategies and reporting
II.A. Healthcare Statistics and Research
1. Indices, databases and registries
2. Vital statistics
3. Healthcare statistics
4. Descriptive statistics (such as means, frequencies, ranges, percentiles, standard deviations)
5. Statistical applications with healthcare data
6. Institutional Review Board (IRB) processes
7. National guidelines regarding human subjects research
8. Research protocol monitoring
9. Data selection, interpretation, and presentation
10. Knowledge-based research techniques (such as library, Medline, Web-based)
II.B. Quality Management and Performance Improvement
1. Quality assessment and improvement (such as process, collection tools, data analysis, reporting techniques)
2. Utilization management, risk management, and case management
3. Regulatory quality monitoring requirements
4. Outcomes measures and monitoring
III.A. Healthcare Delivery Systems
1. Organization of healthcare delivery in the United States
2. Healthcare organizations structure and operation
3. External standards, regulations, and initiatives (such as licensure, certification, accreditation, HIPAA)
4. Payment and reimbursement systems
5. Healthcare providers and disciplines

Table 13.1.   Knowledge cluster content assessment, Associate Degree Program *(continued)*

Knowledge Cluster Content
III.B. Healthcare Privacy, Confidentiality, Legal, and Ethical Issues
1. Legislative and regulatory processes
2. Legal terminology
3. Health information/record laws and regulations (such as retention, patient rights/advocacy, advanced directives, privacy)
4. Confidentiality, privacy, and security policies, procedures, and monitoring
5. Release of information policies and procedures
6. Professional and practice-related ethical issues
IV.A. Information and Communication Technologies
1. Computer concepts (such as hardware components, operating systems, languages, software packages)
2. Communication and Internet technologies (such as networks, intranet, standards)
3. Common software applications (such as word processing, spreadsheet, database, graphics)
4. Health information systems (such as administrative, patient registration, ADT, EHR, personal health record (PHR), laboratory, radiology, pharmacy)
5. Voice recognition technology
6. Health information specialty systems (such as ROI, coding, registries)
7. Application of systems and policies to health information systems and functions and healthcare data requests
IV.B. Data Storage and Retrieval
1. Document archival, retrieval, and imaging systems
2. Maintenance and monitoring of data storage systems
IV.C. Data Security and Healthcare Information Systems
1. System architecture and design
2. System acquisition and evaluation
3. Screen design
4. Data retrieval and maintenance
5. Data security concepts
6. Data integrity concepts
7. Data integrity and security processes and monitoring
8. Data recovery and risk management
9. Work process design (such as ergonomics, equipment selection)
V.A. Organizational Resources
1. Roles and functions of teams and committees
2. Teams/consensus building and committees
3. Communication and interpersonal skills
4. Team leadership concepts and techniques
5. Orientation and training (such as content, delivery, media)
6. Workflow and process monitors
7. Performance monitors
8. Revenue cycle monitors
9. Organizational plans and budgets (framework, levels, responsibilities, and so on)
10. Resource allocation monitors

Source: CAHIIM 2007

Table 13.2.   HIM Associate Degree Entry-level Competencies: Domains, subdomains, and tasks

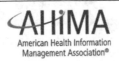

American Health Information
Management Association®

HIM Associate Degree Entry-Level Competencies
Domains, Subdomains, and Tasks
For 2006 and beyond

I. Domain: Health Data Management

   A. Subdomain: Health Data Structure, Content and Standards

     1. Collect and maintain health data (such as data elements, data sets, and databases).

     2. Conduct analysis to ensure documentation in the health record supports the diagnosis and reflects the patient's progress, clinical findings, and discharge status.

     3. Apply policies and procedures to ensure the accuracy of health data.

     4. Contribute to the definitions for and apply clinical vocabularies and terminologies used in the organization's health information systems.

     5. Verify timeliness, completeness, accuracy, and appropriateness of data and data sources for patient care, management, billing reports, registries, and/or databases.

   B. Subdomain: Healthcare Information Requirements and Standards

     1. Monitor and apply organization-wide health record documentation guidelines.

     2. Apply policies and procedures to ensure organizational compliance with regulations and standards.

     3. Report compliance findings according to organizational policy.

     4. Maintain the accuracy and completeness of the patient record as defined by organizational policy and external regulations and standards.

     5. Assist in preparing the organization for accreditation, licensing, and/or certification surveys.

   C. Subdomain: Clinical Classification Systems

     1. Use and maintain electronic applications and work processes to support clinical classification and coding.

     2. Apply diagnosis/procedure codes using ICD-9-CM.

     3. Apply procedure codes using CPT/HCPCS.

     4. Ensure accuracy of diagnostic/procedural groupings such as DRG, APC, and so on.

     5. Adhere to current regulations and established guidelines in code assignment.

     6. Validate coding accuracy using clinical information found in the health record.

     7. Use and maintain applications and processes to support other clinical classification and nomenclature systems (such as ICD-10-CM, SNOMED, and so on).

     8. Resolve discrepancies between coded data and supporting documentation.

Table 13.2.   **HIM Associate Degree Entry-level Competencies: Domains, subdomains, and tasks** *(continued)*

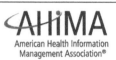

American Health Information
Management Association®

D. **Subdomain: Reimbursement Methodologies**

   1. Apply policies and procedures for the use of clinical data required in reimbursement and prospective payment systems (PPS) in healthcare delivery.

   2. Support accurate billing through coding, chargemaster, claims management, and bill reconciliation processes.

   3. Use established guidelines to comply with reimbursement and reporting requirements such as the National Correct Coding Initiative.

   4. Compile patient data and perform data quality reviews to validate code assignment and compliance with reporting requirements such as outpatient prospective payment systems.

II. Domain: Health Statistics, Biomedical Research, and Quality Management

A. **Subdomain: Healthcare Statistics and Research**

   1. Abstract and maintain data for clinical indices/databases/registries.

   2. Collect, organize, and present data for quality management, utilization management, risk management, and other related studies.

   3. Compute and interpret healthcare statistics.

   4. Apply Institutional Review Board (IRB) processes and policies.

   5. Use specialized databases to meet specific organization needs such as medical research and disease registries.

B. **Subdomain: Quality Management and Performance Improvement**

   1. Abstract and report data for facility-wide quality management and performance improvement programs.

   2. Analyze clinical data to identify trends that demonstrate quality, safety, and effectiveness of healthcare.

III. Domain: Health Services Organization and Delivery

A. **Subdomain: Healthcare Delivery Systems**

   1. Apply information system policies and procedures required by national health information initiatives on the healthcare delivery system.

   2. Apply current laws, accreditation, licensure, and certification standards related to health information initiatives from the national, state, local, and facility levels.

   3. Apply policies and procedures to comply with the changing regulations among various payment systems for healthcare services such as Medicare, Medicaid, managed care, and so forth.

   4. Differentiate the roles of various providers and disciplines throughout the continuum of healthcare and respond to their information needs.

(continued on next page)

Table 13.2.   HIM Associate Degree Entry-level Competencies: Domains, subdomains, and tasks *(continued)*

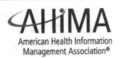

B. Subdomain: Healthcare Privacy, Confidentiality, Legal, and Ethical Issues

1. Participate in the implementation of legal and regulatory requirements related to the health information infrastructure.
2. Apply policies and procedures for access and disclosure of personal health information.
3. Release patient-specific data to authorized users.
4. Maintain user access logs/systems to track access to and disclosure of identifiable patient data.
5. Conduct privacy and confidentiality training programs.
6. Investigate and recommend solutions to privacy issues/problems.
7. Apply and promote ethical standards of practice.

IV. Domain: Information Technology and Systems

A. Subdomain: Information and Communication Technologies

1. Use technology, including hardware and software, to ensure data collection, storage, analysis, and reporting of information.
2. Use common software applications such as spreadsheets, databases, word processing, graphics, presentation, e-mail, and so on in the execution of work processes.
3. Use specialized software in the completion of HIM processes such as record tracking, release of information, coding, grouping, registries, billing, quality improvement, and imaging.
4. Apply policies and procedures to the use of networks, including intranet and Internet applications to facilitate the electronic health record (EHR), personal health record (PHR), public health, and other administrative applications.

B. Subdomain: Data, Information, and File Structures

1. Apply knowledge of data base architecture and design (such as data dictionary, data modeling, data warehousing) to meet departmental needs.

C. Subdomain: Data Storage and Retrieval

1. Use appropriate electronic or imaging technology for data/record storage.
2. Query and generate reports to facilitate information retrieval.
3. Design and generate reports using appropriate software.
4. Maintain archival and retrieval systems for patient information stored in multiple formats.
5. Coordinate, use, and maintain systems for document imaging and storage.

Table 13.2.   **HIM Associate Degree Entry-level Competencies: Domains, subdomains, and tasks** *(continued)*

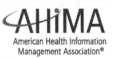

American Health Information
Management Association®

D. **Subdomain: Data security**

1. Apply confidentiality and security measures to protect electronic health information.
2. Protect data integrity and validity using software or hardware technology.
3. Apply departmental and organizational data and information system security policies.
4. Use and summarize data compiled from audit trail and data quality monitoring programs.
5. Contribute to the design and implementation of risk management, contingency planning, and data recovery procedures.

E. **Subdomain: Healthcare Information Systems**

1. Participate in the planning, design, selection, implementation, integration, testing, evaluation, and support for organization-wide information systems.
2. Use the principles of ergonomics and human factors in work process design.

V. **Domain: Organizational Resources**

A. **Subdomain: Human Resources**

1. Apply the fundamentals of team leadership.
2. Organize and contribute to work teams and committees.
3. Conduct new staff orientation and training programs.
4. Conduct continuing education programs.
5. Monitor staffing levels and productivity standards for health information functions, and provide feedback to management and staff regarding performance.
6. Communicate benchmark staff performance data.
7. Prioritize job functions and activities.
8. Use quality improvement tools and techniques to monitor, report and improve processes.

B. **Subdomain: Financial and Physical Resources**

1. Make recommendations for items to include in budgets and contracts.
2. Monitor and order supplies needed for work processes.
3. Monitor coding and revenue cycle processes.
4. Recommend cost-saving and efficient means of achieving work processes and goals.
5. Contribute to work plans, policies, procedures, and resource requisitions in relation to job functions.

6/23/2004 Education Strategy Committee

Source: CAHIIM 2004

Knowledge Base

The HIM professional has a broad range of skills. There are other professions that require some of the same skills an HIM professional holds, but there is no other profession that requires the same depth and breadth of skills. HIM skills include data management, data analysis, system analysis, system implementation, health data structure, documentation requirements, data quality, information system management, privacy and security, coding, and reimbursement among many others. In 2002, AHIMA conducted a workforce study of its members to learn what HIM professionals were currently doing and what they were expected to do in the future. The study identified 16 areas in which the HIM professional needed to be competent in the future. These areas are:

- Establishing and guiding national, local, and state health information policy development and implementation

- Establishing and implementing policies, practices, and procedures governing all aspects of HIM

- Establishing and implementing standards for privacy, security, and confidentiality of health information

- Establishing and implementing policies and standards for monitoring of data integrity, accuracy, validity, authenticity, and version control

- Developing health information format and content standards to ensure the collection of complete, accurate, timely, and compliant health information

- Facilitating communication of health information across organizational healthcare teams and between different entities

- Facilitating the concurrent use of health information for multiple purposes (such as for direct patient care, outcomes measurement and evaluation, wellness and prevention, research, public health, and policy development)

- Managing compliance, regulatory, accreditation, licensure, and (re)certification programs and activities

- Analyzing and synthesizing qualitative and quantitative health information for various and diverse needs and audiences

- Developing, designing, and implementing clinical vocabularies

- Translating and interpreting health information for consumers and their caregivers

- Helping consumers to access and obtain diverse and often complex health information

- Informing and educating consumers about health information issues

- Providing the context to understand, analyze, and interpret health information

- Helping providers understand data flow and reporting requirements within the context of dynamic rules, regulations, and guidelines

- Leading business process redesign efforts (AHIMA e-HIM Task Force 2003):

Most if not all of these skills depend on technology in some way. Some of these skills involve the development or usage of the information system; others rely on the output from the information system to provide the data needed to conduct the analyses. Some of these skill areas and the job roles that use them are illustrated in figure 13.1.

Entry-level skills are validated by the **Registered Health Information Administrator (RHIA)** and **Registered Health Information Technician (RHIT)** certification examinations. The RHIA is for those who graduate from an accredited bachelor or masters program.

Figure 13.1.   HIM skills

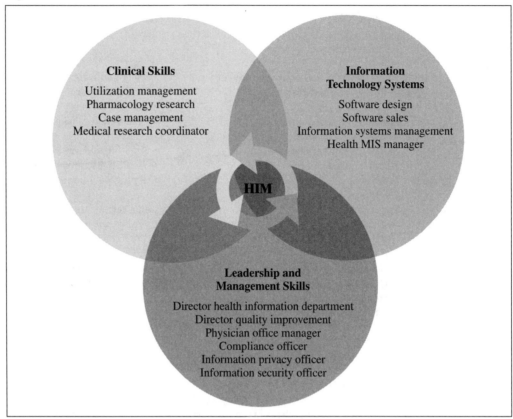

Source: AHIMA 2005

The RHIT is for those who graduate from an accredited associate degree program. These examinations are both entry-level certifications over the entire scope of HIM skills. The HIM professional may take additional specialty certifications such as Certified in Healthcare Privacy and Security (CHPS) that validate advanced knowledge in specific areas rather than the generalist approach of the RHIA and RHIT certifications. In October, 2008 the American Health Information Management Association House of Delegates passed a new certification, Certified in Health Data Analytics (CHDA), which is also an advanced practice certification. (AHIMA 2009a).

Roles by Work Setting

The AHIMA 2002 Workforce Study identified 40 different work settings for HIM professionals. Some of the more common work settings discussed in this chapter include:

- Healthcare facilities
- Vendors
- Consulting firms
- Governmental agencies
- Standards developmental organizations
- Educational facilities (AHIMA 2005)

Figure 13.2 lists some of the additional job settings listed by respondents to the survey.

Figure 13.2.   2002 AHIMA member survey: job settings listed by respondents

In addition to the job settings presented in the instrument, respondents to the surveys listed the following additional settings. These settings are provided as examples of the opportunities for HIM professionals in many healthcare settings.

Settings listed on the survey instrument for selection by respondents:
- Hospital-inpatient/acute care
- Hospital-outpatient/ambulatory
- Rehabilitation hospital
- Skilled nursing facility
- Pharmaceutical company
- Laboratory
- Home health agency
- Physician office/clinic
- Insurance company
- HMO managed care organization
- Consulting firm
- Professional association
- Technology vendor
- Nontechnology vendor
- Educational institution
- Government agency
- Cancer or other registry
- Self employed
- Not employed
- Other _____

Settings listed by respondents in the category "Other":

Behavioral Health
- Psychiatric hospital
- Psychiatric center
- Mental health outpatient facility
- State psychiatric hospital
- Behavioral health for children
- Outpatient substance abuse rehabilitation facility
- Mental health correctional facility
- County mental health organization
- Psychiatric chemical dependency facility
- Chemical dependency treatment facility
- Inpatient mental health
- Hospital inpatient—adult psychiatric
- Acute mental health facility

Legal
- Medical legal firm
- Law firm
- Department of corrections
- Social security law firm
- Correctional facility/prison
- Adoption firm
- Law firm—medical defense

Coding and Billing
- Outsourcing agency
- Remote coding
- Home coding company
- Traveling coding
- Transcription service
- Home transcription company
- Physician billing service

Long-Term Care
- Skilled nursing facility
- PACE Program
- Long-term care hospital
- Long-term ambulatory care facility
- Long-term mental retardation facility
- Assisted living facility
- Geriatric care organization
- Adult day care center
- Nonprofit long-term care network/education organization
- Continuing care retirement community
- Developmental disabilities organization
- Hospice
- Care management organization
- Retirement community

Government
- Social service agency
- Department of Health and Human Services (HHS)
- Public health department
- Indian Health Services (IHS)
- State division developmental disabilities
- Regional health authority
- Department of corrections
- Regional cancer registry
- Department of Defense (DoD)

Peer Review and Professional Organizations
- Accreditation organization
- Medical peer review organization
- State peer review organization
- Quality improvement organization
- Hospital association

Ambulatory Care
- Tribal ambulatory clinic
- Outpatient diagnostic imaging services
- Community health services
- University health center
- College health clinic
- Student health center
- College athletic training department

Figure 13.2.   2002 AHIMA member survey: job settings listed by respondents *(continued)*

Ambulatory Care *(continued)* • Freestanding ambulatory surgery center • Renal dialysis center • Outpatient hemodialysis center • Occupational health • Dental practice • Home infusion provider **Education** • Veterinary teaching hospital • Medical library **Vendors and Consultants** • SNOMED • Medquist • Durable medical equipment company • Occupational medicine corporation • Independent consulting firm • Practice management company • Group purchasing firm • Medical management company • Medical service organization (MSO) • Biotechnology firm • Healthcare corporation • Health information content company • Genomic technology company	• Pharmaceutical company • Application service provider **Staffing** • Human resources company • Locum tenens staffing agency • Physician staffing company • Medical exchange **Research** • Research organization • Clinical research organization • Institutional review board • Contract research organization/clinical trials • Cancer research **Providers** • Integrated delivery system • Physician practice health system • Corporate services tertiary health system • Multispecialty group practice **Insurance** • Independent practice association • Preferred provider organization (PPO) • Electronic claims clearinghouse

Source: AHIMA 2002a.

Healthcare Facilities

In a healthcare facility, the HIM professional may be found in traditional HIM roles such as cancer registry, HIM director, and coder. With the evolving change of the profession and healthcare, HIM professionals may be found in many nontraditional roles such as system implementation, privacy and security officer, project management, and clinical vocabulary manager. HIM professionals are employed in the traditional HIM department, the information systems department, quality improvement department, and other departments throughout the facility. Some of these roles will be described in the roles by function section of this chapter.

Vendors

HIM professionals work in many different types of vendor environments such as HIM equipment/supplies and information systems. In the information systems vendor environment, the HIM professional can be found in system development, customer service, system implementation, training, and other roles. In many of these roles, the HIM professional works with hospitals and other clients around the country to support their information system needs. Many vendor roles require the HIM professional to travel up to 100 percent of the time and may telecommute when not traveling.

Consulting Firms

Many of the vendor roles mentioned in the vendor section may also be found in consulting firms. The consultants are hired by the hospital or other healthcare organization to assist in various HIM roles such as interim management, coding, information systems training and implementation, and other projects the facility does not have time or expertise to handle alone. The specific role will be defined by the needs of the facility and the contract signed between the two parties. As with the vendor environment, the HIM professional may spend a lot of time traveling to customer sites.

Governmental Agencies

The roles in government agencies will vary by the agency in which the HIM professional operates. Roles can be traditional HIM roles, such as director of the HIM department at a Veterans Administration hospital or may include nontraditional roles in agencies across local, state, and federal government, such as data collection, data analysis, standards development, and research. With the focus on quality of care, the EHR, fraud and abuse, and other HIM responsibilities, there is a need for HIM professionals to assume development and oversight roles in these areas.

Standards Developmental Organizations

In standards developmental organizations, the HIM professional will assist in the development, implementation, and testing of standards; educating the public; and ensuring that sound HIM principles are used. They can also participate in data modeling, data warehousing, development of a data dictionary, and data mapping. The HIM professional's input is important because of their knowledge of data quality, data collection, data content, and other related areas. Again, the HIM professional is a valuable part of this team because of the wide range of skills he or she possesses.

Educational Facilities

In colleges and universities, HIM professionals play an important role in the transition from the traditional paper-based environment to the EHR as they prepare future HIM professionals for the new roles that they will encounter. Educators must stay current with all changes in the profession in order to formally educate the student. Most HIM educators come from the "real world" rather than from an academic background. This requires educators to learn about learning styles and teaching strategies. The Domains, Subdomains, Tasks, and Knowledge Clusters provide a guide for educators as they prepare to teach new and evolving roles in HIM. HIM professionals in colleges and universities have generally earned a degree higher than what they are teaching. For example, in an associate in Health Information Management program, the educator should have at least a Bachelor's degree; likewise, an educator in a bachelor in health information management program should have at least a Master's degree.

Check Your Understanding 13.1

1. The organization that accredits HIM educational programs is:

   A. AHIMA
   B. CAHIIM
   C. Joint Commission
   D. CMS

2. The credential for someone who graduates from an accredited associate level HIM program and passes the national examination is:

   A. RHIA
   B. CDA
   C. CHPS
   D. RHIT

3. The work setting that includes system development, customer service, and training as part of its services is:

   A. healthcare facility
   B. vendor
   C. consultant
   D. government

4. Understanding data modeling, data warehousing, data dictionaries, and data mapping is an important part of this organization's role. The organization is a:

A. vendor
B. government agency
C. healthcare facility
D. standards development organization

5. True or False: The skills of the HIM professional are all unique to the HIM profession.

Roles by Function

HIM professionals have been active in many information technology roles for a number of years. With the evolution of technology and informatics, the HIM professional is being found in a wide variety of roles. The 2002 AHIMA Workforce Study identified many new roles for the HIM professional. As expected, many of these are technological in nature and rely on the combination of skills that are unique to the HIM profession (AHIMA 2005).

Job Titles

AHIMA has identified 125 different job titles held by HIM professionals (AHIMA 2005). Many of these positions are related to technology. HIM professionals have long worked in information technology roles within healthcare facilities and vendor sites. These roles have been the more traditional information technology roles of systems analyst, system implementation, project manager, system development, technical support, and sales. A brief description of these roles is as follows:

- The systems analyst identifies the stakeholders of an information system as well as the functionality required of a system. Tasks include data collection, data analysis, and developing data flow diagrams. The system analyst would assist in the reengineering of business processes that would take advantage of the benefits of the system being implemented.

- In system implementation, the HIM professional would assist in many aspects of the process such as systems analysis, developing the request for proposal, selecting systems, setting configurations, training, reengineering, and other steps in the process.

- HIM professionals have been project managers who control the budget, staff, and other resources allocated to ensure it is meeting the goals of the system.

- HIM professionals also work in system development roles, where they add value to the programming staff because they know HIM functions and processes needed. This knowledge allows them to determine if the needs of the facilities and regulatory/accreditation demands are being met.

- Some HIM professionals assist with technical problems that are encountered with an information system. They identify the source of the problems and take the necessary steps to resolve them.

- HIM professionals are valuable in the role as part of a sales team because they are able to talk to the HIM purchasers of information systems with an understanding of the daily issues.

Figure 13.3 lists some of the additional job titles listed by respondents to the survey.

Figure 13.3.   2002 AHIMA member survey: job titles listed by respondents

In addition to the job titles provided as options in the survey instrument, respondents to the survey listed the following job titles. These positions/titles have been loosely grouped to demonstrate the variety of functions across settings. There is overlap across categories.

Titles listed on the survey instrument for selection by respondents:
- CEO/COO/president
- CFO/finance VP
- CIO/information VP
- Other patient care executive/VP
- Clinical data analyst
- Coder/clinical data specialist
- Compliance officer
- Consultant
- Coordinator/registrar
- Data quality manager
- Database administrator
- Division manager

The following titles were included by respondents in "Other":

Clerical Positions
- Appointment clerk
- Answer phones, medical exchange
- Central scheduler, outpatient services
- Admitting and registration
- Patient access/laboratory clerk
- Dictator/auditor, discharge summaries
- Contract transcriptionist
- Hospital transcriber
- Medical transcriber
- Home-based transcriber
- Receptionist
- File clerk in records storage facility
- Secretary
- Physician office billing
- Administrative assistant, chief medical staff
- Release of information clerk
- Food stamps worker
- Unit secretary
- Director/assistant director
- Educator/instructor
- HIM supervisor/manager
- Information system specialist
- Privacy security officer
- Principal/partner of private company
- Project manager
- Release of information coordinator
- QI/UM
- Vendor representative
- Other, HIM _____
- Other, not HIM related _____

Nursing
- Nursing student
- Registered nurse
- Director of nursing
- Staffing nurse
- Nurse practitioner
- Assessment nurse
- ICU nurse
- Clinical director, nursing

Coordinators
- Pediatric services coordinator
- Community medicine specialist liaison
- Coordinator of women's health
- Organ donation requestor
- Coordinator, inpatient transfers

Other Clinical
- Medical assistant
- Laboratory assistant
- Manager, dietary services
- Acupuncture physician

Coding
- Coding team leader
- Ambulatory Patient Classification (APC) coordinator
- Coding audit and training
- Coding products and services
- Concurrent coding/utilization review
- Chargemaster coordinator
- Chargemaster analyst
- Chargemaster maintenance
- Supervisor, coding department
- Coding quality coordinator
- Owner, coding agency
- Corporate director clinical coding
- Coordinator, field operations, coding consulting company
- Nosologist
- Ambulatory Patient Classification (APC) coordinator, manager
- Medicare Severity Diagnostic Related Group (MS-DRG) coordinator
- National coding manager
- Physician order management team leader

Finance/Revenue
- Medical billing
- Reimbursement clerk
- Collections
- Auditor, revenue int

Figure 13.3.   2002 AHIMA member survey: job titles listed by respondents (*continued*)

Finance/Revenue (*continued*)
- Accounts payable clerk
- Reimbursement chargemaster
- Revenue specialist
- Reimbursement coordinator
- Payment posting
- Physician office billing
- Central billing manager
- Medical business manager
- Business analyst
- Director revenue
- Reimbursement contracting
- Physician liaison to coding and billing
- Director, manager, business office
- Owner, billing company
- Director, provider compensation
- Director, third-party payment
- Financial services representative
- Healthcare services contract monitor
- Internal auditor
- Prospective payment systems manager

Insurance
- Insurance and billing receivable clerk
- Appeals, Medicare denials
- Health claims processor
- Insurance follow-up, correspondence
- Provider relations manager
- Benefit recovery specialist
- Policy analyst reimbursement
- Corporate director, risk management
- Claims analyst
- Risk manager
- Manager clinical appeals
- PPO owner, CEO
- Claims editor/special projects
- Managed care coordinator
- Managed care project facilitator
- Managed care operations officer

Personnel
- Personnel manager
- Manager, human resources
- Recruiter, HIM

Patient Services
- Patient support representative
- Patient relations
- Manager, patient access center
- Administrative assistant—care management
- Patient rights representative
- Recipient's rights officer
- Patient accounts manager
- Case management
- Discharge planning
- Patient care associate
- Patient safety/risk management
- Patient administrative services manager

Administrative
- Radiology film room supervisor
- Radiology office manager
- X-ray film management
- Medical office manager
- Office manager, pediatric practice
- Word processing supervisor
- Medical staff coordinator
- Executive assistant
- Protocol specialist
- Transcription unit coordinator
- Emergency room admitting supervisor
- Management II supervisor of clerical
- Clinic manager, administrator
- Admissions supervisor
- Ambulatory care manager

Other Managerial
- Foundations coordinator, hospital
- Medical business manager
- Director strategic operations
- Operations manager, large group practice
- Regional director of operations
- Area manager for ROI company
- Assist. VP, finance
- Assist. VP, imaging
- Assistant executive director
- District manager
- Executive director clinical affairs
- Partner, public company

Long-Term Care
- LTC consultant
- Nursing home administrator
- Geriatric case manager
- Coding analysis long-term care and rehabilitation
- Administrator residential care

Other Settings
- Dental practice manager
- Executive director of care consortium
- Self-employed consultant
- Management, program analyst-government
- HIM state mental retardation institution
- Investigator, Office for Citizens with Developmental Disabilities
- Social services counselor
- Employee health record administrator, aerospace corporation
- Account manager, consultant
- Product analyst
- Product development manager, vice president
- Product safety associate, endocrine products
- Implementation manager, vendor
- Clinical technical editor
- Central office coordinator for state HIM professional association

(*continued on next page*)

Figure 13.3.   2002 AHIMA member survey: job titles listed by respondents *(continued)*

Other Settings *(continued)*
- Global business development
- District manager
- Implementation analyst for vendor
- Marketing manager
- Marketing analyst
- Vice president, client operations

Information Systems
- Systems administrator
- Database manager
- Information system director
- Information system manager, acute care
- Director, information services
- Clinical applications coordinator for CPR
- Computer programmer
- Computer software trainer for clinical staff
- Senior programmer
- Product development computer software
- Software QA test engineer
- Software engineer, specialist
- Systems analyst, software company
- Systems development administrator
- Transplant database coordinator, manager
- Healthcare IT analyst
- Application analyst/project manager
- Care management decision support system specialist
- Computer specialist
- Consultant—database development
- Decision support analyst, coordinator
- Director health information systems
- Director of product development
- Director of IS, customer service and operations
- EMR software support
- Knowledge engineer
- Manager, applications development
- Manager, network operations

Legal
- Paralegal
- Freedom of information officer
- Lawyer, alternative dispute resolution
- Legal assistant
- Law clerk
- Manager, legal department
- Legal specialist

Privacy/Security
- HIPAA privacy officer
- HIPAA manager
- Health information security officer
- HIPAA compliance officer

Compliance
- Professional billing compliance
- Documentation compliance

- Physician record, corporate compliance
- Revenue cycle manager, compliance
- Regulatory compliance specialist
- Compliance consultant, analyst
- Compliance auditor
- Coding compliance auditor
- Compliance training manager
- Corporate compliance team
- State surveyor regulatory compliance
- Compliance officer
- Performance improvement, regulatory coordinator
- Investigator

Quality
- Quality review, endovascular and endoscopy
- Director of quality, risk management
- Quality improvement specialist I
- Quality improvement director
- Quality management
- Quality resource specialist
- Consultant QA, privacy
- Utilization review
- Data quality auditor
- Quality assurance coding
- Local medical review policy specialist
- Administrative director health information quality and risk management, utilization review, and so on
- Quality assurance birth records and vital records
- Process improvement coordinator

Medical Records
- Nuclear records
- Chart analysis
- Independent contractor—data abstraction
- Business systems analyst for medical records
- LMRP coordinator
- Medical records coordinator for clinical division
- Coordinator, record retention center
- Health Information coordinator, manager, and so on
- Information management governance team

Education
- Advisory committee for HIM students
- Professor
- Proctor
- Continuing medical education
- Certified public educator
- Faculty, medical school
- Associate dean, academic affairs
- CME coordinator, specialist
- Course scheduling administrator

Figure 13.3.   2002 AHIMA member survey: job titles listed by respondents *(continued)*

Registries	• Data quality control editor
• Public health representative, state cancer registry	• Data manager, quality management
• Atlas abstractor	• Corporate manager, cancer data
• Editor, cancer registry	• Outpatient/inpatient data validation
• Tumor registrar	
• Trauma registrar	**Research**
• Birth certificate registrar	• Research study coordinator
• Registrar of vital statistics	• Cancer clinical trials supervisor
	• Contract/grant administrator
Libraries	• Research assistant
• Medical librarian	• Research analyst
• National archives	• Principal investigator
• Supervisor, USAF Central ECG Library	• Institutional review board
	• Administration, outcomes research
Data	
• Abstractor	**Credentialing**
• Abstraction program coordinator	• Credentials verification specialist
• Biostatistician	• Health facility evaluator
• Oncology data specialist	• Accreditation administrator
• ECU statistical reporting	• Credentialing specialist
• Data integrity analyst	• Healthcare facility surveyor

Source: AHIMA 2002b.

Newer Roles by Function

HIM professionals are going beyond the traditional information system roles they have played for years. They are now working in roles such as clinical vocabulary manager, data analyst, and other new and evolving roles. Some of these roles are listed next and are described in this section.

- Clinical vocabulary manager

- Data analyst

- Terminology asset manager

- Data miner

- Data navigator

- Data quality and integrity monitor

- Data resource manager

- Data security, privacy, and confidentiality manager

- Data translator

- Information system designer

- Work and data flow analyst (AHIMA e-HIM Task Force 2003)

Clinical Vocabulary Manager (Clinical Terminology Manager)

Some people believe that the **clinical vocabulary manager's** role is the same as or similar to that of the coding supervisor. The reality is that these two roles are very different. The coding supervisor evaluates the coding to determine if the proper code is utilized. The role of the clinical vocabulary manager is to:

- Create, maintain, and implement terminologies, validation files, and maps for a variety of use cases in the EHR

- Perform ongoing review of the auto and manual encoder systems for terminology and classification systems, including methods and processes, and implement recommendations for improving and optimizing the encoding process

- Assist in the analysis of the enterprise's classification and grouping system assignment trends and use data from classification and grouping systems to assist in decision making

- Proactively monitor developments in the field of clinical terminologies and medical vocabularies

- Recommend the most appropriate classification or terminology systems to meet all required information reporting needs

- Possess expertise in clinical terminology, medical vocabulary, classification systems and skill in mining, and deriving or engineering clinical ontologies (Giannangelo, Greene, Perron and Cook)

To be successful in the clinical vocabulary manager role, the HIM professional must have many skills including knowledge of medical terminologies, data modeling, data mining, linguistics, and data warehouses. To completely fulfill the needs of this role, the HIM professional may need a graduate degree in medical informatics.

Data Analyst

The **data analyst** is responsible for turning data into meaningful information. The data analyst manipulates data and generates reports using structured query language (SQL) or statistical software, and other tools. The data analyst will be responsible for the display of data in graphs, tables, or other appropriate formats. The data analyst will need to understand data and how it is collected, descriptive statistics, inferential statistics, and research methodologies. Some data analysts may work with data warehouses or other clinical databases whereas others focus more on the quality of the data. In the role of monitoring quality, the data analyst is frequently responsible for the integrity of the master patient index. Other responsibilities may include audits, developing policies and procedures for data quality, and notifying users of problems encountered.

Terminology Asset Manager

This position develops **data sets, nomenclatures, and classification standards**, and in order to do so the HIM professional must understand the data needs of all stakeholders. Stakeholders include public health agencies, government agencies, and healthcare facilities. The developer must be detail oriented in order to maintain the integrity of the system as it changes over time. This role is required for systems such as ICD-10-CM as the system is developed, implemented, and revised. The HIM professional in this role must also be able to develop the system in such a way as to reach expected goals.

Data Miner

The role of the **data miner** is to convert information into knowledge that can be used for decision making. A data miner must be able to use data mining tools such as online analytical processing (OLAP) to drill down into data and transform buried data into logical information. The data miner must have strong math skills and be able to analyze statistical data to identify patterns within data. The data miner must ensure that the data necessary to make decisions and identify patterns are available in a timely manner. The data miner must also understand the different types of data mining models available to ensure that the proper model is selected for the analysis to be performed. An example of the type of request a data miner may address is to determine why the healthcare facility is losing money on cardiology patients. It may be because of expensive drugs, poorly negotiated contracts, recent equipment purchases, a failure to follow evidence-based medicine, or some other cause. The financial and clinical data would be run through OLAP or another tool to identify the root cause of the losses.

Data Navigator

A **data navigator** would be part of the information system development team. The person in this role would specialize in the development of the graphical user interface used to capture and navigate through the EHR and other systems. The data navigator would utilize human-computer interfaces such as drop-down menus, speech recognition, templates, and natural language processes to interact with the user. The data navigator would need to understand the system and how it will be used in order to ensure that the navigation is appropriate and user-friendly. The data navigator would be looking for ways to efficiently move from one function to another using a minimum of keystrokes or mouse clicks. The data navigator would also look for ways to quickly enter data while achieving and maintaining quality.

Data Quality and Integrity Monitor

The person in the **Data Quality and Integrity Monitor** role is responsible for the quality of the information collected and stored by the facility. This individual would work with the information system department to ensure that quality is built into the system as much as possible through the use of logic or structured data. An example of logic edits to ensure data quality could be that a patient's temperature cannot be below 85°F or above 115°F. An example of structured data would be forcing the user to choose between male or female when entering the patient's gender. The data quality and integrity monitor would also audit and report on data quality, reliability, and validity in the information systems. Patterns identified would then be reported to the appropriate entities to be addressed within the facility.

Data Resource Manager

Information is key to the success of a healthcare organization. The **data resource manager** (also referred to as "data resource administrator") is responsible for managing the data. To manage the data, the data resource manager must understand the sources of data and the individual data elements. The data resource manager should know the data collected by the facility and propose a plan to fill in gaps in the data. The data resource manager uses technology to obtain the information needed to provide care. The technology includes the EHR, data repositories, and data warehouses.

The data resource manager uses data management tools such as SQL and data mining to convert the abundance of data into meaningful information. The data resource manager is also responsible for data integrity and access to the information. This person must maintain the integrity of historical data collected for as long as the facility decides to retain it to meet research, patient care, and legal needs. For example, the data resource manager will still have to maintain ICD-9-CM data long after ICD-10-CM and ICD-10-PCS have been implemented. He or she helps the organization use the data collected and stored in many ways. For example, they must be able to convert patient-specific data into aggregate data to facilitate analysis. The data resource manager must also be able to convert patient-specific data into comparative data. According to Mon, Herbst, and Nunn, the uses of data should include:

- Support for point-of-care processes
- Quality improvement, outcomes measurement, performance measurement
- Basic and applied clinical research
- External reporting (for example, ORYX, HEDIS, HCFA (now CMS)
- Strategic planning, competitive strategy, and market trend analysis
- Health services, management, and clinical decision support
- Process reengineering
- Outreach to patient, professionals, and other consumers (Mon et al. 1998)

As shown by this list of uses for data, the data are used to make strategic as well as operational decisions; therefore, data must be managed for as long as they are retained.

Figure 13.4 shows a sample job description for a data resource administrator (also referred to as "data resource manager")

Privacy Officer and Security Officer

The **privacy officer** and **security officer** are responsible for protecting the data from unauthorized access, alteration, or destruction. These roles may be combined, or it may be divided into two or more positions within the facility. The HIM professional in this role may have the title of Chief Privacy Official/Privacy Officer or Chief Security Officer/ Security Officer, or at least perform the duties of these roles as defined by HIPAA. These individuals would be responsible for developing and establishing a compliance program including policies and procedures to control the management of health information privacy and security. Additionally, these professionals would be responsible for monitoring state, federal, and local laws to ensure the facility's compliance with privacy and security legislation both now and in the future. Finally, the privacy officer and security officer will have to monitor trends and make the necessary changes to policies to ensure optimal patient privacy protection and overall compliance.

Specifically, the privacy officer oversees the activities related to privacy and access to protected health information (AHIMA e-HIM Work Group on Health Information in a

Figure 13.4.   Sample job description: data resource administrator

---

Position Title: Data Resource Administrator

Immediate Supervisor: Director of Information Services

General Purpose: The data resource administrator provides overall leadership for data resource management in the organization and is responsible for developing, communicating, and monitoring data resource management policies and procedures to ensure that the organization's data are secure, accessible, accurate, and reliable for business and patient care uses

Responsibilities:
- Works with health information management (HIM), legal services, and other departments to develop and maintain the organization's data resource management policies and procedures
- Monitors compliance with the organization's data resource management policies and procedures
- Works with data analysts and database managers from the information services department to develop and manage the organization's data repository and data warehouse
- Works with data quality managers and other HIM professionals to ensure the quality of the organization's health information
- Develops and maintains the organization's data sets, data dictionary, data standards, and data model
- Works with HIM, legal services, information security, and information services staff to develop access and release of information policies and procedures
- Forecasts the organization's future information system requirements
- Participates in the planning and negotiation of acquisitions of new information system software and hardware
- Manages the functions, staff, and budget of the data resource department
- Performs strategic planning activities for the data resource department and participates in strategic planning for the organization
- Assesses training needs among data users and coordinates training activities
- Monitors advancements in information technology and HIM
- Monitors changes in laws, regulations, and accreditation standards as they apply to data resource management

Qualifications:
- Baccalaureate degree in HIM or a related field; advanced degree or coursework in computer science desirable
- Certification as an RHIA
- Knowledge of health information systems, database management and design, spreadsheet design, and computer technology

---

Source: AHIMA (nd)

Hybrid Environment 2003). Although these individuals may protect all patient identifiable health information, including paper records, the use of technology has increased the need and responsibilities of this role.

Figure 13.5 shows a sample job description for a privacy officer that was published in the *Journal of the American Health Information Management Association*.

Among the security officer's specific responsibilities would be performing or delegating the responsibility for audits to ensure that policies are being followed and that

Figure 13.5.   Sample job description: privacy officer

Privacy Officer

Sample Position Description

General Purpose: The privacy officer oversees all activities related to the development, implementation, maintenance of, and adherence to the organization's privacy program in compliance with federal and state laws. Activities include developing policies and procedures, as well as workforce educational activities that address access, use, and disclosure of patient health information.

Reports to: Chief Information Officer or Vice President of Corporate Compliance

Responsibilities:
Oversight of the Privacy Program
- Develop, implement, and maintain the organization's protected health information privacy and security policies, procedures and guidelines in compliance with federal and state laws, as well as accreditation standards, and in coordination with organization leadership, the Privacy/HIPAA compliance oversight structure, and legal counsel
- Set the direction and provide the vision for the privacy compliance program
- Plans, implements, and directs ongoing privacy and data security risk activities
- Report on the status of the privacy and data security program
- Measure effectiveness, performance, and quality of the program to the board, system leadership, and HIPAA/compliance oversight structure as well as provide input, recommendations, and guidance on privacy and security issues
- Coordinate an ongoing compliance auditing and monitoring program of workforce members, business associates, trading partners, etc, to ensure that organizational privacy and security policies and procedures are up-to-date and maintained addressing concerns, requirements, and responsibilities

Compliance
- Establishes, resolves, and administers a process for the receipt, documentation, receiving, tracking, and investigation of compliance violations against the organization's privacy and data security practices as well as provide recommendations and execute actions for said violations
- Investigates and monitors all complaints to ensure the consistent application of sanctions for failure to comply with privacy practices
- Reviews all organizational information security and privacy plans to ensure alignment between security and privacy practices
- Collaborates with leadership, key departments, and committees/structures to ensure the implementation, maintenance, enforcement, and update of appropriate documentation (e.g., NPP, authorization forms, investigation forms, etc.) as needed in compliance with federal laws, state laws, and relevant accreditation standards
- Performs/directs risk assessments (i.e., protected information privacy and security audits, policies and procedures, trend analyses, audits, projects, and violation investigations) to ensure organizational compliance
- Ensures organizational compliance with legal, ethical, regulatory, accreditation, licensing, certification requirements, and other administrative requirements regarding privacy and data security, and implementation of supporting administrative, physical, and technical safeguards
- Cooperates with the Office for Civil Rights and/or other investigative agencies in coordination with organization officers in responding to external compliance reviews or investigations

(continued on next page)

Figure 13.5.   Sample job description: privacy officer *(continued)*

Daily Operations
- Facilitates privacy and security training through awareness activities providing education on organizational policies, procedures, and practices
- Serves on various committees and projects in a leadership role for the planning, design, and evaluation of privacy, and data security; coordinates development of strategic teams, work groups, and resources
- Delegates responsibility and authority to individuals to act as privacy and data security coordinators as needed
- Directs and manages the daily operations of privacy and data security compliance
- Develops job descriptions, manages budgets and performs financial processes, strategic planning, and staff management functions
- Provides leadership, strategic direction, and affirms that the workforce of the organization adheres to regulatory mandates regarding privacy and confidentiality

Exchange of Information
- Directs the development and management of the organization's authorization forms and release of information policies, procedures, and practices for disclosure of PHI; Responds to requests to exercise individual's privacy rights (i.e. inspection, amendment, account of disclosures, and restriction of access to PHI);
- Ensures the efficiency and efficacy of the organization's processes with respect to the electronic exchange of data and patient information in compliance with state and federal laws.
- Designs, implements, and manages role-based access control; oversees audits of access to PHI; recommends appropriate action necessary as a result of audit activities

Privacy and HIPAA Expertise
- Serves as a liaison to the community on HIPAA Privacy, IRB, clinical & administrative systems, and Data Security topics and as an internal resource/consultant to the organization on privacy and security compliance related activities
- Works with organization leadership, legal counsel, and other related parties to represent the organization's information privacy and security interests with external parties who undertake to adopt or amend privacy legislation, regulations, or standards
- Maintains current knowledge of applicable federal and state health information privacy and security laws and accreditation standards
- Monitors advancements in information privacy technology to ensure organizational adaptation and compliance
- Provides community support for privacy and security initiates that impact the organization and its stakeholders

Other Skills
- Proficient in Microsoft Office: PC-based spreadsheet programs (i.e., Power Point, Excel, Word)
- Knowledge of and the ability to apply the principles of HIM, project management, and change management; knowledge of health care industry
- Demonstrates organization, facilitation, communication, and presentation skills
- Experience in information systems and data risk management
- High degree of personal and professional integrity

Requirements:
- Bachelor's degree in health information management, healthcare administration, or related field required.
- Master's degree preferred
- CHPS, RHIA, or RHIT credential preferred
- At least 5 years in healthcare operations, clinical care, health information management, research, or a related field

Notes:
1. The title for this position will vary from organization to organization, and may not be the primary title of the individual serving in the position. "Chief" would most likely refer to very large integrated delivery systems. The term "privacy officer" is specifically mentioned in the HIPAA Privacy Regulation.
2. The reporting structure for this position will vary depending on the institution and its size. Since many of the functions are already inherent in the health information or medical records department or function, many organizations may elect to keep this function in that department.

Source: AHIMA 2009b.

breaches have not occurred. This individual would also be responsible for risk assessment and ensuring that the current privacy and security plans are working.

Data Translator

The healthcare delivery system is a complicated maze of forms, jargon, rules and regulations, and other concepts. This makes it difficult for patients to know what to do or how to obtain their health information, and to understand their patient information once they have it. A **data translator** works as the liaison between the patient and his or her health data. Data translators assist the patient in understanding their rights, such as the right to control access to their protected health information. They work with patients to help overcome barriers such as translating medical terminology into understandable terms.

Work and Data Flow Analyst

The **work and data flow analyst** must be able to study the flow of data into the system and its associated processes and look for ways to improve it. The work and data flow analyst must be able to use data flow diagrams and other tools to document the various flows of data within the facility. This role is important as the transition to the EHR will change workflows and tasks through the elimination of paper and manual processes using the creation of electronic ones. This individual must be able to work well with people because they will need to identify how work is being done and then be able to envision how it will change in the electronic environment to develop an efficient and effective new workflow.

Check Your Understanding 13.2

1. The role that identifies the information system functions needed is a:

    A. System developer
    B. Project manager
    C. Systems analyst
    D. Data analyst

2. The HIM role in which the individual must be knowledgeable in medical terminology, data modeling, data mining, linguistics, and data warehousing is:

    A. Clinical vocabulary manager
    B. Data analyst
    C. Terminology asset manager
    D. Data resource manager

3. Which HIM role works with patients to help them understand health data?

    A. Resource manager
    B. Data translator
    C. Data analyst
    D. Data security, data privacy, and confidentiality manager

4. The HIM role that protects data from unauthorized use is:

    A. Resource manager
    B. Data translator
    C. Data analyst
    D. Data security, data privacy, and confidentiality manager

5. I am using a data flow diagram to identify ways to improve a process. I must be a:

    A. Clinical vocabulary manager
    B. Data analyst
    C. Terminology asset manager
    D. Work and data flow analyst

References

AHIMA e-HIM Task Force. 2003. A Vision of the e-HIM Future: A Report from the AHIMA e-HIM Task Force. http://library.ahima.org/xpedio/groups/secure/documents/ahima/bok1_020835.hcsp?dDocName=bok1_020835

AHIMA e-HIM Work Group on Health Information in a Hybrid Environment. 2003. Practice brief: Complete medical record in a hybrid EHR environment: Part I: Managing the transition. http://library.ahima.org/xpedio/groups/public/documents/ahima/bok1_021581.hcsp?dDocName=bok1_021581.

AHIMA HIM Practice Transformation Work Group. 2005. EHR career opportunities: Sample HIM job descriptions. *Journal of AHIMA* 76(6):56A–D.

American Health Information Management Association. nd. Data resource administrator sample job description. http://library.ahima.org/xpedio/groups/secure/documents/ahima/bok1_013528.pdf.

American Health Information Management Association. 2002a. 2002 AHIMA member survey: Job settings listed by respondents. Data gathered for AHIMA Workforce Study.

American Health Information Management Association. 2002b. 2002 AHIMA member survey: Job titles. Data gathered for AHIMA Workforce Study.

American Health Information Management Association. 2005. AHIMA Workforce Study. Embracing the Future: New Times, New Opportunities for Health Information Managers. 2005. Summary Findings from the HIM Workforce Study.

American Health Information Management Association. 2009a. Certified Health Data Analyst (CHDA). http://www.ahima.org/certification/chda.asp.

American Health Information Management Association. 2009b. Privacy officer: Sample position description. http://campus.ahima.org/Campus/courses/SA/PrivacyOfcr/po_sample_jobdesc.pdf.

Commission on Accreditation for Health Informatics and Information Management Education. 2004. HIM associate degree entry-level competencies domains, subdomains, and tasks for 2006 and beyond. http://cahiim.org/resources/documents/HIM_AEC.pdf.

Commission on Accreditation for Health Informatics and Information Management Education. 2007. Knowledge cluster content assessment associate degree program. http://www.cahiim.org/resources/documents/HIMASSOCIATEDEGREEKNOWLEDGECNov2007.doc.

Health Information Careers. 2007. http://himcareers.ahima.org/.

Giannangelo, K., M. Greene, K. Perron, and J. Cook. 2006. Evolving roles for the clinical terminology manager. *Proceedings from the American Health Information Management Association's 78th National Convention and Exhibit* (October 2006).

Mon, D., M.R. Herbst, and S. Nunn. 1998. Practice brief: Data resource administration: The road ahead. *Journal of AHIMA* 69(10).

Chapter 14
The Future of Computers in Healthcare

Objectives

- Differentiate between the two types of computer-assisted coding.

- Recommend when natural language processing should be used.

- Support the need for the personal health record.

- Assist in the selection of the type of personal health record to be used.

- Describe the role of the Office of the National Coordinator in the development of the health information exchange.

- Address the issues related to the development of the health information exchange.

- Assist patients in the use of consumer health informatics.

- Discuss the attributes of open software.

- Justify the need for certification for the electronic health record.

Key Terms

Certification Commission on Health Information Technology (CCHIT)
Computer-assisted coding (CAC)
Consumer awareness campaign
Consumer health informatics
Electronic prescribing (e-prescribing)
Free and open source software
General equivalence mapping
Health information exchange

Health record banking
International Classification of Diseases, 10th Revision, Clinical Modification
International Classification of Diseases, 10th Revision, Procedural Coding System
MyPHR.com
Natural language processing (NLP)

Office of the National Coordinator for Health Information Technology (ONCHIT)
Open code
Personal health record (PHR)
Proprietary software
Public domain software
Regional health information organization (RHIO)

What Next?

Technology is an ever-evolving field that has changed and will continue to change the healthcare industry. Healthcare facilities have and will continue to implement the electronic health record (EHR), allowing patients various forms of online access (such as scheduling an appointment) and giving physicians tools such as clinical decision support systems to help diagnose patient conditions. Some of the changes come from current technologies that will grow into a very sophisticated system of the future. This chapter will discuss many of these evolving and emerging technologies.

Evolving Technologies

Evolving technologies are not necessarily new but, rather, existing technologies that are becoming more mature, more sophisticated, and therefore more useful. The evolving technologies discussed in this chapter are:

- Natural language processing
- Computer-assisted coding
- Personal health record
- ICD-10 Clinical Modifications and Procedure Coding System (ICD-10-CM and ICD-10-PCS)

Natural Language Processing

Natural language processing (NLP) is the conversion of unstructured data into structured data through the use of computer algorithms or statistical methods (Johns 2006). NLP requires the ability to "process the commands, instructions or other input when provided by sentences as spoken in normal human discourse" (LaTour and Eichenwald Maki 2006, 559). Uses of NLP include dictation and computer-assisted coding. NLP is sophisticated enough to consider the different meanings of terms in order to correctly classify the spoken word (LaTour and Eichenwald Maki 2006). NLP assigns code numbers to the data used for data storage. As stated earlier, one use of NLP is automated coding of diagnoses and procedures. NLP can analyze data entered and apply algorithms or statistical methods to the data to determine the correct code from either the ICD-9-CM or other coding systems. To be successful, automated coding must be able to understand the relationships between the terms. For example, the ICD-9-CM code for hypertensive heart disease is different from hypertension and heart disease; thus, algorithms must be able to understand these differences. NLP may also be utilized in clinical information systems and the EHR to convert narrative text into data that can be easily analyzed.

Computer-Assisted Coding

Much of coding is very routine. Many codes are used over and over again. This routine work can be performed by **computer-assisted coding (CAC)**. CAC is "the use of computer software that automatically generates a set of medical codes for review, validation, and use based upon clinical documentation provided by healthcare practitioners" (AHIMA e-HIM Work Group on Computer-Assisted Coding 2004, 48A). CAC has been in the developmental or infancy stage for a number of years, but has not been mainstreamed into HIM departments. CAC will assign an ICD-9-CM, Current Procedural Terminology (CPT), or other code from various coding systems to an episode of care. These codes must be reviewed by a credentialed HIM professional to validate the accuracy of the codes before they are released for billing, research, and other purposes.

The current manual coding process is very expensive and problematic. The accuracy of coding is frequently not up to the desired level. Problems with coding quality may result in improper billing that in turn may result in fraud and abuse charges. Hospitals and other healthcare facilities frequently find themselves with staffing shortages due to resignations, vacations, sick time, and other reasons. The shortage of coders frequently creates a backlog in the coding process, which in turn creates an increase in discharged not final billed reports and problems with cash flow, among many others for the facility.

CAC is supported by the steady implementation of the EHR. The electronic data stored in the EHR along with NLP provide the infrastructure needed for CAC. There are two forms of CAC. The first form uses NLP to abstract data from narrative text. This text is then converted into the codes necessary to document diagnoses and procedures associated with the patient's encounter. The second form utilizes structured data, also called codified data, which are input into a clinical information system and then used for CAC. Structured data are mapped to a code that describes the data selected from the structured drop-down boxes or other structured data entry options (AHIMA e-HIM Workgroup on Computer-Assisted Coding 2004).

The AHIMA e-HIM Workgroup on Computer-Assisted Coding identified advantages and barriers to CAC. The advantages of CAC include:

- Increased coding productivity

- Increased efficiency frees professional from mundane tasks

- Comprehensive code assignment

- Consistent application of rules

- Electronic coding audit trail (AHIMA e-HIM Workgroup on Computer-Assisted Coding 2004, 48B)

Barriers to CAC include:

- Cost of CAC hardware and software

- Complexity, quality, and format of health record documentation

- User resistance to change

- Technological limitations

- Potential increase in errors in the coding process

- Lack of industry standards (AHIMA Workgroup on Computer-Assisted Coding 2004, 48B-48C)

CAC is currently used in a limited number of medical specialties. This technology does not replace human coders but, rather, is a tool to support coders. As technology evolves and as ICD-10-CM and ICD-10-PCS are implemented, CAC will be advanced into more and more areas, including inpatient records (AHIMA e-HIM Workgroup on Computer-Assisted Coding 2004).

Personal Health Record

AHIMA defines the **personal health record (PHR)** as "an electronic, universally available, lifelong resource of health information needed by individuals to make health decisions. Individuals own and manage the information in the PHR, which comes from healthcare providers and the individual. The PHR is maintained in a secure and private environment, with the individual determining rights of access. The PHR is separate from and does not replace the legal record of any provider" (AHIMA e-HIM Personal Health Record Work Group 2005, 64A). The PHI contains health information that comes from both the physician and the patient but the PHR is controlled by the patient. The PHR is important because it will link health information from all of the patient's care providers into one central location, which will help to improve the overall quality of the care provided. The PHR can also improve communications between providers since the merging of the patient's health information ensures that they know all of the medications that a patient is on, the treatments they are experiencing, and other information that can stop contraindicated medication from being ordered, reduce or eliminate duplication of tests, and speed up treatment (Quinsey et al. 2005).

The PHR can be as simple as a folder with copies of records or it can be a sophisticated Web-based information system. There are currently four common methods of PHRs. These are: paper, personal computer, Internet, and portable devices. Obtaining copies of medical records and organizing them into a folder or a three-ring binder is a great way to start a PHR. It is relatively quick and everyone is comfortable with the paper. However, accessibility is limited to the one source. The health information can also be scanned documents on a USB drive, PDA, or other portable device. While much more portable than a folder or three-ring binder, it still limits accessibility. A PC-based product uses the patient's computer for storage that can be printed or copied to a portable device to take to the care provider. The Internet PHR provides access 24/7/365 from anywhere. Internet PHRs can be obtained by the patient in several ways. One way is for the patient to purchase a PHR service from a vendor who stores the data and provides basic services to the user. In this case, the patient must collect records from their physicians and other providers and enter the information into the PHR. The patient's healthcare provider or insurer may provide the service automatically, populating it with clinical information and/or claims data (Quinsey et al. 2005).

Suggested categories of common data elements in a PHR include:

- Personal demographic information
- General medical information
- Allergies and drug sensitivities
- Conditions
- Hospitalizations
- Surgeries
- Medications
- Immunizations
- Clinical tests
- Pregnancy history (AHIMA e-HIM Personal Health Record Work Group 2005)

AHIMA views the PHR as a significant and useful tool of technology. In 2003, AHIMA created the MyPHR Web site (**www.myphr.com**) to promote and educate the public about the PHR and to provide guidance on how to create one (AHIMA e-HIM Personal Health Record Work Group 2005). MyPHR provides a variety of resources to the public including the definition of what a PHR is, the different types of formats available, the value of a PHR, health forms, and how to create a PHR. Figure 14.1 shows the MyPHR Web site.

AHIMA also started a **consumer awareness campaign**, which, as of November 2008, had trained 975 HIM professionals on the PHR and on how to speak and educate the public in churches, community centers, various clubs, and other neighborhood groups (AHIMA 2008). As of September 2009 more than 600 additional HIM professionals had been trained (May 2009).

With the interest in the PHR, standardization has become critical to its success. This standardization of the PHR must address operability, security, content, and other issues.

Figure 14.1.   The home page of AHIMA's PHR resource—MyPHR.com

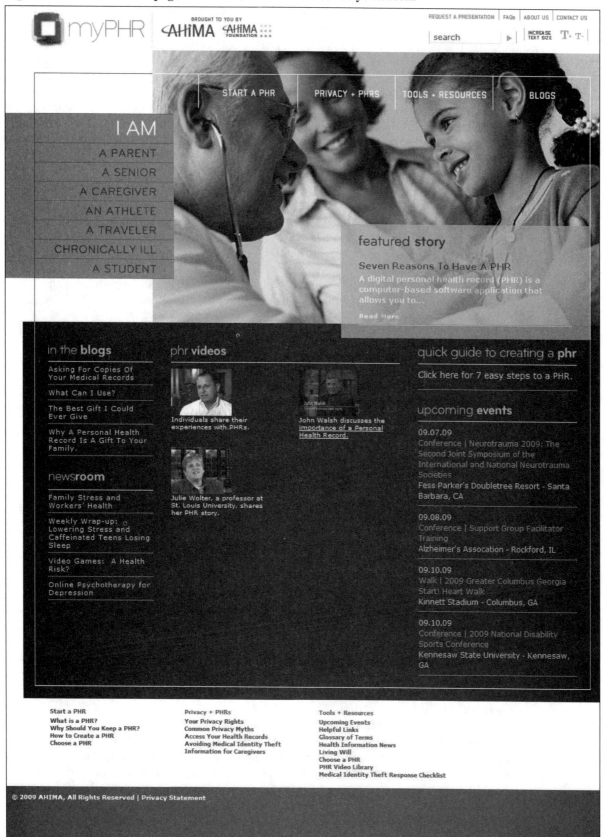

Standardization of PHRs is important and Health Level 7 (HL7) has developed the PHR System Functional Model. This proposed standard lists the functionalities that a PHR should have in order to enhance communication between patient, care provider, and other stakeholders. The model addresses integration issues, connectivity issues, and interoperability.

PHRs have caught the attention of big businesses such as Google, Microsoft, and other Fortune 500 companies entering the PHR market. The different philosophies among these companies are reflected in their respective versions of the PHR. For example, Microsoft's Health Vault allows patients to search for health information as well as store their medical information. Health Vault and many other products such as Revolution Health (founded by the founder of America Online) are open to the general public. Dossia, which is sponsored by AT&T, Intel, BP, and Wal-Mart, is a closed system for employees, their families, and retired employees (Dimick 2008b).

Initially two major PHR models were utilized. The first was when healthcare providers used data from their EHR to populate the PHR. The other model was the freestanding PHR. This model is considered the most likely to be a longitudinal record as the patient can store information from all of their care providers (Mon 2005). Currently there are a number of different models. Rode (2008) identified the following:

- Provider-based "tether" models, which offer a combination of provider- and consumer-entered data, along with functions such as appointment scheduling and record requests

- Health plan models, similarly tethered, which offer claims and secondhand provider data, along with consumer-entered data

- Provider or health plan portals, offering a view of certain provider or plan information

- Employer-based models that offer benefit information and allow consumer-submitted data

- Employer-sponsored models such as Dossia

- Internet models such as those announced by Microsoft and Google

- Health record banks that offer a centralized data bank controlled by the individual

- Consumer-held PHRs in a variety of desktop, flash drive, and other configurations (Rode 2008, 18)

While there are similarities between many of these models, they vary in level of control by the consumer, use of claims data, identification of source of information, and more.

A key player in the PHR initiatives is Connecting for Health. This organization was developed in September of 2002. It is a public-private organization with representatives from more than 100 organizations. Their mission is to make the changes necessary to implement health information technology. They are actively involved in the PHR, health information networks, privacy, and other related topics. With regard to the PHR, they developed a framework for the PHR and addressed issues related to privacy and security (Connecting for Health 2008).

It is expected that PHRs will be populated by physicians in the future. Barriers to physicians populating the PHR include privacy, liability, and ownership. The concern regarding privacy and security of the PHR is an ongoing topic of debate. A PHR must be available and solely managed by the patient, including access to the data contained within. The PHR should be available at any time and from anywhere, especially in event of an emergency. Privacy and security standards must be created along with content standards and other standards to address these issues before the PHR can fully realize the benefits (Rhodes 2007).

PHR Issues

Figure 14.2 identifies some issues raised by the PHR.

Health Information Exchange

Health information exchange (HIE) is a term used to refer to a "plan in which health information is shared among providers" (AHIMA 2010, 128). Over the years, a number of different terminologies have been used to describe data exchange. These include national health information infrastructure, health information network, and **regional health information organization (RHIO)** (Bloomrosen and Heubusch 2006). RHIOs are defined by AHIMA as "an organization that manages the local deployment of systems promoting and facilitating the exchange of healthcare data within a national health information network (AHIMA 2010, 251). The terms "RHIO" and "HIE" are frequently used interchangeably.

HIEs look and operate very differently, but generally they bring stakeholders together to develop, implement, and manage patient information. The exchange of data in an HIE must be interoperable and secure. There are a number of models of HIEs in use. These are:

- Federated model with shared repositories

- Federated model with peer-to-peer network

- Nonfederated peer-to-peer network (co-op model)

- Centralized database or data warehouse

The goal of all of the models is the same; however, the models vary in how data is collected and/or stored. As demonstrated in figure 14.3, some models utilize a centralized database, whereas others connect the databases of the participants.

Privacy and other operational issues are some of the holdups in developing an HIE. The HIE would be subject to the HIPAA requirements thus requiring them to meet minimum necessary standard, proper access controls, notice of privacy practices, and more. The

Figure 14.3.　Models of HIE

Federated model with shared repositories. This model uses a network of networks connected through the Internet. Participants submit data to a regional repository responsible for patient identification, storage, system management, security, and privacy. The regional repositories are interconnected.

Federated model with peer-to-peer network. This model employs a peer-to-peer network of participant networks connected through the Internet. Participants maintain their own health information network with no centralized repositories. A national or regional entity maintains a master patient index for the HIE. Using this index, participants can obtain patient data from the other individual participant networks. This can be done peer to peer by direct communication to the participant holding the data or through a national or regional entity that manages the index as an intermediary.

Nonfederated peer-to-peer network (co-op model). This approach uses a peer-to-peer network of participant networks connected through the Internet. The network may be smaller and more community-based (e.g., a hospital system and affiliated clinics with point-to-point communication). Participants maintain their own health information network, and there is no centralized repository. All communications are direct from participant to participant. There is no national or regional entity maintaining a master patient index for the HIE, so a mechanism to identify the location of records is required.

Centralized database or data warehouse. This model employs a regional centralized repository of health information accessed through the Internet. A database or data warehouse may be a component or building block of other models. Storage, system management, patient identification, security, and privacy are all managed at a central site. Participants submit data to and request data from this central site.

Source: Carter et al. 2006

HIE may need to offer an opt-in or opt-out option for patients to choose whether or not to include their protected health information in the HIE. The HIE must also ensure that the information contained in the HIE is accurate, thus requiring data standards for content and definitions. The HIE should be able to correctly identify the patient without improperly releasing information on other patients. These and other issues must be addressed before the HIE is operational.

Many states are working to develop HIEs through various methods. State involvement is important as they create the laws and regulations to control privacy, security, retention, and other issues facing the development and maintenance of an HIE. The state level HIE (SLHIE) consensus project has researched the projects occurring around the country. This project looked for consensus in the functions of an HIE as well as evaluating the state-level projects to be leaders in the HIE development for the state. These initiatives may be developed by the state government, but is commonly led by other entities who are leading the efforts for the geographic area (Dierker 2008).

Creating HIEs requires a large investment on the part of the stakeholders. The American Hospital Association reports that the cost of development and implementation could cost from $3 to $10 million. This is after an investment in the planning process of $300,000 to $1,000,000. Prior to the commitment of this type of investment, legal issues related to who pays the expenses, ownership of the data, privacy, security, and other HIE issues must be addressed (AHA 2006).

Certification Commission on Health Information Technology

In 2004, the **Certification Commission on Health Information Technology (CCHIT)** was developed by the American Health Information Management Association (AHIMA), the Health Information Management Systems Society (HIMSS), and the National Alliance for Health Information Technology (NAHIT). These organizations committed money to support this voluntary, private-sector organization. The CCHIT Web site states that the purpose was "to accelerate the adoption of robust, interoperable health information technology by creating a credible, efficient certification of process" (CCHIT 2008a). CCHIT obtained a contract from HHS to develop and evaluate certification criteria and to develop a process to be used to certify vendor products (CCHIT 2008a). The first products were certified in July 2006.

The goals of CCHIT are to

- Reduce risk of physician and provider investment in health IT

- Facilitate interoperability between EHRs, health information exchanges, and other entities, with the goal of making patient records portable and making measurement and improvement of quality possible

- Enhance availability of adoption incentives and regulatory relief

- Protect the privacy of personal health information (CCHIT HIE Work Group 2008, 2)

CCHIT now has standards for inpatient, ambulatory, and emergency room EHR products. The ambulatory EHR has additional certification that a vendor may choose to apply for, such as child health and cardiovascular medicine. All of these standards include specific functionality, interoperability, and security criteria. Vendors who are certified in all three domains may choose to become certified at the enterprise level, which validates interoperability of the three components. The first criteria published and certified were for the ambulatory setting. This certification process provides assurance that the EHR products meet the minimum requirements by CCHIT. The requirements used by CCHIT are updated each year to meet increasing expectations of the EHR. CCHIT works in an open environment and asks for input from stakeholders. Although CCHIT does not create standards, it is responsible for ensuring compliance with the standards (CCHIT 2008a).

Certification is useful to the many stakeholders of the EHR. Physicians, hospitals, and other healthcare providers can be assured that the EHR under consideration meets minimum requirements. Some insurers pay incentives to healthcare providers who implement the EHR. With certified EHRs, these insurers can be confident that they are paying for systems that provide the expected benefits (Leavitt and Gallagher 2006). Other stakeholders include the standards development organizations, vendors, and consumers (CCHIT 2008a).

To become certified, vendors must complete a documentation review of their product and its functionality. CCHIT jury members will then observe demonstrations of the product to confirm the presence of the functionality, interoperability, and security required for certification. The product will also be subjected to technical testing. Once these three stages are completed with 100% compliance with the standards, the vendor is certified (CCHIT 2008b).

According to CCHIT, EHRs with CCHIT certification improve the quality of patient care and patient safety. Some of the reasons for this include the presence of clinical decision support, prevention of adverse effects, use of alerts, and research. Certified EHRs also assist in the defense of the physician in court. This occurs through the use of evidence-based medicine, a legible record, documentation of informed consent, and providing a justification for the alteration of the EHR (CCHIT 2007).

Check Your Understanding 14.2

1. The two goals for ONC are:

   A. Patient-focused health care and population health
   B. Patient-focused health care and personal health record
   C. Population health and consumer health informatics
   D. Consumer health informatics and health information exchange

2. The model of HIE that interconnects regional repositories through the Internet is the:

   A. Federated model with shared repositories
   B. Federated model with peer-to-peer network
   C. Nonfederated peer-to-peer network
   D. Centralized database of data warehouse

3. The term used to describe a secure means of communication with patients in a manner customized for that patient is:

   A. Consumer health informatics
   B. Patient-portal
   C. Health information exchange
   D. Regional health information exchange

4. The organization that certifies EHRS is:

   A. CCHIT
   B. HIE
   C. SDOs
   D. CHI

5. Which of the following statements is true regarding certification of EHRs?

   A. CCHIT only certifies inpatient EHRs
   B. CCHIT does not ask for the input from the stakeholders such as hospitals, standard development organizations, and more
   C. CCHIT was started by three organizations including the American Hospital Association
   D. CCHIT has additional certifications for the ambulatory EHR in child health and cardiovascular medicine

ICD-10-CM and ICD-10-PCS

The World Health Organization (WHO) developed *International Classification of Diseases and Related Health Problems*, Tenth Revision (ICD-10). Many countries across the world use ICD-10 to document diagnoses and procedures. At the time of the writing of this book, the United States only uses ICD-10 for mortality coding. Because the United States uses this classification for reimbursement and because of the needs of the healthcare system, ICD-10 has been modified. The modified systems are called ***International Classification of Diseases*, Tenth Revision, Clinical Modification (ICD-10-CM)** and ***International Classification of Diseases*, Tenth Revision, Procedural Coding System (ICD-10-PCS)** (Hazelwood and Venable 2009). ICD-10-CM is controlled by the National Center for Health Statistics (NCHS), whereas ICD-10-PCS is controlled by Centers for Medicare and Medicaid Services. On January 16, 2009, HHS published a final rule for the adoption of ICD-10-CM and ICD-10-PCS code sets to replace the currently used ICD-9-CM code. Under this rule, implementation of ICD-10-CM and ICD-10-PCS would occur for all encounters and discharges occurring on or after the compliance date, which is October 1, 2013 (45 CFR 160, 162, and 164).

The implementation of ICD-10-CM and ICD-10-PCS will have a major impact on information systems. The current systems that utilize ICD-9-CM may not be compatible with ICD-10-CM and may have to be replaced or upgraded. Systems to be upgraded will include billing, decision support, encoders, abstracting, and other systems that accept ICD-9-CM codes (Bowman 2008).

The new ICD-10-CM codes are very different in structure from the ICD-9-CM codes. In ICD-9-CM, codes are numeric except for the use of the letters "E" and "V". The ICD-9-CM codes are also 3–5 digits for diagnosis codes and 3–4 digit codes for procedures. All ICD-10-CM codes begin with an alphabetic character and have 5–7 digits. In ICD-10-CM, there may be up to four characters past the decimal point rather than the current two. ICD-10-PCS codes are seven characters and are alphanumeric, utilizing letters and numbers with the exceptions of the letters I and O. The differences will require changes in the number of characters and formats accepted. Information systems will require changes in edits and logic. For example, the current systems know what codes are nonspecific codes and which are complications/comorbidities and major complications/comorbidities. In ICD-9-CM, the encoder alerts the coders to the need for additional codes. Not only would the codes change but due to the differences in coding, the logic would change as well (Hazelwood and Venable 2009).

Healthcare facilities will have to work closely with the information system vendors to assess their readiness for the conversion. If new installations are necessary, the healthcare facility will need to start early because it can take one year or longer to select and implement an information system.

The implementation of ICD-10-CM does not negate the fact that healthcare facilities have years of existing data coded in ICD-9-CM. To address this issue, **general equivalence mapping (GEM)** between ICD-9-CM and ICD-10-CM is used. GEMs were developed by the National Center for Health Statistics, Centers for Medicare and Medicaid Services, AHIMA, the American Hospital Association, and 3M Health Information Systems. Rather than a crosswalk between the two systems, GEM is more like a two-way translation dictionary, much like a Spanish-English and English-Spanish dictionary. The same formatting is used for the diagnoses and procedures (Butler 2007).

Emerging Technologies

Emerging technologies are new technologies that are and may continue to make an impact on the future of healthcare. The emerging technologies discussed in this section are:

- Health record banking
- Open EHR

- Technology to improve patient safety
- Role of cell phones in health information

Health Record Banking

Health record banking is a new concept that is making headlines. This PHR model would allow patients and healthcare providers to share information by making deposits of health information into a bank. The health record bank would have to protect the privacy and security of the health information. This model allows patients to deposit health information much like an individual deposits money into a financial bank account. The patient would control the bank account, and thus control who has access and what can be accessed. Researchers and public health officials could request access to the charts of patients who have previously agreed to allow review of their health information for these purposes (Wolter 2007).

Interoperability would be required so that health information could be shared between banks. There would need to be standards controlling what and how data are transmitted from the healthcare providers to the bank (Dimick 2008a).

Open EHR

The term **open code** refers to software that is available to the general public and can be modified by anyone. **Proprietary software** refers to software where the company that developed it maintains all rights to the software and will provide it to the user for a fee. Proprietary software cannot be modified without the expressed written agreement by the owner. One type of open software is **free and open source software (FOSS)**. FOSS is software that is available to the public for little or no cost to the user. Generally a license agreement is not required for FOSS software. Users can freely use, modify, and distribute the software to other users. Examples of FOSS are OpenOffice and Firebox Web Browser. A number of major vendors such as Hewlett Packard and IBM are involved in FOSS development (Goldstein et al. 2007).

Another type of free software that has no restrictions is **public domain software**. Although there is no copyright for the software (and unlike FOSS), public domain software does not come with the source code. An example of public domain software is the VistA EHR developed by the Veterans Administration (VA) for use in their hospitals and other facilities. VistA can be used in inpatient, ambulatory, and long-term settings. The software is available to any facility thanks to the Freedom of Information Act. The VA will provide the application code upon request. VistA contains both management and clinical modules for use throughout a facility.

A number of other open software products have been developed for the healthcare system, including ambulatory EHRs. These open EHR products include OpenEMR, FreeMED, and CHLCare and vary widely in the functionality provided.

Technology to Improve Patient Safety

In 1999, the Institute of Medicine report, *To Err is Human*, reported that one of the leading causes of deaths in the United States was preventable adverse reactions to medications. Their research found that a minimum of 44,000 people die each year in the United States hospitals because of medical errors These errors cost at least $17 billion dollars (Kohn et al. 1999). Since that time, using technology to improve patient safety has been a priority. Much of the focus has been on medication errors. A number of technological measures assist in the reduction of medication errors including the EHR, computerized physician order entry (CPOE), electronic prescribing (e-prescribing), barcoding, and Web-based reporting. The role of the EHR, CPOE, and barcoding in the reduction or errors has been previously discussed in chapter 10.

Web-based reporting allows nurses and other healthcare professionals to report medication errors quickly and easily. In one study, the facility identified three key findings: the need to improve investigation of medication error; the involvement of the chief executive officer in patient safety encouraged others to focus on patient safety issues; and an increased awareness of patient safety.

E-prescribing

The CMS defines **e-prescribing** as "a prescriber's ability to electronically send an accurate, error-free and understandable prescription directly to a pharmacy from the point-of-care" (CMS 2008). The Medicare Modernization Act of 2003 required drug plans participating in Medicare Part D to offer e-prescribing. Standards were implemented January 1, 2006 for:

- Transactions between prescribers (who write prescriptions) and dispensers (who fill prescriptions) for new prescriptions; refill requests and responses; prescription change requests and responses; prescription cancellation, request, and response; and related messaging and administrative transactions.

- Eligibility and benefits queries between prescribers and Part D sponsors.

- Eligibility queries between dispensers and Part D sponsors (CMS 2008).

In addition to these basic standards, the Medicare Modernization Act required CMS to conduct pilot studies on five more standards. The standards are:

- Formulary and benefit information

- Prior authorization

- Medication history

- Structured and codified SIG

- RxNorm (CMS 2008)

The final rule was published in the *Federal Register* in April 2008; it went into effect in April, 2009 (42 CFR 423). The final rule calls for formulary and benefit transactions to notify the prescriber as to which drugs are covered under the Part D plan and also be notified of other drugs that the patient is currently taking. The rule also requires pharmacies to notify the prescriber if the patient picks up some or all of the prescription.

E-prescribing improves patient safety and the quality of care by eliminating illegible prescriptions, using warnings and alerts, and providing access to the patient's medical history. It reduces or eliminates the need for the physician and pharmacies to call each other to clarify the dosage, drug, or other pertinent details of the prescription. E-prescribing eliminates the need to fax prescriptions or other information to the pharmacy. The refill process is more efficient because the online interface allows routine prescriptions to be reordered automatically and other nonroutine prescriptions to be completed with just a few clicks. Patients may be more likely to fill a prescription when it is sent automatically. In addition, e-prescribing makes it more likely for the prescriber to prescribe drugs from the formulary. From a patient viewpoint, e-prescribing simplifies the process for the patient, reducing the steps taken to two: submitting the prescription (new or nonroutine); and receiving it, either by picking it up at the pharmacy or by mail order. Handheld devices allow prescribers to submit prescriptions electronically from any location. Finally, e-prescribing allows the prescriber or facility to run reports on medication practices. These reports can be used to identify patients taking a medication that has been recalled. They also can be used to monitor prescribing practices (Pennell 2005). It should be noted that controlled substances cannot be prescribed electronically; however, there are initiatives in place to try to change this.

To encourage adoption of e-prescribing, CMS will pay eligible providers two percent more in 2009 and 2010. This incentive is reduced to one percent in 2011 and 2012, and further reduced to one-half of a percent in 2013. Prescribers who do not utilize e-prescribing will receive a reduction in payment starting in 2012. CMS will allow exemptions to this reduction on a case-by-case basis (PSQH 2008b).

Transfusion Safety Management Systems

Unfortunately mistakes in transfusion administration do occasionally occur. To help prevent these mistakes, facilities use a patient safety technology known as transfusion safety management systems. These systems use wireless handheld devices and barcodes to control the accuracy in drawing blood samples and the administration of blood and blood products (PSQH 2008a). This technology would also document adverse reactions. These systems address the administration cycle, which includes "blood product labeling and tracking, the transportation of blood products to the correct patient, the accurate identification of the patient at the point of transfusion, and the appropriate utilization of blood products" (LaRocco and Brient 2008). Transfusion safety management systems support blood collection, management, and administration (LaRocco and Brient 2008). Barcodes on the patient's armband along with barcodes on the blood packaging can be used to prevention errors in transfusion administration. Radiofrequency identification (RFID) tags may also be used in managing transfusion safety by tracking blood and identification of the blood product (Dzik 2005)

Role of Cell Phones in Health Information

Cell phones and other handheld devices are becoming more sophisticated. With the ongoing increase of hard drive storage capacity, personal health information may be stored on a patient's cell phone. Data can be shared with healthcare providers and others at the discretion of the user. The patient can also receive reminders of appointments, tests, and other healthcare related issues. Cell phones can also be used to access knowledge-based systems designed for the consumer. The Medical Records Institute has developed an organization called the Center for Cell Phone Applications in Healthcare. The purpose of this organization is to evaluate the possibilities that cell phones provide for the future (Merrill 2008).

Check Your Understanding 14.3

1. Health record banking is a form of:

   A. EHR certification
   B. personal health record
   C. open software
   D. e-prescribing

2. e-prescribing improves patient safety by:

   A. using alerts
   B. educating pharmacists
   C. educating physicians
   D. having a second physician review the prescription

3. To prepare information systems for ICD-10-CM and ICD-10-PCS, these issues must be addressed:

   A. Must modify system to accept the differences in the code
   B. Must modify system to accept ICD-10
   C. Must modify system to be HL-7 compliant
   D. Must modify system to utilize FOSS

(continued on next page)

Check Your Understanding 14.3 (continued)

4. GEM is a(n) _____ for ICD-10-CM and ICD-10-CM/ICD-10-PCS.

   A. crosswalk
   B. open software product
   C. translation dictionary
   D. edit check

5. The Medicare Modernization Act requires which drug plans to offer e-prescribing:

   A. Ones that are subject to HIPAA
   B. Ones that participate in the Medicaid program
   C. Ones that participate in the Veterans Administration
   D. Ones that participate in the Medicare part D program

References

45 CFR 160, 162, and 164. 2008 (Aug. 22). HIPAA administrative simplification: modification to medical data code set standards to adopt ICD-10-CM and ICD-10-PCS. http://edocket.access.gpo.gov/2008/E8-19298.htm

42 CFR 423. 2008 (April 7). Medicare program; standards for e-prescribing under Medicare Part D and identification of backward compatible version of adopted standard for e-prescribing and the Medicare Prescriptions Drug Program (Version 8.2); Final rule. http://edocket.access.gpo.gov/2008/pdf/08-1094.pdf.

AHIMA e-HIM Personal Health Record Work Group. 2005. The role of the personal health record in the EHR. *Journal of AHIMA* 76(7):64A–D.

AHIMA Workgroup on Computer-Assisted Coding. 2004. Delving into computer-assisted coding. *Journal of AHIMA* 75(10):48A–H.

American Health Information Management Association. 2008. The power of PHR. *AHIMA Advantage* 12(3).

American Health Information Management Association. 2010. *Pocket Glossary of Health Information Management and Technology*, 2nd ed. Chicago: AHIMA.

American Hospital Association. 2006. Health information exchange projects: What hospitals and health systems need to know. http://www.aha.org/aha/content/2006/pdf/AHARHIOfinal.pdf.

Bloomrosen, M. and K. Heubusch. 2006. Language of health data exchange. *Journal of AHIMA* 77(4):34–37.

Bowman, S. 2008. ICD-10 preparation checklist. *Journal of AHIMA* 79(3):32.

Bush, George W. 2004. Address before a Joint Session of the Congress on the State of the Union, January 20, 2004. *Public Papers of the Presidents of the United States*. Washington, DC: Government Printing Office.

Butler, R. 2007. The ICD-10 general equivalence mappings: Bridging the translation gap from ICD-9. *Journal of AHIMA* 78(9):84–86.

Campbell, R. 2005. Getting to the good information: PHRs and consumer health information. *Journal of AHIMA* 76(10):46–49.

Carter, P., C, Lemery, and D. Mikels. 2006. Privacy and security in health information exchange. *Journal of AHIMA* 77(10):64A–C.

Centers for Medicare and Medicaid Services. 2008. E-prescribing overview. http://www.cms.hhs.gov/eprescribing.

Certification Commission for Healthcare Information Technology. 2007. CCHIT certified electronic health records reduce malpractice risk: The case for offering liability insurance premium credits to physicians who use them. http://www.cchit.org/files/wpCCHITPhysicianBusinessCaseforCertEHR.pdf.

Certification Commission for Health Information Technology. 2008a. http://www.cchit.org.

Certification Commission for Healthcare Information Technology. 2008b. Certification handbook: CCHIT certified 08 programs version 08-1.0. http://www.cchit.org/handbook/materials/.

Certification Commission for Healthcare Information Technology HIE Work Group. 2008. Certification future directions. http://www.cchit.org/files/comment/09/02/cchitfuturedirectionshie20081222.pdf.

Connecting for Health. 2008. http://www.connectingforhealth.com.

Department of Health and Human Services. 2008. Office of the National Coordinator. http://www.hhs.gov/healthit/onc/mission.

Dierker, L. 2008. The state connection: State-level efforts in health information exchange. *Journal of AHIMA* 79(5):40–43.

Dimick, C. 2008a. Taking medical records to the bank. *Journal of AHIMA* 79(5):24–29.

Dimick, C. 2008b. The great PHRontier: Private business stakes a claim in personal health records. *Journal of AHIMA* 79(6):24–28.

Dzik, W.H. 2005. Technology for enhanced transfusion safety. *Hematology*. 2005 (1):476–482.

Goldstein, D, P.J. Groen, S. Ponkshe, and M. Wine. 2007. *Medical Informatics 20/20: Quality and Electronic Health Records through Collaboration, Open Solutions, and Innovation*. Boston: Jones & Bartlett Publishers.

Hazelwood, A.C. and C.A. Venable. 2009. *ICD-10-CM and ICD-10-PCS Preview*. Chicago: AHIMA.

Johns, M.L., ed. 2006. *Health Information Management Technology: An Applied Approach*. Chicago: AHIMA

Kohn, L.T., J.M. Corrigan, and M.S. Donaldson, eds. 2000. *To Err Is Human: Building a Safer Health System*. Washington, DC: National Academies Press. http:// www.nap.edu/catalog/9728.html.

LaRocco, M. and K. Brient. 2008. An interdisciplinary approach to safer blood transfusion. *Patient Safety and Quality Healthcare*. http://www.psqh.com/marapr08/transfusion.html.

LaTour, K. and S. Eichenwald Maki, eds. 2006. *Health Information Management: Concepts, Principles and Practice*, 2nd edition. Chicago: AHIMA.

Leavitt, M. and L. Gallagher. 2006. EHR seal of approval: CCHIT introduces product certification to spur EHR adoption. *Journal of AHIMA* 77(5):26–30.

May, C. 2009 (September 3). Email message to editor.

Merrill, M. 2008. New organization studies role of healthcare applications on cell phones. *Healthcare IT News*. http://www.healthcareitnews.comp/printSotry.cms?id=9820.

Mon, D.T. 2005. PHR and EHR: What's the difference? Records differ in span and legality. *Journal of AHIMA* 76(10):60–61.

Office for the National Coordinator of Health Information Technology. 2008. The ONC-coordinated federal health IT strategic plan: 2008–2012. http://www.hhs.gov/healthit/resources/reports.html.

Patient Safety and Quality Healthcare. 2008a. FDA approves IntelliDOT® Blood product administration™. http://www.psqh.com/products/prodja8.html#idot.

Patient Safety and Quality Healthcare. 2008b. HHS takes new steps to accelerate adoption of electronic prescribing. http://www.psqh.com/enews/0808f.html.

Pennell, U. 2005. What is E-prescribing and what are the benefits? 2005. http://www.emrconsultant.com/emr_ePrescribing.php.

Quinsey, C., B. Friedman, and J. Wolter. 2005. Everything you wanted to know about the PHR and more! *Proceedings from the American Health Information Management Association's 77th National Convention and Exhibit*.

Rhodes, H.B. 2007. The PHR quandary: Despite the benefits, issues of technology and trust slow adoptions. *Journal of AHIMA* 78(4):66–67, 69.

Rode, D. 2008. PHR debates: The personal record gets political, but there is danger in rushing legislation. *Journal of AHIMA* 79(6):18, 20.

Shams Group. 2007. Portals. *Proceedings from the American Health Information Management Association's 79th National Convention and Exhibit*.

The White House Office of the President. 2004 (April). *Transforming Health Care: The President's Health Information Technology Plan*. Washington, DC: The White House.

Wolter, J. 2007. Health record banking: An emerging PHR Model. *Journal of AHIMA* 78(9):82–83.

Appendix A

E-mail as a Provider-Patient Electronic Communication Medium and its Impact on the Electronic Health Record (AHIMA Practice Brief)

Background

The American Medical Association defines provider-patient e-mail (electronic mail) as computer-based communication between providers and patients within a professional relationship, in which the provider has taken on an explicit measure of responsibility for the patient's care.[1] Electronic communications have been shown to be effective in facilitating communication among providers and patients, thereby allowing for greater continuity of care and more timely interventions.[2]

Provider-patient electronic communications, such as e-mail and text messaging, are healthcare organizational business records and are therefore subject to the same storage, retention, retrieval, medicolegal, privacy, security, and confidentiality provisions as any other patient-identifiable health information.[3] As such, organizations need to develop policies to manage e-mail records just as they manage any other medical records.[4]

Approximately 19 percent to 38 percent of providers currently use electronic communications with their patients.[5] Growth in e-mail use is being hampered by the lack of reimbursement for these types of communications for Medicare patients. However, some third-party payers have begun to reimburse in some instances, with demonstrated improvements in both cost and workflow. If Medicare reimbursement for electronic provider-patient

Source: AHIMA e-HIM Work Group on E-mail as a Provider-Patient Electronic Communication Medium and Its Impact on the Electronic Health Record (October 2003).

Copyright ©2003 American Health Information Management Association. All rights reserved. All contents, including images and graphics, on this Web site are copyrighted by AHIMA unless otherwise noted. You must obtain permission to reproduce any information, graphics, or images from this site. You do not need to obtain permission to cite, reference, or briefly quote this material as long as proper citation of the source of the information is made. Please contact Publications at permissions@ahima.org to obtain permission. Please include the title and URL of the content you wish to reprint in your request.

communications occurs, electronic communications between provider and patient are likely to increase.[5]

Examples of provider-patient e-mail applications include

- Appointment scheduling
- Prescription refill
- Transferring lab reports or results
- Patient education

Although e-mail communication is most common, other means of provider-patient electronic communications include

- PDA text messaging
- Online consultations
- Online prescribing
- Web messaging
- Digital transfer of lab reports or results

Benefits

Time/production/workflow efficiencies: Electronic communication can reduce interruptions caused by phone calls, reduce nonessential office visits, and save time relative to communication by telephone. Traditional telephone calls are not always a practical means of communication. Often, one of the parties is not available to communicate or does not have the time or appropriate information at hand to complete the communication. Telephone messages are not always private or confidential. Many telephone messaging systems do not allow enough time to leave complete messages. E-mail allows both parties to read and respond to the message when it is convenient to do so. E-mails allow for enough space in the document to send a complete message. Finally, because e-mail messages allow for attachments of supporting documentation, Web site and e-mail addresses can be added to complete the communication.

Improved quality of care: E-mail can improve communication between provider and patient by documenting instructions, educational materials, or interpretation of lab results, or it can allow for more timely communication of test results to patients. E-mail allows both the provider and the patient more options than traditional face-to-face, written, and telephone interaction so communication is enhanced.

- **Cost efficiencies:** Using e-mail for provider-patient communications can result in cost savings as compared to a face-to-face encounter.

- **Provides a business record of the conversation and transaction:** Unlike face-to-face conversations or telephone conversations, e-mail communication provides a ready-made record of the communication.

- **Liability protections:** An e-mail message documents the precise communication between provider and patient.

- **Convenience:** Providers and patients can schedule time to send or answer e-mail messages.

Risks

Security and Privacy Risks

- An e-mail message may be intercepted and threaten patient privacy. E-mail message content can be altered and/or forwarded to unintended recipients.

- Numbers and letters in an e-mail address can be easily transposed, and e-mail may be delivered to the wrong person or not delivered at all.

- Difficulty can arise in establishing or confirming the identity of the patient in an e-mail request. A patient name without other identifiers may be insufficient to establish the identity of the patient. Accepting e-mail messages containing only the patient name and/or e-mail address without other identifiers can result in confusion with other patients with like names and e-mail addresses. The individual sending the e-mail may not be the patient, but an imposter using the patient's e-mail.

- Group e-mail messages present a risk for loss of confidentiality. Individual confidentiality is not protected when recipients are able to see the names and/or e-mail addresses of other group e-mail recipients.

- Word documents sent as attachments that stay on a hard drive present a risk for unauthorized access and breach of confidentiality.

- Clinicians answering patient e-mail messages from an unsecured location such as home computers could present a problem. Protected health information would be retained on private personal computers and in files maintained by Internet service providers.

- Opening an attachment with a virus may cause serious damage.

Administrative and Medicolegal Risks

- Delays in turnaround time could nullify the benefits of the electronic medium. Work flow efficiencies potentially gained from e-mail are lost if a patient does not receive a response and initiates either further e-mail messages or telephone calls that require a response as well. E-mail can serve as a protection against liability because precise communication between the provider and patient is documented. This can become a liability, however, if the provider's documentation is not complete or lacks timeliness.

- Misfiles or lost communications can nullify the benefit of an electronic medium. E-mail messages provide precise documentation between the provider and patient only if the documentation can be easily referenced and retrieved.

- Electronic communication can be misinterpreted due to lack of verbal and nonverbal cues. Electronic communication requires a certain level of patient e-mail/health literacy. It may be difficult for the provider to determine if the patient is able to understand the medical terms and concepts contained in the e-mail messages.

- Web pages used as links that are not "active" or contain information that is not credible present problems.

- E-mails are returned to the sender when addresses are incorrect or outdated.

- There is a lack of documentation that the intended recipient received and read the e-mail message sent by the provider.

- E-mail may overburden provider schedules.

- Laws may vary between states on use of e-mail for patient care or provider licensure requirements.

- Inappropriate utilization by patients, such as an emergency situation, could result in an adverse outcome for patients.

Recommendations

Security and Privacy

- Security is a primary concern. The e-mail system security must be sufficient to ensure, to the highest degree possible, the following:

  — Nonrepudiation

  — Messages are read only by their intended recipients

  — Verification of delivery/receipt

  — Labeling of sensitive material

  — Control of access by those other than the provider

  — Security of computer hardware

  — Completeness

  — Trustworthiness[4]

- Strive to retain the integrity of the message and authentication of source.

- Whenever feasible, instruct users to copy and paste addresses or use the e-mail reply button.

- The availability of secured (encrypted) e-mail transmission will be the determining factor limiting the content and use of e-mail.

- Browser-based communication with patients has advantages because it provides additional security as compared to e-mail. For example, log-ins are required and audit trails are accessible. Security/encryption, physical security, structured messaging, approval/revocation options, and group access versus single access are more characteristics of browser-based communication.

- Maintaining a secure mail server is an ongoing process. A critical role in a secure mail server is an extensive network infrastructure (firewalls, routers, intrusion detection systems). Internet/intranet issues must be addressed. E-mail may be secure on an intranet and not secure on the Internet.

- Encryption software is available for wired and wireless communication. Configuration management is an essential part of maintaining a secure system. The complex mathematic algorithms involved in the highest levels of confidentiality increase e-mail size and slow servers. Also, encryption may interfere with virus scanning and mail content filtering. Administrative overhead is often required. Software must be monitored even after installation for upgrades, patches, and correct versus default settings, especially after a server crash.

- The HIPAA security rule provides guidelines as to the appropriate use of transmission security.[6] The associated risk to electronic protected health information should drive the decision to use transmission security tools. Following is the Department of Health and Human Services response to comments and questions regarding the use of encryption tools to secure protected health information transmitted from one point to another.[7]

Response: In general, we agree with the commenters who asked for clarification and revision. This final rule has been significantly revised to reflect a much simpler and more direct requirement. The term "Communications/network controls" has been replaced with "Transmission security" to better reflect the requirement that, when electronic protected health information is transmitted from one point to another, it must be protected in a manner commensurate with the associated risk.

We agree with the commenters that switched, point-to-point connections, for example, dial-up lines, have a very small probability of interception.

Thus, we agree that encryption should not be a mandatory requirement for transmission over dial-up lines. We also agree with commenters who mentioned the financial and technical burdens associated with the employment of encryption tools. Particularly when considering situations faced by small and rural providers, it became clear that there is not yet available a simple and interoperable solution to encrypting e-mail communications with patients. As a result, we decided to make the use of encryption in the transmission process an addressable implementation specification. Covered entities are encouraged, however, to consider use of encryption technology for transmitting electronic protected health information, particularly over the Internet.

As business practices and technology change, there may arise situations where electronic protected health information being transmitted from a covered entity would be at significant risk of being accessed by unauthorized entities. Where risk analysis showed such risk to be significant, we would expect covered entities to encrypt those transmissions, if appropriate, under the addressable implementation specification for encryption.

We do not use the term "open network" in this final rule because its meaning is too broad. We include as an addressable implementation specification the requirement that transmissions be encrypted when appropriate based on the entity's risk analysis.

From Sec. 164.312, Technical Safeguards:

(e)(1) Standard: Transmission security. Implement technical security measures to guard against unauthorized access to electronic protected health information that is being transmitted over an electronic communications network.

(2) Implementation specifications:

(i) Integrity controls (Addressable). Implement security measures to ensure that electronically transmitted electronic protected health information is not improperly modified without detection until disposed of.

(ii) Encryption (Addressable). Implement a mechanism to encrypt electronic protected health information whenever deemed appropriate.

- Cryptosystems provide a means to ensure confidentiality, authenticity, nonrepudiation, and integrity of e-mail messages. Three common types of cryptographic hardware and/or software systems are:

   — **Symmetric cryptography:** A single key is shared by the sender and the recipient. The encryption algorithm (e.g., data encryption standard [DES], 3DES) is much simpler and thus faster.

   — **Asymmetric cryptography (e.g., public key infrastructure):** Each user owns a pair of keys, one public and one private. The public key is given to the sender to encrypt the messages, and the corresponding private key is used by the recipient to decrypt messages. The encryption algorithm (e.g., Rivest-Shamir-Aldeman, a public-key cryptographic algorithm that hinges on the assumption that the factoring of the product of two large primes is difficult) has to match the decryption algorithm, which makes it very complex and thus much slower.

— **Hybrid cryptography (e.g., pretty good privacy [PGP]):** This is a combination of symmetric and asymmetric cryptography. A session key is randomly generated for each message. The plain text is then encrypted with this session key. The public key-encrypted session key is then transmitted, along with the session key-encrypted cipher text, to the recipient. In this method, the encryption (session) key is securely distributed by the public key and the plain text is encrypted by faster symmetric cryptography.

- Virtual private networks (VPN) allow use of the public Internet to securely connect remote offices and employees at a fraction of the cost of dedicated, private telephone lines such as frame relay. A VPN supports at least three different modes of use:

— **LAN-to-LAN internet working** connects two or more geographically separated networks, such as those at a main office and a remote branch office.

— **Remote access client connections** allow telecommuters to safely log into company networks.

— **Controlled access within an intranet** can also use VPN technology to implement controlled access to individual subnets on the private network.

The most important component of a VPN is the gateway. The symmetric encryption (e.g., 3DES) is done between gateways of two networks.

With the hype that has surrounded VPNs historically, the potential pitfalls or "weak spots" in the VPN model can be easy to forget. These four concerns with VPN solutions are often raised:

1. VPNs require an in-depth understanding of public network security issues and taking proper precautions in VPN deployment.

2. The availability and performance of an organization's wide-area VPN (over the Internet in particular) depend on factors largely outside of the organization's control.

3. VPN technologies from different vendors may not work well together due to immature standards.

4. VPNs need to accommodate protocols other than IP and existing ("legacy") internal network technology.

- Web e-mail with a domain name and secure socket connection provides a higher level of security than standard secured e-mail messages.[8] A secure Web server is purchased and managed by system security professionals.

- Hard drives used by providers for patient e-mail communication must be cleaned using a "wipe" utility before the processor is surplused or reassigned to another person.

Administrative and Medicolegal Recommendations

- Create a policy that establishes **criteria for the provider-patient e-mail communication** and consent process before initiating electronic communication with the patient. The provider and patient should have an established relationship. Differentiate among preexisting conditions, ongoing treatment, follow-up questions related to a previous discussion, and a new diagnosis and treatment addressed exclusively online. New diagnosis and treatment of conditions addressed exclusively online may increase liability.

- Develop procedures for the **patient's authorization/agreement** to use e-mail as a communication medium. The procedures must outline where patient authorization will be filed, how it will be retrieved, and what indicators or flags in the patient record, if any, show that the patient wishes to participate in electronic communication with the provider.

- Develop policies addressing issues that require the e-mail documentation to become **part of the patient record.**

- Establish and enforce **retention policies.** Original e-mail, with reply, should be filed in the electronic health record or printed for the paper record. The provider should initial and date the paper copy for the paper record.

- **Develop policies and procedures to guide the use of group e-mail messages** that describe the necessity of protecting the identities of individual group members from other members in the group and provide instructions to users (i.e., blind copy [bcc] feature).

- Develop criteria to **determine a patient's health literacy level** and ability to use an e-mail application.

- Establish procedures to **instruct the patient** to follow up in person or by phone for requests that do not meet content guidelines. Lengthy e-mail messages or prolonged correspondence with a patient may necessitate scheduling an appointment with the patient or calling the patient.

- Establish a policy for e-mail **turnaround time.** The policy should prioritize e-mail messages by type of request, clearly identifying what may constitute an urgent or emergent request. It should also include actions to take when the turnaround time is not met.

- Develop a policy and educate patients about **appropriate types of e-mail** (e.g., prescription refills, appointment scheduling, lab results).

- Laws regarding e-mail communication may vary between states. **Research** your state's laws and those of surrounding states regarding the use of e-mail for medical treatment. (Alllaw.com is a Web site for researching state laws regarding the use of e-mail for medical treatment.)

- Develop a policy that addresses **security issues** when using remote access. Providers must not communicate with patients in the context of their professional relationship using personal e-mail accounts such as America Online, Earthlink, or any other nonemployer e-mail system.

- Develop a policy that addresses the following **topics that should not be discussed in e-mail** transactions and procedures that include a response to patients whose e-mail addresses these issues:

  — Protected diagnoses or treatments such as mental health or chemical health (based on state or federal privacy regulations)

  — HIV status

  — Workers' compensation injuries and disability

  — Urgent health conditions

- Develop and enforce policies defining and prohibiting emergency e-mail messages.

- Develop procedures addressing a **workable documentation mechanism** for responding to an e-mail via telephone call and responding to a telephone call via e-mail.

- Develop a policy and procedure to guide **termination** of a patient from e-mail communication (e.g., patient notice, registration indicator).

- Establish a methodology to **audit** all e-mail correspondence to ensure appropriate

  — Customer service

  — Quality of care provided via the e-mail communication

  — Quality of the response provided to the patient via e-mail

  — Review for possible legal risk issues

  — Patient privacy and confidentiality

  — Tracking e-mail messages returned because of incorrect address

- Organizational procedures for **cleaning computer hard drives** must be established and enforced.

- **Update current confidentiality policies** to incorporate references to e-mail if they are not already in place.

(See Appendix A, "HIM Managers Tasks and Skills with Regard to Administrative-Medicolegal Risks at http://library.ahima.org/xpedio/groups/public/documents/ahima/bok1_021590.hcsp?dDocName=bok1_021590")

E-mail Recommendations

- The provider's e-mail signature block should contain the provider's full name, contact information, response time, instructions for when response time is not met, and instructions for handling patient emergencies.

- Web pages used as links (or given to patients) should be credible, and links should be active. Links should be monitored often and updated as needed.

- One method of controlling misdirected e-mail is to not allow providers to initiate e-mail messages. The patient initiates the e-mail, and the provider responds by using the reply button.

- Use e-mail system functionality (e.g., automatic reply to acknowledge receipt, return receipt to confirm patient receipt, blind copy feature to uphold patient privacy).

- Establish a central patient registration database that will serve as a systemwide directory. A central directory will prevent duplications and errors in the patient's e-mail information. A central directory will allow for greater control, with prompt and easy updating of patient e-mail addresses and identifying information. Verify patients' e-mail addresses during appointment scheduling and/or patient registration.

- Patients must register e-mail addresses and provide identifying information in e-mail messages.

- Patient identifiers other than name are important (duplicate names). Medical record numbers will not be a relevant identifier if e-mail is being forwarded to another healthcare facility (e.g., referral).

- A healthcare entity should have a standardized template for e-mail in place to ensure the appropriate information is communicated and captured. This will also keep e-mail concise.

- Educate staff on appropriate e-mail etiquette. Sarcasm, anger, harsh criticism, and libelous references to third parties in e-mail messages are not appropriate.

- Whenever feasible, instruct users to copy and paste addresses or use the e-mail reply button.

- Patients should be informed of the e-mail policies and procedures in advance. The patient should knowingly authorize to communicate via e-mail in advance. (See Appendix B, "Documentation of Authorization to E-mail Discussion" at http://library.ahima.org/xpedio/groups/public/documents/ahima/bok1_021591. hcsp?dDocName=bok1_021591 and Appendix C, "Patient Authorization for E-mail Communication at http://library.ahima.org/xpedio/groups/public/documents/ahima/bok1_021592.hcsp?dDocName=bok1_021592")

- When communicating confidential medical information via e-mail, a banner similar to the one below should be displayed prominently at the beginning of the e-mail message:

  THIS CONFIDENTIAL COMMUNICATION CONTAINS INFORMATION PROTECTED BY PROVIDER-PATIENT PRIVILEGE.

- A statement of confidentiality should be posted on all e-mail correspondence such as:

  The contents of this e-mail message and any attachments are confidential and are intended solely for addressee. The information may also be legally privileged. This transmission is sent in trust, for the sole purpose of delivery to the intended recipient. If you have received this transmission in error, any use, reproduction, or dissemination of this transmission is strictly prohibited. If you are not the intended recipient, please immediately notify the sender by reply e-mail or (area code) (phone number) and delete this message and its attachments, if any.

Patient Education: Confidentiality Recommendations

- **Inform patients** regarding practices of screening e-mail (e.g., if office personnel screen e-mail for the provider). Point out the need for the patient to develop privacy practices. Point out that patients are charged with the responsibility to handle their information in a secure manner.

- **Instruct patients** regarding the type of information that must be included in the e-mail message. The subject line should include the category or type of request to facilitate prioritizing and routing messages (e.g., appointment, prescription refill, lab results). The specific provider's name should be included as well.

- **Define patient identifiers,** besides the patient's full legal name, that will be used to verify patient identity and facilitate filing in the electronic or paper medical record. Suggested patient identifiers are

  — Date of birth

  — Last four to six digits of social security number

  — Phone number

  — Mother's maiden name

  — Password created by the patient

  Organization **procedures must support the retention** of these data elements in the patient registration system, and e-mail templates may include these items on the form as prompts to the patient.

- Inform patients that the provider will **terminate** e-mail correspondence with patients who repeatedly do not adhere to the written e-mail guidelines.

- It is a commonly accepted axiom that communication is 7 percent words, 38 percent voice, and 55 percent body language. If this axiom is true, e-mail must be considered to be a communication media with **limited effectiveness.** Providers communicating via e-mail must be aware of its limitations and adjust their communication accordingly.

- Inform patients about the **risk** of loss of confidentiality when using their employer's e-mail account.

- Inform patients in advance if e-mail messages may be **forwarded** to other clinics/ providers (e.g., referrals).

- Inform patients that e-mail communications are **retained** as part of the patient's permanent legal medical record.

- Inform the patient about **indemnity** for information loss due to technical failures.

- Patients should be educated about the **appropriate types** of transactions for e-mail communications. E-mail templates may be created to assist the patient in identifying the type of request (e.g., check boxes). Examples of when e-mail is appropriate include

  — Prescription renewals

  — Nonurgent medical advice

  — Test results, based on professional judgment

  — Insurance inquiries

  — Benefit information

  — Provider network information

  — Billing information

  — Scheduling/canceling/rescheduling appointments

  — Clinic/provider changes

  — Other nonurgent communication

- **Document** patient education in the patient's medical record and reference education materials given to the patient.

Electronic Document Management Recommendations

E-mail must be treated like any other healthcare organizational business record (e.g., patient medical record, patient financial record, employee record) because it is subject to the same course of evidentiary discovery and has a life cycle that requires management guidelines (i.e., it is created, indexed, searched, retrieved, routed, stored, and purged).

E-mail management is an enormous, complex problem. This problem is expected to get worse as the numbers and types of senders and receivers (e.g., providers and patients) increase exponentially. Therefore, the following guidelines are recommended:

- Identify existing, **enterprise-wide repositories** that securely store (or should store) e-mail records and attachments that merit evidentiary handling.

- Develop or acquire an easy-to-use yet **functionally robust e-mail management system** that includes a centralized archive. The e-mail management system should

  — Have **intuitive methods for identifying** e-mail classifications and retention rules. For example, one classification might be healthcare-related information that is linked directly to the master patient index. Another classification might be meetings and general business communication information. Different retention rules could be linked to each classification group.

— Include dependable **search capabilities** as well as fast and efficient access to archives.

— Have an "open architecture" allowing for **compatibility** with popular e-mail systems.

— Enforce e-mail **archiving** policies. For example, when an individual closes an e-mail and is ready to discard or save it, a prompt should appear with a yes-or-no choice asking if the user would like to make this a part of any of the healthcare organization's "business" records (e.g., classification of patient medical records). This "opt in/out" e-mail capture function can be eliminated if the healthcare organization declares ahead of time that the e-mail must always be retained to comply with a regulatory, legal, or business need (e.g., an e-mail correspondence between a provider and a patient). In addition, this function can be managed in the background using Web technology so that, for example, each new patient added to the master patient index triggers a domain name, with all inbound and outbound e-mail captured for patientname.com.

— Include **retention rules** that are triggered automatically by actions. This includes automatically deleting or encrypting a "patient class" of e-mail after X number of days/months/years so it cannot be accessed. (Note: Never archive encrypted e-mail records for fear of losing the algorithms or keys.)

- **Create** appropriate rules, policies, and procedures specific to each organization upon system deployment to eliminate the risk of purging e-mail attachments in a storage crisis. These systems quickly become overwhelmed by metadata and attachments.

- Establish a methodology to meet **HIPAA's** requirement for providing an accounting of disclosures.

(See also Appendix D, "Summary of Best Practices for Provider-Patient E-mail Communication at http://library.ahima.org/xpedio/groups/public/documents/ahima/bok1_021593. hcsp?dDocName=bok1_021593")

Notes

1. American Medical Association. "Guidelines for Physician-patient Electronic Communication." Available at www.ama-assn.org/ama/pub/category/2386.html.

2. Institute of Medicine. "Key Capabilities of an Electronic Health Record System: Letter Report." Available at http://books.nap.edu/books/NI000427/html/index.html.

3. Kohn, D. "E-mail: Treat It as Just Another Record." *Advance for HIM Professionals.* Available at www.advanceforhim.com/common/editorialsearch/viewer.aspx?FN=02oct28_hip33.html&AD=10/28/2002&FP=hi.

4. Kahn, R. "Beyond HIPAA: The Complexities of Electronic Records Management." *Journal of AHIMA* 74, no. 4 (2003). Available in the FORE Library: HIM Body of Knowledge at www.ahima.org.

5. "Handhelds Hot, E-mail Not for US Physicians." Press release issued Nov. 4, 2002, by the Healthcare Information and Management Systems Society. Available at http://www.himss.org/ASP/ContentRedirector.asp?ContentId=23146.

6. "Health Insurance Portability and Accountability Act of 1996." Public Law 104–191. August 21, 1996. Available at http://aspe.hhs.gov/admnsimp/.

7. "Final Rule for Security Standards." *Federal Register* 68, no. 34 (February 20, 2003). Available at http://www.access.gpo.gov/su_docs/fedreg/a030220c.html.

8. Rognehaugh, A., and R. Rognehaugh. *Healthcare IT Terms.* Chicago: Healthcare Information and Management Systems Society, 2001.

References

American College of Physicians. "The Changing Face of Ambulatory Medicine-Reimbursing Physicians for Computer-based Care." Available at www.acponline.org/hpp/e-consult.pdf.

Bowman, B. "Beyond the Telephone: Electronic Tools for Patient-provider Communications." *Group Practice Journal* 51, no. 1 (2002). Available at www.amga.org/Publications/gpj/articles/CoverStories/coverStoryJan02_gpj.pdf.

Burrington-Brown, J., and G. Hughes. "AHIMA Practice Brief: Provider-Patient E-mail Security" (Updated June 2003). Available in the FORE Library: HIM Body of Knowledge at www.ahima.org.

California Health Care Foundation. "E-encounters." Available at www.chcf.org/documents/ihealth/EEncounters.pdf.

HealthyEmail. "Email and Clinical Practice." Available at www.healthyemail.org/and www.healthyemail.org/toolkit.php.

Kane, B., and D. Z. Sands. "Guidelines for the Clinical Use of Electronic Mail with Patients. *JAMIA* 5, no. 1 (1998): 104–111.

Manhattan Research. "The Future of Medicine Is in the Hands of 205,000 Physicians." Available at www.manhattanresearch.com/thepulse.htm.

Medem. "eRisk Working Group for Healthcare: Guidelines for Online Communication." Available at www.medem/com/phy/phy_eriskguidelines.cfm.

Medem. "eRisk Working Group for Healthcare: Guidelines for Online Communication [Addendum]." Available at www.medem.com/corporate/corporate_Addendum_A_eRiskGuidelines.cfm.

Medem. "Secure Messaging and Online Consultation FAQ for Physicians." Available at www.medem.com/phy/phy_faq_physician.cfm.

Murphy, G. "Patient-centered E-mail: Developing the Right Policies." *Journal of AHIMA* 71, no. 3 (2000). Available in the FORE Library: HIM Body of Knowledge at www.ahima.org.

Patt, M. et al. "Doctors Who Are Using E-mail with Their Patients: A Qualitative Exploration." *Journal of Medical Internet Research* 5, no. 2 (2003). Available at www.jmir.org/2003/2/e9/index.htm.

Sands, D. Z. "Guidelines for the Use of Patient-centered E-mail." Available at www.mahealthdata.org.

Techencyclopedia. Available at www.techweb.com/encyclopedia/.

Tracey, M., W. Jansen, and S. Bisker. *Guidelines on Electronic Mail Security.* Washington, DC: National Institute of Standards and Technology, US Department of Commerce.

Prepared by

This practice brief was developed by the following AHIMA e-HIM work group:

- Marti Adkins, RHIA
- Nancy Russell Cardamone, RHIA
- Ray Chien, MS
- Angela Clark, RHIA
- Lynn Crothers, RHIT
- Carmella Jackson, MS, RHIA, NMCC

- Stephanie John, RHIA
- Bassam Kawwass, RHIA
- Sandra Kersten, RHIA
- Gail Kraft, RHIA
- Catherine Krawetz, RHIT, CCS
- Lynda Mitchell, RHIA, CPHQ
- David Mozie, PhD, RHIA
- Deborah Nieves, RHIA
- Harry Rhodes, MBA, RHIA, CHP (staff)
- Mary Stanfill, RHIA, CCS, CCS-P (staff)
- David Sweet (staff)

Acknowledgements

For assistance in the development of this practice brief: Deborah Kohn, MPH, RHIA, CHE, CPHIMS, FHIMSS.

Appendix B
RFI/RFP Template

The RFI/RFP process is vital to procuring a system that meets organizational and user needs. Because of this, it is imperative that adequate time be allotted for the process.

This template is provided as a tool to assist healthcare providers as they issue a request for information or a request for proposal for electronic health record or component systems. It is meant to be used in conjunction with the June 2007 practice brief titled "The RFP Process for EHR Systems."

Healthcare providers should utilize the components of this template that are applicable for their needs, deleting those that are not.

Sections 1 and 2 should be completed by the facility.

1. Introduction (introducing the facility to the vendor)

   a. Brief Description of the Facility

   b. Facility Information

      i. Complete Address

      ii. Market (acute, ambulatory, long-term care, home health)

      iii. Enterprise Information: The organizations should provide all relevant information including if the facility is a part of a healthcare delivery system and the facilities that are included in the project.

      iv. Size: The organization should provide any information that will be relevant to the product such as the number of discharges, visits, beds, etc.

      v. General Description of Current Systems Environment: The organization should provide general information regarding current information systems structure (i.e., hardware and operating systems).

   c. Scope

      The organization should provide a brief narrative description of the project that the RFP covers and the environment sought (e.g., total EHR, phased approach, hybrid support).

Source: American Health Information Management Association. 2007. RFI/RFP template. *Journal of AHIMA* 78(6): web extra. http://library.ahima.org/xpedio/groups/public/documents/ahima/bok1_034278.hcsp?dDocName =bok1_034278.

2. Statement of Purpose

    a. Overall Business Objectives/Drivers

       The organization should list high-level business goals it is looking to achieve by implementing the software.

    b. Key Desired Functionality

       When requesting information for the facility-wide solution (e.g., EHR), the organization should list the various features and functions of the system it is looking for, as well as any pertinent details.

       i. Document Imaging

       ii. Clinical Repository

       iii. Clinical Documentation

       iv. Computerized Physician Order Entry (CPOE)

       v. Ancillary Support (e.g., lab, radiology, pharmacy, etc.)

       vi. Picture Archiving Communication System (PACS)

       vii. Other

    c. e-HIM Process Support

       When requesting information for the HIM solution (e.g., document imaging system), the organization should list the various processes and functions of the system it is looking for, as well as any pertinent details.

       i. Chart Analysis/Deficiency Management

       ii. Coding/Abstracting

       iii. Release of Information

       iv. Disclosure Management

       v. Forms Management

       vi. Support for Mandated Reportable Data Sets

       vii. Other

    d. System Administration and Management

       This functionality is applicable or used for all components or modules of an application. Facility requirements for this functionality should be specified in the detailed system requirements.

       i. User Administration

       ii. Access Privilege Control Management

       iii. Logging Capabilities

       iv. Auditing Functions

       v. Digital Signature Functions

       vi. Archiving Functions

       vii. Support for Back-up/Recovery

       viii. Customizable Workflow Management

    e. Future Plans

       General description of long-term plans, including identified future systems environment and projected timetables.

Sections 3 and 4 should be completed by the vendor,

3. Requirements

Vendors should provide availability and timelines for development of software to fulfill requirements not available at this time.

a. User Requirements

Sample questions related to HIM functional user requirements and features are provided below. This table is a *sample only*. Organizations must customize this to meet their needs. Each functional area is expected to have its own set of user requirements.

Functional User Requirements/Features (refer to CCHIT requirements and HL7's EHR System Functional Model)	Available	Custom Developed	Future Development	Not Available
Chart Completion/Deficiency Analysis				
Can the organization define the intervals for aging analysis (e.g., 7-days, 14-days, 21-days, etc.)?				
Does the system allow for standard and ad-hoc reporting for chart deficiency/delinquency analysis?				
Can delinquency reports be sent to physicians/ clinicians in electronic (e.g., e-mail or fax) and in paper format (letters)?				
Does the system allow you to define or detail all deficiencies by provider, by area of deficiency, or other combinations (e.g., group practices, etc.)?				
Does the system allow the organization to list all records (charts) by the deficiency type?				
Can deficiency analysis be conducted at the time the patient is prepared for discharge from the facility?				
Does the system support most industry standard dictation systems to allow transcribed reports to be easily and efficiently completed?				
Coding Completion/Analysis				
Can the user assign cases based on special attributes (e.g., VIP, dollars, or by type of case such as cancer or trauma, etc.)?				
Can coders and supervisors communicate online?				
Does the system support most industry standard encoders/groupers?				
Does the system support both on-site and remote coding activities?				
Does the system support assignment of high-risk coding to supervisory staff or allow coding verification as staff complete cases?				
Can the system support ICD-10-CM and/or ICD-10-PCS?				

(continued on next page)

Functional User Requirements/Features (refer to CCHIT requirements and HL7's EHR System Functional Model)	Available	Custom Developed	Future Development	Not Available
Disclosures and Release of Information				
Does the system support HIPAA management of non-TPO disclosures?				
Does the system support accounting for disclosures to patients?				
Can users receive automatic alerts of disclosure limitations and potential HIPAA violations?				
Does the system generate invoices with user-defined pay scales?				
Does the system allow tracking of payments received?				
Does the system support requests for amendments or corrections by patients?				
Does the system generate template letters for standard correspondence (e.g., patient not found, date of service not valid, etc.)?				
Patient Financial Support				
Is your proposed solution fully integrated, offering users an electronic form of the business office?				
Can patient information be placed in folders to easily identify those details that refer to the patient (guarantor) account(s)?				
Can you electronically capture, store, and retrieve computer-generated documents and reports, such as the UB-04 or the CMS 1500?				
Data Reporting				
Does the system allow for real-time data collection and progress measurement against preset targets?				
Does the system produce reports on turnaround days, dollars pending, costs per chart by process, days to billing, and so on, as related to AR?				
Can your system interface with other disparate systems that collect quality measurement data (e.g., CMS quality measurement requirements, Joint Commission ORYX measurement, etc.)?				

b.   System Requirements

Organizations should provide a list to vendors of what current technology needs to be supported. Vendors should then provide information on their system's available requirements.

Sample questions related to system requirements and features are provided below. This table is *a sample only*. Organizations must customize this to meet their needs.

System Requirements/Features (refer to CCHIT requirements and HL7's EHR-S Functional Model)	Met Fully	Custom Developed	Under Development	Not Available
General System Requirements				
Is the system integrated or interfaced?				
Does the system provide the ability to archive via tape, CD, DVD? Describe any other options.				
Are the COLD data streams available in ASCII?				
Does the system support audit trails at the folder level for managing access, editing, and printing of documents?				
Does the system make audit trail logs available to the organization, including the date, time, user, and location?				
Does the system support an online help function/ feature?				
Is the proposed solution scalable (e.g., can it support 50–800 workstations, etc.)?				
Can the system identify or distinguish the facility location in a multi-entity environment?				
Can the system support a centralized database across multiple facilities?				
How compliant is your product with the HL7's EHR System Functional Model and EHR profiles? (Please provide us with your HL7 EHR System Functional Model and profile conformance statements.)				
System Security				
Does the system prevent users from accessing functions when they have not been granted user rights?				
Does the system monitor security attempts for those without user rights, and those logged in the audit trail/log?				
Does the system track all activity/functions, including where it changes the database, and can it be managed through the audit trail/log?				
Technical Requirements and Industry Standards				
Is the operating system Window's 2000 or NT based?				
Do the communication components include TCP/IP?				
Does the system utilize CCITT Group III, IV for compression schemes?				
Does the system support standard HL7 record formatting for all in/output?				
Does the system support SQL for communication?				
Does the system support thin–client PCs?				
Is the system sized for capacity to allow for planning? Describe your recommendations.				
Does the system support disk shadowing and system redundancy provisions? Please describe.				
Can your solution be supported as an ASP (hosted) model?				
Does the system support browser-based options?				

c. Interfaces

Organizations should provide a list of existing interfaces that will need to be supported, as well as new interfaces that will have to be created and supported, including any pertinent interoperability information that exists and will be needed in the future. Vendors should provide information regarding their system's ability to meet the organization's interface requirements.

4. Vendor Questionnaire

The organization should request information about the vendor and the product that will help it make a decision about the vendor and its product.

a. Vendor Background and Financial Information

i. Company Name and Geography

The organization should request an address of a branch close to the facility as well as the headquarters. Staff may want to visit both.

ii. Company Goals

iii. Year the Company Was Established, Significant Company Merges, Acquisitions, and Sale-Offs

iv. Whether the Vendor Is Public or Privately Owned

v. Bankruptcy/Legal Issues (including under which name the bankruptcy was filed and when. Organizations should also find out if there are there any pertinent lawsuits, closed or pending, filed against the company.)

vi. Research and Development Investment (expressed in a total amount or percentage of totals sales)

vii. Status of CCHIT Certification

b. Statement of Key Differentiators

The vendor should provide a statement describing what differentiates it products and services from its competitors.

c. Customer Base and References

i. Customer List (or total number of customers per feature or function, if a list of customers cannot be provided due to confidentiality/ privacy concerns)

ii. References that Can Be Contacted

The vendor should provide references the facility can contact/visit based on product features and functions most suitable to the facility as well as those using the latest versions of the software.

d. User Participation

i. User Groups

Organizations should provide a list of the user groups and ask whether it can attend a meeting or a call for review purposes.

ii. Requirements Gathering

The vendor should request information regarding customer participation in requirements gathering stages of system development. How is customer feedback, such as requests for new requirements, handled?

e. Technology

The vendor should describe the technology that supports the product. (e.g., database, architecture, operating system, ASP vs. in-house, etc.)

f. Services

The vendor should describe the services offered by the vendor

    i. MPI Clean-Up

    ii. Legal Health Record Definition

    iii. Process Re-engineering

    iv. Other

g. Training

The vendor should outline the training provided during and after implementation

h. Documentation

The vendor should specify the documentation that is available and their formats

i. Implementation/Migration

The vendor should provide detailed information about the implementation such as the timelines and resources required

j. Data Conversion

k. Maintenance

    i. Updates/Upgrades

    The vendor should provide information on how the system is maintained, including how often the updates/upgrades are applied and which methods are utilized

    ii. Expected Product Lifetime

    The vendor should outline the expected time frame for the next version requiring a different platform or operating system upgrade

    iii. Vendor Support

    The vendor should outline the methods of support offered, such as the help desk or tickets, and the tools used (e.g., 800 number, email, web-based, etc.)

    iv. Expected Facility Support

    The vendor should outline the number of FTEs expected to support the product at the facility

l. Pricing Structure

    i. Product Software Pricing

        1. Price

        The vendor should provide the price of the proposed solution, broken down by the component, including licensing fees.

        2. Cost of Ownership (breakdown over 'x' number of proposed contract years)

        3. Other Costs (maintenance, upgrades, consultation and support fees, post-implementation training and services)

        4. Discounts (available discounts such as those based on participating as a beta site)

      ii. Invoicing (fee schedule and terms)

      iii. Return on Investment

      iv. Acceptance Period

          The vendor should outline the terms for validating the product after implementation and the refund policy

  m. Warranty

      The organization should request a copy of the warranty as well as how it is affected by maintenance and support agreements after the implementation period

Sections 5 and 6 are to be completed by the facility.

5. Vendor Requirements and Instructions

  a. RFP Questions

      The facility should list those staff members at the facility to contact with RFP questions. Generally, questions about the RFP must be submitted in writing within a given time frame, and the questions and answers are distributed to all vendors responding the RFP. Provide the preferred method of contact such as fax number or e-mail.

  b. Response Format, Deadline, and Delivery

6. Terms and Conditions

  a. Confidentiality (state confidentiality rules in regards to the information the facility disclosed in the RFP as well as the rules pertaining to the information provided by the vendor)

  b. Information Access

      The organization should describe who will have access to the returned RFP and for what purpose

  c. General Conditions

      i. Contract Duration (how long the returned information will be considered valid)

  d. Bid Evaluation and Negotiation

      The facility should briefly describe the evaluation process and the deadlines and provide the appropriate information if vendors are allowed to negotiate after the evaluation is complete

  e. Formal Presentation

      The facility should describe the process and format of presentation if the vendor is invited

  f. Acceptance or Rejection

      The facility should describe how the vendor will be notified regardless of whether the product is selected or not

  g. Contract Provisions

      The facility should note the sections of the RFP response that can be included in the final contract

Appendix C
Answer Key: Check Your Understanding

Chapter 1

Check Your Understanding 1.1

1. C
2. C
3. A
4. D

Check Your Understanding 1.2

1. A
2. D
3. C
4. C

Check Your Understanding 1.3

1. D
2. B
3. D
4. D

Check Your Understanding 1.4

1. B
2. A
3. A
4. A

Check Your Understanding 1.5

1. B
2. B
3. D
4. A

Chapter 2

Check Your Understanding 2.1

1. C
2. B
3. D
4. B

Check Your Understanding 2.2

1. A
2. C
3. B
4. A

Check Your Understanding 2.3

1. B
2. A
3. C
4. D

Check Your Understanding 2.4

1. C
2. D
3. A
4. D

Chapter 3

Check Your Understanding 3.1

1. C
2. D
3. A

Check Your Understanding 3.2

1. C
2. D
3. C

Check Your Understanding 3.3

1. A
2. A
3. D

Check Your Understanding 3.4

1. C
2. B
3. B

Chapter 4

Check Your Understanding 4.1

1. C
2. A
3. C
4. B
5. A

Check Your Understanding 4.2

1. A
2. B
3. C
4. A
5. C

Check Your Understanding 4.3

1. A
2. A
3. A
4. C
5. C

Check Your Understanding 4.4

1. D
2. A
3. C
4. D
5. C

Chapter 5

Check Your Understanding 5.1

1. F
2. A
3. D
4. B
5. A

Check Your Understanding 5.2

1. C
2. B
3. B
4. A
5. A

Check Your Understanding 5.3

1. B
2. D
3. D
4. False
5. False

Check Your Understanding 5.4

1. D
2. C
3. A
4. B
5. False

Check Your Understanding 5.5

1. True
2. C
3. A
4. True
5. C

Chapter 6

Check Your Understanding 6.1

1. A
2. B
3. C
4. C
5. A

Check Your Understanding 6.2

1. C
2. B
3. B
4. B
5. D

Check Your Understanding 6.3

1. B
2. B
3. A
4. A
5. B

Check Your Understanding 6.4

1. D
2. B
3. B
4. C
5. C

Check Your Understanding 6.5

1. D
2. A
3. D
4. A
5. D

Check Your Understanding 6.6

1. C
2. B
3. A
4. C
5. B

Check Your Understanding 6.7

1. C
2. A
3. A
4. C
5. B

Check Your Understanding 6.8

1. A
2. D
3. B
4. B
5. D

Chapter 7

Check Your Understanding 7.1

1. A
2. A
3. D
4. B
5. A

Check Your Understanding 7.2

1. B
2. C
3. B
4. B
5. D

Check Your Understanding 7.3

1. C
2. A
3. D
4. A
5. C

Chapter 8

Check Your Understanding 8.1

1. A
2. B
3. A
4. D
5. B

Check Your Understanding 8.2

1. A
2. C
3. D
4. B
5. B

Check Your Understanding 8.3

1. B
2. A
3. A
4. D
5. A

Chapter 9

Check Your Understanding 9.1

1. C
2. C
3. B
4. A
5. D

Check Your Understanding 9.2

1. C
2. A
3. B
4. D
5. B

Chapter 10

Check Your Understanding 10.1

1. B
2. B
3. D
4. B
5. D

Check Your Understanding 10.2

1. A
2. C
3. B
4. B
5. D

Check Your Understanding 10.3

1. A
2. B
3. A
4. D
5. B

Check Your Understanding 10.4

1. C
2. B
3. D
4. A
5. D

Check Your Understanding 10.5

1. D
2. D
3. D
4. A
5. C

Chapter 11

Check Your Understanding 11.1

1. A
2. B
3. C
4. B

Check Your Understanding 11.2

1. A
2. A
3. D
4. True

Chapter 12

Check Your Understanding 12.1

1. A
2. C
3. D
4. B
5. A

Check Your Understanding 12.2

1. B
2. C
3. B
4. B
5. A

Check Your Understanding 12.3

1. C
2. B
3. D
4. D
5. A

Check Your Understanding 12.4

1. C
2. A
3. A
4. C
5. B

Check Your Understanding 12.5

1. A
2. C
3. C
4. C
5. B

Check Your Understanding 12.6

1. D
2. B
3. A
4. B
5. D

Check Your Understanding 12.7

1. A
2. C
3. A
4. D
5. D

Check Your Understanding 12.8

1. D
2. A
3. B
4. C
5. A

Chapter 13

Check Your Understanding 13.1

1. B
2. D
3. B
4. D
5. False

Check Your Understanding 13.2

1. C
2. A
3. B
4. D
5. D

Chapter 14

Check Your Understanding 14.1

1. B
2. D
3. B
4. B
5. D

Check Your Understanding 14.2

1. A
2. A
3. B
4. A
5. D

Check Your Understanding 14.3

1. B
2. A
3. A
4. C
5. D

Glossary

.bmp: The file extension that identifies raster graphics stored in bit map file format (Microsoft Corporation 2002).

.jpg: The file extension that identifies graphic images encoded in the JPEG File Interchange Format, as originally specified by the Joint Photographic Experts Group (Microsoft Corporation 2002).

.tif: The file extension that identifies bitmap images in Tagged Image File Format (Microsoft Corporation 2002).

Accelerated Graphics Port (AGP):   A high-performance bus specification designed for fast, high-quality display of 3-D and video images (Microsoft Corporation 2002).

Access controls: 1. A computer software program designed to prevent unauthorized use of an information resource; 2. The process of designing, implementing, and monitoring a system for guaranteeing that only individuals who have a legitimate need are allowed to view or amend specific data sets (AHIMA 2010).

Ad hoc report: Ad hoc reports are needed only once. They may be used for a special report, a research program, or other purpose.

Address bus: A bus consisting of 20 to 64 separate hardware lines that is used to carry the signals specifying memory locations for data (Microsoft Corporation 2002).

Administrative data: Coded information contained in secondary records, such as billing records, describing patient identification, diagnoses, procedures, and insurance (AHIMA 2010).

Administrative information systems: A category of healthcare information systems that supports human resources management, financial management, executive decision support, and other business-related functions (AHIMA 2010).

Administrative safeguard: A set of nine standards defined by the HIPAA Security Rule including security management functions, assigned security responsibility, workforce security, information access management, security awareness and training, security incident reporting, contingency plan, evaluation, and business associate contracts and other arrangements (AHIMA 2010).

Administrative simplification: The section of HIPAA that deals with privacy and security as well as standardization of electronic transactions and code sets (Abdelhak et al. 2007).

Admission, discharge, transfer (ADT):   The administrative information system that stores basic demographic information and performs those functions related to admitting, discharging, and transferring a patient (Abdelhak et al. 2007).

Adoption: The decision to purchase, implement, and utilize an information system such as the EHR.

Aggregate data: Data extracted from individual health records and combined to form de-identified information about groups of patients that can be compared and analyzed (AHIMA 2010).

AHIMA Data Quality Model: A managerial process that ensures the integrity (accuracy and completeness) of an organization's data during data collection, application, warehousing, and analysis (AHIMA 2010).

Alert: A message triggered by an information system to notify the healthcare provider of information required to provide quality care (Amatayakul 2009).

Alpha site: An alpha site is the first healthcare facility to implement the information system.

American Health Information Community (AHIC):   A public-private federal advisory committee associated with the Office of the National Coordinator that makes recommendations to the secretary on how to accelerate adoption of interoperable electronic health information technology (AHIMA 2010).

American National Standards Institute (ANSI):   An organization that governs standards in many aspects of public and private business; developer of the Health Information Technology Standards Panel (AHIMA 2010).

Annotation: Annotation is the ability to alter the image in some way. Because the images may be a legal document, the image itself cannot be altered; however, an overlay to the document will show the annotation.

Application service provider (ASP):   A third-party service company that delivers, manages, and remotely hosts standardized applications software via a network through an outsourcing contract based on fixed, monthly usage or transaction-based pricing (AHIMA 2010).

Arrow keys: Any of four keys labeled with arrows pointing up, down, left, and right, used to move the cursor vertically or horizontally on the display screen, or in some programs to extend the highlight (Microsoft Corporation 2002).

Artificial neural networks (ANN):   A computational technique based on artificial intelligence and machine learning in which the structure and operation are inspired by the properties and operation of the human brain (AHIMA 2010).

ASC X12 format: The ASC X12 format is used primarily for processing of financial data, such as claims billing (McWay 2008, 174).

ASC X12 standard: A committee of the American National Standards Institute (ANSI) responsible for the development and maintenance of electronic data interchange (EDI) standards for many industries. The ASC "X12N" is the subcommittee of ASC X12 responsible for the EDI health insurance administrative transactions such as 837 Institutional Health Care Claim and 835 Professional Health Care Claim forms (AHIMA 2010).

Asynchronous: Occurring at different times (AHIMA 2010).

Audit controls: A method for monitoring attempts to gain access to a computer information system (AHIMA 2010).

Audit reduction tool: Audit reduction tools review the audit trail and compare it to facility-specific criteria and eliminate routine entries such as the periodic back-ups (Amatayakul, 2004b).

Audit trail: A chronological record of electronic system(s) activities that enables the reconstruction, review, and examination of the sequence of events surrounding or leading to each event and/or transaction from its beginning to end. Includes who performed what event and when it occurred (AHIMA 2010).

Automated codebook encoder: A type of encoder that mimics the codebook.

Back-end speech recognition (BESR):   By definition, back-end speech recognition is the "specific use of SRT in an environment where the recognition process occurs after the completion of dictation by sending voice files through a server" (AHIMA and MTIA Joint Task Force on Standards Development 2008, p. 18).

Backscanning: Backscanning is the process of scanning past medical records into the system so that there is an existing database of patient information, making the system valuable to the user from the first day of implementation.

Backspace key: The key that is used to delete any character that is to the left of the cursor.

Barcode: A type of data entry that uses a computer-readable identifier (Abdelhak et al. 2007).

BASIC: Beginner's All-purpose Symbolic Instruction Code, a high-level programming language developed in the mid-1960s by John Kemeny and Thomas Kurtz at Dartmouth College. It is widely considered one of the easiest programming languages to learn (Microsoft Corporation 2002).

Best of breed: A vendor strategy used when purchasing an EHR that refers to system applications that are considered the best in their class (AHIMA 2010).

Best of fit: A vendor strategy used when purchasing an EHR in which all the systems required by the healthcare facility are available from one vendor (AHIMA 2010).

Beta site: Beta sites are the next few healthcare facilities who subsequently implement the system.

Bigram: In the language model, an example of a bigram might be the "word pair 'world affairs' over 'whirled affairs' because 'world' occurs more frequently than 'whirled', giving it a higher unigram probability; and because 'world affairs' occurs more frequently than 'whirled affairs' in the speech and writing of target users, resulting in a higher bigram probability" (Voice Perfect Systems 2008).

Biometrics: The physical characteristics of users (such as fingerprints, voiceprints, retinal scans, iris traits) that systems store and use to authenticate identity before allowing the user access to a system (AHIMA 2010).

Birth certificate information system: This software reports births occurring in the healthcare facility to the state health agency. The birth certificate information system software may be developed by the state or by a vendor.

Bit: The level of voltage (low or high) in a computer that provides the binary states of 0 and 1 that computers use to represent characters (AHIMA 2010).

Bitmaps: A data structure in memory that represents information in the form of a collection of bits (Microsoft Corporation 2002).

Bluetooth port: An access port that uses radio waves as its signals rather than using infrared waves.

Blu-Ray disc: A disc similar to a CD or DVD except these hold more data (White 2008, 185).

Boolean search: An advanced search feature where the user can specify to add descriptive terms to the search such as "and, or, and not" to the search to help limit the search fields.

Broadband: A type of communications medium that can transmit multiple channels of data simultaneously (AHIMA 2010).

Broadband bandwidth: A type of communications medium that can transmit multiple channels of data simultaneously (AHIMA 2010).

Browser: A program that provides a way to view and read documents available on the World Wide Web (AHIMA 2010).

Bus network: In a bus network the computers that are networked together are lined up on a single cable.

Business associate: According to the HIPAA privacy rule, an individual (or group) who is not a member of a covered entity's workforce but who helps the covered entity in the performance of various functions involving the use or disclosure of patient-identifiable health information or disclosure of individually identifiable health information (AHIMA 2010).

Business continuity planning (BCP):   A program that incorporates policies and procedures for continuing business operations during a computer system shutdown; sometimes called contingency and disaster planning (AHIMA 2010).

Byte: A string of eight numbers is called a 'byte' of information (Joos et al. 2006, 15).

Cable: The coaxial cable within the television network where a copper wire is used that is shielded by plastic and braided copper (White 2008, 320).

Cable television modem: A modem that connects to a PC and a cable-ready television using the cable television pathway.

Cache memory: Cache memory is located on the CPU and can also be on a part of the processor. Thus when data is copied from RAM it is placed into the cache memory and can be retrieved faster from the cache memory than from the RAM (White 2008, 50).

Cancer registry information system: The cancer registry information system tracks information about the patient's cancer from the time of diagnosis to the patient's death. The cancer registry information systems are extremely complex and track very detailed information regarding diagnosis and treatment.

Centers for Medicare and Medicaid Services (CMS):   The division of the Department of Health and Human Services that is responsible for developing healthcare policy in the United States and for administering the Medicare program and the federal portion of the Medicaid program and maintaining the procedure portion of the International Classification of Diseases, 9th revision, Clinical Modification (ICD-9-CM); called the Health Care Financing Administration (HCFA) prior to 2001 (AHIMA 2010).

Central processing unit (CPU):   The CPU is the computer's brain or the circuits that make the electrical parts function.

Certification Commission on Health Information Technology (CCHIT):   An independent, voluntary, private-sector initiative organized as a limited liability corporation that has been awarded a contract by the U.S. Department of Health and Human Services (HHS) to develop, create prototypes for, and evaluate the certification criteria and inspection process for electronic health record products (EHRs) (www.cchit.org) (AHIMA 2010).

Certified in Healthcare Privacy and Security (CPHS):   AHIMA credential that recognizes advanced competency in designing, implementing, and administering comprehensive privacy and security protection programs in all types of healthcare organizations; requires successful completion of the CHPS exam sponsored by AHIMA (AHIMA 2010).

Certified Information Systems Security Professional (CISSP):   The Certified Information Systems Security Professional (CISSP) certification is sponsored by the International Information Systems Security Certification Consortium (ISC). It is a generic security certification and therefore is not healthcare specific. To be eligible, an individual must have 5 years full-time experience in security.

Chargemaster: A financial management form that contains information about the organization's charges for the healthcare services it provides to patients; also called charge description master (CDM) (AHIMA 2010).

Chart deficiency system: If the medical record comes to the HIM department with a deficiency, then the documentation omission is recorded and tracked in the chart deficiency system. The deficiencies can be in paper, imaged, and/or electronic records depending on the system used.

Chart locator system: The chart locator system is designed to track the paper medical record.

Chief information officer: The senior manager responsible for the overall management of information resources in an organization (AHIMA 2010).

Classification systems: 1. A system for grouping similar diseases and procedures and organizing related information for easy retrieval; 2. A system for assigning numeric or alpha-numeric code numbers to represent specific diseases and/or procedures (AHIMA 2010).

Client/server network: A type of network in which some of the processing is performed on the client (PC) and the remaining on the server.

Clinical data: The special identification code printed as a set of vertical bars of differing widths on books, grocery products, and other merchandise (Microsoft Corporation 2002).

Clinical data repository (CDR):   A central database that focuses on clinical information (AHIMA 2010).

Clinical decision support system (CDSS):   A special subcategory of clinical information systems that is designed to help healthcare providers make knowledge-based clinical decisions (AHIMA 2010).

Clinical information system (CIS):   A category of a healthcare information system that includes systems that directly support patient care (AHIMA 2010).

Clinical messaging: The function of electronically delivering data and automating the work flow around the management of clinical data (AHIMA 2010).

Clinical provider order entry (CPOE):   The CPOE contains preprogrammed clinical decision support designed to assist the user through making an entry appropriately.

Clinical vocabulary manager: The HIM role that manages classification systems and vocabularies for the organization.

COBOL: Common Business-Oriented Language. A verbose English-like compiled pro-gramming language developed between 1959 and 1961 and still in widespread use today, espe-cially in business applications typically run on mainframes (Microsoft Corporation 2002).

Code 39:   The recommended bar code symbology or format is Code 39, also known as Code 3 of 9.

Code sets: Under HIPAA, any set of codes used to encode data elements, such as tables of terms, medical concepts, medical diagnostic codes, or medical procedure codes; includes both the codes and their descriptions (AHIMA 2010).

Commission on Accreditation of Health Information and Informatics Management Education (CAHIIM):   The accrediting organization for educational programs in health informatics and information management (AHIMA 2010).

Compact disc (CD):   Plastic encased discs that use a finely focused laser beam to write and read data.

Computer output to laser disk (COLD):   Enterprise report management (ERM), also known as computer output to laser disk (COLD) technology is frequently used in place of scanning. ERM/COLD is the transfer of data from a computer directly into the document imaging system.

Computer-aided software engineering (CASE) software: Computer-aided software engineering (CASE) software is designed to create many of the diagrams and other tools used in the data model. CASE software can develop tools such as the entity-relationship diagrams described above as well as data flow diagrams (DFDs).

Computer-assisted coding (CAC):   The process of extracting and translating dictated and then transcribed free-text data (or dictated and then computer-generated discrete data) into ICD-9-CM and CPT evaluation and management codes for billing and coding purposes (AHIMA 2010).

Computer-assisted instruction: CAI is a software program designed to use multimedia and interactive technology to teach a topic.

Consumer awareness campaign: The AHIMA campaign that educates the consumer about the importance of and need for a personal health record.

Consumer health informatics (CHI):   The branch of health informatics that addresses the needs of the consumer.

Contingency plan: Documentation of the process for responding to a system emergency, including the performance of backups, the line-up of critical alternative facilities to facilitate continuity of operations, and the process of recovering from a disaster (AHIMA 2010).

Continuity of care record (CCR):   The CCR is a snapshot of data from the EHR and includes basic information such as diagnoses, allergies, medications, and future treatment. The CCR should be available to all healthcare providers so as to improve the continuity of patient care as well as reduce medical errors.

Continuous speech recognition: A computer technology that automatically translates voice patterns into written language in real time (AHIMA 2010).

Covered entity: Under HHS HIPAA regulations, any health plan, healthcare clearinghouse, or healthcare provider that transmits specific healthcare transactions in electronic form (AHIMA 2010).

Current Procedural Terminology: The American Procedural Association's Current Procedural Terminology (CPT) are the terms used in professional billing.

Cursor: A special on-screen indicator, such as a blinking underline or rectangle, that marks the place at which a keystroke will appear when typed (Microsoft Corporation 2002).

Daisy chain network: Computers in a network where each computer is connected to the next in a series.

Data accuracy: The extent to which data are free of identifiable errors (AHIMA 2010).

Data analyst: The data analyst is responsible for turning data into meaningful information. The data analyst manipulates data and generates reports using structured query language (SQL) or statistical software, and other tools.

Data bus: A bank of electrical bits; basically, these are the actual data. A bus is like a traffic cop within the computer, directing the electrical traffic so that it does not stop or slow down. The more buses that are used to direct traffic flow, the faster the data flow within the computer.

Data collection: The process by which data are gathered (AHIMA 2010).

Data content standards: Data content standards is defined as the "clear guidelines for the acceptable values for specified data fields" (Fenton et al. 2007).

Data conversion: The task of moving data from one data structure to another, usually at the time of a new system installation (AHIMA 2010).

Data definition: The specific meaning of a healthcare-related data element (AHIMA 2010).

Data definition language (DDL):   A special type of software used to create the tables within a relational database, the most common of which is structured query language (AHIMA 2010).

Data Elements for Emergency Department Systems (DEEDS):   A data set designed to support the uniform collection of information in hospital-based emergency departments (AHIMA 2010).

Data flow diagram (DFD):   A DFD is a diagram of how data flows within the database. The DFD is a good way to show management and other nontechnical users the system design.

Data integrity: 1. The extent to which healthcare data are complete, accurate, consistent, and timely; 2. A security principle that keeps information from being modified or otherwise corrupted either maliciously or accidentally; also known as data quality (AHIMA 2010).

Data manipulation: Data manipulation allows the user to add and delete rows in a table and to sort, find, and compare (>, <, =).

Data manipulation language (DML):   A special type of software used to retrieve, update, and edit data in a relational database, of which the most common is structured query language (AHIMA 2010).

Data miner: The role of the data miner is to convert information into knowledge that can be used for decision making. A data miner must be able to use data mining tools such as online analytical processing (OLAP) to drill down into data and transform buried data into logical information.

Data mining: The process of extracting information from a database and then quantifying and filtering discrete, structured data (AHIMA 2010).

Data modeling: The process of determining the users' information needs and identifying relationships among the data (AHIMA 2010).

Data navigator: A data navigator would be part of the information system development team. The person in this role would specialize in the development of the graphical user interface used to capture and navigate through the EHR and other systems.

Data projector: Used to display a presentation on a screen to a large audience or classroom. The projector is connected to a computer and the projector uses the same principle as the LCD display of a laptop.

Data quality and integrity monitor: The person in the Data Quality and Integrity Monitor role is responsible for the quality of the information collected and stored by the facility. This individual would work with the information system department to ensure that quality is built into the system as much as possible through the use of logic or structured data.

Data quality indicator system: The data quality indicator system is an abstracting system that records information about the patient and the care provided to the patient.

Data recovery: The restoration of lost data or the reconciliation of conflicting or erroneous data after a system failure. Recovery is often achieved using a disk or tape backup and system logs (Microsoft Corporation 2002).

Data reliability: The stability, repeatability, or precision of data (AHIMA 2010).

Data repository: An open-structure database that is not dedicated to the software of any particular vendor or data supplier, in which data from diverse sources are stored so that an integrated, multidisciplinary view of the data can be achieved; also called a central data repository or, when related specifically to healthcare data, a clinical data repository (AHIMA 2010).

Data resource manager: A role that ensures that the organization's information systems meet the needs of people who provide and manage patient services (AHIMA 2010).

Data retention: Each facility must decide how long patient-specific data will be retained. This decision must be made based on the needs of the organization, regulations, and laws.

Data security, privacy, and confidentiality manager:　The HIM role that safeguards protected health information from inappropriate use.

Data set:　A list of recommended data elements with uniform definitions that are relevant for a particular use (AHIMA 2010).

Data sources:　The location from which data originates.

Data standards:　Standards used to control the data elements, how the data is entered, and how data is shared (Giannangelo 2006).

Data translator:　A data translator works as the liaison between the patient and his/or her health data.

Data warehouse:　A database that makes it possible to access data from multiple databases and combine the results into a single query and reporting interface (AHIMA 2010).

Database:　An organized collection of data, text, references, or pictures in a standardized format, typically stored in a computer system for multiple applications (AHIMA 2010).

Database management system (DBMS):　Computer software that enables the user to create, modify, delete, and view the data in a database (AHIMA 2010).

Decision support system:　A computer-based system that gathers data from a variety of sources and assists in providing structure to the data by using various analytical models and visual tools in order to facilitate and improve the ultimate outcome in decision-making tasks associated with nonroutine and nonrepetitive problems (AHIMA 2010).

Degaussing:　The process of removing or rearranging the magnetic field of a disk in order to render the data unrecoverable (AHIMA 2010).

Delete key:　The key used to eliminate any text or characters to the right of the cursor's position.

Denial of service:　Denial of service attack is a type of malware that is designed to overload a Web site or other information system so that the system cannot handle the load and eventually shuts down (Joint NEMS/COCIR/JIRA Security and Privacy Committee 2003).

Department of Health and Human Services (DHHS):　The cabinet-level federal agency that oversees all the health- and human-services–related activities of the federal government and administers federal regulations (AHIMA 2010).

Designated standard maintenance organizations (DSMOs):　Organizations designated by HIPAA to control standards used in the electronic transmission used in healthcare (Giannangelo 2006).

Desktop publishing:　A desktop publishing application is professional software that is highly specialized word processing software. This software performs many other features in addition to the basic features of word processing. Desktop publishing gives the user more control over moving text and images in a document and is a general-purpose design tool for projects such as greeting cards, banners, calendars, and other flyers that are of value to business and to the home user.

Deterministic algorithm:　Deterministic algorithms look for exact matches. The algorithm looks at data elements such as name, birth date, gender, and Social Security number. The accuracy rate of identifying potential duplicates with this type of algorithm is only 20 to 40 percent.

Device driver:　A specific type of software that is made to interact with hardware devices. A device driver basically acts as a communication device.

Dial-up modem:　Used for computers with a telephone connection only and Internet service through the local telephone company. The original modem connections were managing data at 28.8 kilobits per second, but most dial-up modems now use a V.90 rate.

Dictation system: The dictation system is used by physicians and transcription staff to dictate various medical reports such as the operative report, history and physical, and the discharge summary.

Digital camera: Used to take still pictures that are then converted to a digital format. When the pictures are uploaded, the images can be read by the computer. Most pictures are able to be viewed as a .jpg file. Once a picture is digitized, it can be saved on the computer's hard drive or any secondary storage device such as flash drive, CD, or DVD.

Digital Imaging and Communications in Medicine (DICOM): A standard that promotes a digital image communications format and picture archive and communications systems for use with digital images (AHIMA 2010).

Digital signature: An electronic signature that binds a message to a particular individual and can be used by the receiver to authenticate the identity of the sender (AHIMA 2010).

Digital subscriber line (DSL) modem: A modem that uses the telephone lines but also uses pure digital signals.

Digital video disc (DVD): Similar to a CD except these hold more data. Whereas the CD holds up to 700 MB of information, the DVD holds up to 8.6 GB of information (White 2008, 185).

Digitized signature: The digitized signature is a scanned image of an individual's actual signature. This method is very insecure because anyone who has access to the image can use the signature.

Disclosure management system: A disclosure management system tracks the disclosures made throughout the healthcare organization. This tracking is required by the Health Information Portability and Accountability Act (HIPAA).

Discrete speech: Older voice recognition applications require each word to be dictated slowly and distinctly by the user. This allows "the software to determine where one word begins and the next stops" (ATRC 2009, p. 2). This is known as discrete speech.

Docking station: A device that smaller computer devices such as PDAs or palmtops will rest in as the data are uploaded into the workstation PC.

Document imaging: The practice of electronically scanning written or printed paper documents into an optical or electronic system for later retrieval of the document or parts of the document if parts have been indexed (AHIMA 2010).

Domain name: An address of a network connection that identifies the owner of that address in a hierarchical format: server.organization.type. For example, www.whitehouse. gov identifies the Web server at the White House, which is part of the U.S. government (Microsoft Corporation 2002).

Domains, subdomains, and tasks: The competencies that accredited health information programs must cover in their curriculum.

Dot-matrix printer: A printing mechanism that makes a series of dots per inch (DPI), and these tiny dots create the text letters or image.

Dots per inch (DPI): A measure of screen and printer resolution that is expressed as the number of dots that a device can print or display per linear inch (Microsoft Corporation 2002).

DRG (diagnosis-related group) groupers: A unit of case-mix classification adopted by the federal government and some other payers as a prospective payment mechanism for hospital inpatients in which diseases are placed into groups because related diseases and treatments tend to consume similar amounts of healthcare resources and incur similar amounts of cost; in the Medicare and Medicaid programs, one of more than 500 diagnostic classifications in which cases demonstrate similar resource consumption and length-of-stay patterns. Under the prospective payment system (PPS), hospitals are paid a set fee for treating patients in a single DRG category, regardless of the actual cost of care for the individual (AHIMA 2010).

DSL: The DSL line is a coaxial line but uses a twisted set of wiring comprising four pairs of insulated wires to help with noise reduction (White 2008, 320). DSL uses a phone line so that would probably tie up a phone line for incoming phone calls, but it doesn't do that! Actually DSL uses the twisted copper wires that the signals are carried within. With DSL, the user does not dial in; the DSL connection is always connected.

Dummy terminal: Dummy terminals consist of a monitor, keyboard, and the minimum hardware needed to connect them to the server to perform their functions.

Edit check: Edit checks are preprogrammed definitions of each data field set up within the software application. So, as data are entered, if any data are different from what has been preprogrammed, an edit message appears on the screen.

Electronic data interchange (EDI):   A standard transmission format using strings of data for business information communicated among the computer systems of independent organizations (AHIMA 2010).

Electronic document management systems (EDMS):   A storage solution based on digital scanning technology in which source documents are scanned to create digital images of the documents that can be stored electronically on optical disks; See document management technology (AHIMA 2010).

Electronic health record (EHR):   A health record in an information system designed to provide access to complete and accurate clinical data, practitioner alerts and reminders, clinical decision support systems, and links to medical knowledge (AHIMA 2010).

Electronic medication administration record (EMAR):   A system designed to prevent medication errors by checking a patient's medication information against his or her barcoded wristband (AHIMA 2010).

Electronic prescribing (e-prescribing):   When a prescription is written from the personal digital assistant and an electronic fax or when an actual electronic data interchange transaction is generated that transmits the prescription directly to the retail pharmacy's information system (AHIMA 2010).

Electronic protected health information (ePHI):   Under HIPAA, all individually identifiable information that is created or received electronically by a healthcare provider or any other entity subject to HIPAA requirements (AHIMA 2010).

Electronic signature: 1. Any representation of a signature in digital form, including an image of a handwritten signature; 2. The authentication of a computer entry in a health record made by the individual making the entry (AHIMA 2010).

Emergency access procedures: A process required by HIPAA that provides access in an emergency situation to healthcare providers even if they do not normally have access to the information.

Encoder(s):   Specialty software used to facilitate the assignment of diagnostic and procedural codes according to the rules of the coding system (AHIMA 2010).

Encryption: The process of transforming text into an unintelligible string of characters that can be transmitted via communications media with a high degree of security and then decrypted when it reaches a secure destination (AHIMA 2010).

Enter key: A primary key that is used to signal to the computer the end of a paragraph and the end of any command.

Enterprise master patient index (EMPI):   Integrated delivery systems (IDS) typically have an enterprise master patient index (EMPI). An EMPI allows all of the components of the IDS to share information about the patient. The medical record number assigned may be the same for all hospitals, ambulatory settings, and other components of the system.

Enterprise report management (ERM):   Enterprise report management (ERM), also known as computer output to laser disk (COLD) technology is frequently used in place of scanning. ERM/COLD is the transfer of data from a computer directly into the document imaging system.

Enterprise software: The term typically used when an application is used for the entire facility, such as applications involving e-mail, network, security issues, and the Internet.

Entity-relationship diagram: A specific type of data modeling used in conceptual data modeling and the logical-level modeling of relational databases (AHIMA 2010).

ESC key: The key used when the user wants to move a step back within a screen or program or quit a screen or program entirely.

Escrow: Escrow is where a third party holds a copy of the software in case the vendor goes bankrupt (AHIMA, 2006).

Essential Medical Data Set (EMDS):   A recommended data set designed to create a health history for an individual patient treated in an emergency service (AHIMA 2010).

Executive information system (EIS):   The executive information system (EIS) is a type of decision support system that is designed to be used by healthcare administrators. As such, it must be easy to use and have access to a wide range of data. With the EIS, a lot of graphs and charts generally are used as part of the results.

Expander: Expanders allow transcriptionists to type an acronym such as "CHF" and the full phrase "congestive heart failure" will automatically be spelled out, thus saving keystrokes and time. The expanders can typically be controlled by the facility (3M 2009).

Extensible Markup Language (XML):   A standardized computer language that allows the interchange of data as structured text (AHIMA 2010).

External bus: Allows communication with external devices such as a printer or scanner.

External data: External data come from outside the facility and can be used to compare the facility with other similar facilities.

Extranet: A system of connections of private Internet networks outside an organization's firewall that uses Internet technology to enable collaborative applications among enterprises (AHIMA 2010).

Facility access controls: Facility access controls limit physical access to authorized information system staff to the data centers where the hardware and software for the electronic information systems are held.

Feasibility study: A feasibility study determines if a proposed information system is an appropriate option to meet the objectives of the organization (Englebardt and Nelson, 2002).

Fiberoptic: The fiberoptic cables connect directly to a network or the Internet and are small hairlike fibers covered by silica glass covered by cladding with light pulses that carry the data along the wires (White 2008, 320).

Field: Within the structure of the database, a hierarchy must be used in order for the computer to recognize the database structure. The lowest level (smallest) is the field. The field is one attribute.

File Transfer Protocol (FTP):   A communications protocol that enables users to copy or move files between computer systems (AHIMA 2010).

Financial applications: The administration system that manages the financial activities of a healthcare facility. May also be called financial information systems.

Financial information system: The administration system that manages the financial activities of a healthcare facility. May also be called financial applications.

Firewall: A computer system or a combination of systems that provides a security barrier or supports an access control policy between two networks or between a network and any other traffic outside the network (AHIMA 2010).

Firewire port: Similar to a USB port in that several devices can be attached to it. These ports can handle 63 devices and are typically used for camcorders, DVD players, and digital audio equipment plug-ins (Joos et al. 2006, 26).

Flash drive: Sometimes referred to as a jump drive, a flash drive is a small, lightweight, removable data storage device to which data can be written and inserted into a USB port, a flash drive offers a dense form of storage that is impervious to scratches and dust (McWay 2008, 314).

Flowchart: A graphic tool that uses standard symbols to visually display detailed information, including time and distance, of the sequential flow of work of an individual or a product as it progresses through a process (AHIMA 2010).

Footer: One or more identifying lines printed at the bottom of a page (Microsoft Corporation 2002).

Force majeure: Force majeure is a legal term that refers to an "act of God" (Merriam-Webster, 2009). This contract clause is designed so that the parties of the contract cannot be held accountable to a deadline if there was an "act of God" that prevented compliance.

Foreign key: A key attribute used to link one entity/table to another (AHIMA 2010).

Forensics: Forensics "is the process used to gather intact and validated evidence" (Derhak, 2003, p 2) and is the process that should be used to gather evidence of the security incident.

Formula translation (FORTRAN):   Short for formula translation. The first high-level computer language (developed over the period 1954–58 by John Backus) and the progenitor of many key high-level concepts such as variables, expressions, statements, iterative and conditional statements, separately compiled subroutines, and formatted input/output (Microsoft Corporation 2002).

Free and open source software (FOSS):   Software, complete with source code, that is distributed freely to users who are in turn free to use, modify, and distribute it, provided that all alterations are clearly marked and that the name and copyright notice of the original author are not deleted or modified in any way (Microsoft Corporation 2002).

Front-end speech recognition (FESR):   FESR is "the specific use of speech recognition technology in an environment where the recognition process occurs in real time (or near real time) as dictation takes place" (AHIMA and MTIA Joint Task Force on Standards Development 2008, p. 18).

Function keys: Function keys perform various tasks within the computer and with certain software. The function keys are not used as much, since the addition of the mouse and drop-down selection boxes.

Functional requirements: A statement that describes the processes a computer system should perform to derive the technical specifications, or desired behavior, of a system (AHIMA 2010).

Gantt chart: A graphic tool used to plot tasks in project management that shows the duration of project tasks and overlapping tasks (AHIMA 2010).

General equivalence mapping (GEM):   A type of mapping that can be used to link a code in one classification system to the comparable code in a different classification system.

Gigabyte (Gb):   A gigabyte is equal 1,000 megabytes.

Go-live: Go-live is the official time and date that the facility beings begins using the new system. The go-live is generally scheduled for a time when the facility is the least busy.

Graphical user interface (GUI):   A style of computer interface in which typed commands are replaced by images that represent tasks; for example, small pictures [icons] that represent the tasks, functions, and programs performed by a software program (AHIMA 2010).

Grouper: The grouper assigns the codes entered into the encoder into the appropriate Medicare severity diagnostic-related groups (MS-DRG) or other diagnosis-related group (DRG). The grouper uses the appropriate grouping software for the insurer assigned to the patient.

Hard drive: The brain of the standard PC and performs all functions of the computer, as this is where the system files are located (White 2008 12).

Header: In word processing or printing, text that is to appear at the top of pages (Microsoft Corporation 2002).

Headphones: A computer accessory that covers the user's ears to allow him or her to listen to audio without disrupting others.

Health information exchange: A plan in which health information is shared among providers (AHIMA 2010).

Health information exchanges (HIEs):   The "seamless exchange of health information across disparate organizations" (Amatayakul 2009).

Health information technology: The technical aspects of processing health data and records, including classification and coding, abstracting, registry development, storage, and so on (AHIMA 2010).

Health Information Technology Standards Panel (HITSP):   HITSP works collaboratively with public and private sectors to achieve what they call "widespread interoperability among healthcare software applications." HITSP membership is available to anyone interested in participating, which includes standards development organizations. HITSP publishes their work products prior to approval in order to obtain public feedback.

Health Insurance Portability and Accounting Act of 1996 (HIPAA):   The Health Insurance Portability and Accounting Act of 1996 (HIPAA) impacts many areas of healthcare such as insurance portability, code sets, privacy, security, and national identifier standards.

Health Level 7 (HL7):   An international organization of healthcare professionals dedicated to creating standards for the exchange, management, and integration of electronic information (AHIMA 2010).

Health Plan Employer Data and Information Set (HEDIS):   A set of performance measures developed by the National Commission for Quality Assurance that are designed to provide purchasers and consumers of healthcare with the information they need to compare the performance of managed care plans (AHIMA 2010).

Health record banking: Health record banking is a new concept that is making headlines. This PHR model would allow patients and healthcare providers to share information by making deposits of health information into a bank. The health record bank would have to protect the privacy and security of the health information.

Hidden Markov model: An algorithm used in voice recognition (Bliss 2005).

Hierarchical database model: A system structured with broad groupings that can be further subdivided into more narrowly defined groups or detailed entities (AHIMA 2010).

Hierarchical model: A system structured with broad groupings that can be further subdivided into more narrowly defined groups or detailed entities (AHIMA 2010).

HL7 format: An international organization of healthcare professionals dedicated to creating standards for the exchange, management, and integration of electronic information (AHIMA 2010).

Home and End keys: Two keys on the standard keyboard. The home key takes the cursor to the beginning of the line and the end key moves the cursor to the end of the line.

Hospital information system: The comprehensive database containing all the clinical, administrative, financial, and demographic information about each patient served by a hospital (AHIMA 2010).

Hot spot: A 'hot spot' is triggered when the mouse is placed on top of a data field. The mouse changes to another symbol, such as a hand, that for a particular vendor indicates another level of choices from which the user can select.

Hub computer: The hub computer can serve numerous workstation computers at a single site or remotely.

Human resources information system (HRIS):   The human resources information system (HRIS) tracks employees within the organization. This tracking includes promotions, transfers, performance appraisal due dates, and absenteeism, for example.

Hybrid network: A hybrid network would basically be any combination of the types of network that can work together.

Hybrid record: A combination of paper and electronic records; a health record that includes both paper and electronic elements (AHIMA 2010).

Hypertext: Text linked together in a complex, nonsequential web of associations in which the user can browse through related topics (Microsoft Corporation 2002).

Hypertext Markup Language (HTML):   A standardized computer language that allows the electronic transfer of information and communications among many different information systems (AHIMA 2010).

Hypertext Transfer Protocol (HTTP):   A communications protocol that enables the use of hypertext linking (AHIMA 2010).

Hypertransport: "[T]he accelerated graphics port (AGP) is the internal bus between the graphics controller and the main memory in the computer. It is specifically designed for a video system" (Joos et al. 2006, 29).

Information system activity review: An information system activity review is the periodic review of the security controls (Rada 2003).

Information systems project steering committee: The information system project steering committee is responsible for every information system acquisition project in the facility (Wager, Lee, and Glaser, et al. 2005). Each project team will report back to the steering committee.

Information systems strategic planning: The process of identifying and assigning priorities to the various upgrades and changes that might be made in an organization's ISS (Johns 2007).

Infrared Data Association (IrDA) port: Used to transmit data by infrared light waves (Joos et al. 2006, 27).

Ink jet printer: {Printers that} use tiny nozzles to spray the ink (whether black or various colors) onto the sheet of paper.

Insert key: A toggle switch key in many programs. It can insert and replace text if it is toggled between an on/off mode.

Integrity: The state of being whole or unimpaired 2. In the context of data security, data integrity means the protection of data from accidental or unauthorized intentional change (Joint Commission 2004 IM-12).

Interactive voice response system: An automated call handler that can be configured to automatically dial a log of callers and deliver appointment reminders, lab results, and other information when a person answers the phone (AHIMA 2010).

Interface: The zone between different computer systems across which users want to pass information; for example, a computer program written to exchange information between systems or the graphic display of an application program designed to make the program easier to use (AHIMA 2010).

Interface engine: An interface engine allows "two applications to exchange information without having to build a customized interface for each application" (Abdelhak et al. 2007, p 280). The interface engine has to convert the data so that it can be accepted by the system receiving the information.

Internal bus: The internal bus permits the communication inside the computer's components; that is, within the memory.

Internal data: Internal data comes from within the facility and include the administrative and clinical data previously discussed.

International Classification of Diseases, 10th Revision, Clinical Modification: The planned replacement for ICD-9-CM, volumes 1 and 2, developed to contain more codes and allow greater specificity (AHIMA 2010).

International Classification of Diseases, 10th Revision, Procedural Coding System: A separate procedure coding system that would replace ICD-9-CM, volume 3, intended to improve coding accuracy and efficiency, reduce training effort, and improve communication with physicians (AHIMA 2010).

International Classification of Diseases, Ninth Edition, Clinical Modification: A coding and classification system used in the United States to report diagnoses in all healthcare settings and inpatient procedures and services as well as morbidity and mortality information (AHIMA 2010).

Internet: An international network of computer servers that provides individual users with communications channels and access to software and information repositories worldwide (AHIMA 2010).

Internet Protocol (IP) address: An Internet Protocol (IP) address is "an identifier for a computer or a device on a TCP/IP network" (White 2008, 312).

Internet service provider (ISP):   A company that provides connections to the Internet (AHIMA 2010).

Interoperability: The ability of different information systems and software applications to communicate and exchange data (AHIMA 2010).

Intranet: A private information network that is similar to the Internet and whose servers are located inside a firewall or security barrier so that the general public cannot gain access to information housed within the network (AHIMA 2010).

Intrusion detection and response: Intrusion detection and response "is the act of monitoring systems or networks for unauthorized users or unauthorized activities and the actions taken for correction to these acts." (Ruano 2003, p 5).

Java: Java is a very popular programming language that was developed by Sun Microsystems as an offshoot from the programming languages of C and C++ (White 2008, 96).

Jukebox: A jukebox holds and retrieves the individual disks just as the traditional a jukebox holds records or CDs.

Junk e-mail: Junk e-mail is unwanted and unsolicited mail that is similar to the junk mail that comes to a person's home mailbox.

Keyboard: A hardware unit with a set of switches that resembles a typewriter keyboard and that conveys information from a user to a computer or data communications circuit (Microsoft Corporation 2002).

Keystoning: When the power is turned on to the projector, the image is shown on the screen; if the angle of the image is projected slightly tilted in any direction, an effect known as keystoning can occur.

Key-word spotting: Key-word spotting is used in call routing systems by a client who when prompted by the system will speak a name or key word and the system will route the caller to the appropriate area or department for phone assistance. This is currently used in many companies with large client bases for directory assistance.

Kilobyte (Kb):   1,000 bytes.

Knowledge clusters: Competencies that accredited HIM programs must teach their students.

Laboratory information system (LIS):   The laboratory information system (LIS) collects, stores, and manages laboratory tests and their respective results. The LIS can speed up access to test results through improved efficiency from various locations, including anywhere in the hospital, the physician's office, or even the clinician's home.

Laptop computer: A small, portable personal computer that runs on either batteries or AC power, designed for use during travel (Microsoft Corporation 2002).

Laser printer: Laser printers use energy from a fast, flashing laser light source to create the images on a special drum; from static electricity, the ink powders (whether black or various colors) are transferred to the sheet of paper.

LCD screen: These monitor screens have become very commonplace in the market. An LCD screen also uses pixels; however, these are wedged between thin plastic layers of electric current or electrodes, making the pixels translucent and resulting in a bright image (White 2008, 201). LCD screens are seen in computers, but are more popular in television screens.

Light pen: A light pen basically emits an electronic signal and an image on the screen at the exact spot where the pen point touches (Joos et al. 2006, 22).

Listserv: A listserv is a professional mailing list organized by an association for its members or interested persons. Anyone may join a listserv by contacting an agency that maintains a listserv, as these are typically nonprofit agencies.

Local area network (LAN):   A network that connects multiple computer devices via continuous cable within a relatively small geographic area (AHIMA 2010).

Logical Observation Identifiers Names and Codes (LOINC):   A database protocol developed by the Regenstrief Institute for Health Care aimed at standardizing laboratory and clinical codes for use in clinical care, outcomes management, and research (AHIMA 2010).

Macro: A macro is similar to a template in the SRT. It basically uses "a series of keystrokes and/or commands that are executed on command;" macros are especially suited to generating "large amounts of text using only a few commands that are easily recognized" (AHIMA 2003 e-HIM Work Group on Speech Recognition in the EHR 2003, p.7).

Mainframe computers: A computer architecture built with a single central processing unit to which dumb terminals and/or personal computers are connected (AHIMA 2010).

Malicious software: Malicious software or malware is designed to harm a computer. The specific damage varies by virus or other malware. Some of these viruses or malware are more of a nuisance, whereas others destroy data or other files that may prevent the computer from operating. HIPAA mandates that the covered entity take steps to protect the data and information system from malware.

Mapping: Creation of a cross map that links the content from one classification or terminology scheme to another (AHIMA 2010).

Markup: The term 'markup' in computer languages simply means this is the way a computer encodes text (White 2008, 356).

Master patient index (MPI):   A patient-identifying directory referencing all patients related to an organization and which also serves as a link to the patient record or information, facilitates patient identification, and assists in maintaining a longitudinal patient record from birth to death (AHIMA 2010).

Materials management information system: Materials management information systems manage the supplies and equipment within the facility.

MEDCIN: A proprietary clinical terminology developed as a point-of-care tool for electronic medical record documentation at the time and place of patient care (AHIMA 2010).

Medical transcriptionists (MTs):   A medical language specialist who types or word-processes information dictated by providers into written form (AHIMA 2010).

Megabyte (Mb):   1,000 kilobytes.

megahertz (MHz):   A measure of frequency equivalent to 1 million cycles per second (Microsoft Corporation 2002).

Megapixel: A megapixel is one million pixels.

Memory chip: Memory chips contain only memory for storage capacity.

Messaging standards: Messaging standards may also be called interoperability standards or data exchange standards. The purpose of messaging standards is to support communications between information systems.

Microphone: A computer accessory that inputs audio.

Middleware: A bridge between two applications or the software equivalent of an interface (AHIMA 2010).

Minimum Data Set for Long Term Care (MDS LTC):   A federally mandated standard assessment form that Medicare- and/or Medicaid-certified nursing facilities must use to collect demographic and clinical data on nursing home residents; includes screening, clinical, and functional status elements (AHIMA 2010).

Mitigation: The Privacy Rule (45 CFR 164.530(f)) requires covered entities to lessen, as much as possible, harmful effects that result from the wrongful use and disclosure of protected health information; possible courses of action may include an apology; disciplinary action against the responsible employee or employees (although such results will not be able to be shared with the wronged individual); repair of the process that resulted in the breach; payment of a bill or financial loss that resulted from the infraction; or gestures of goodwill and good public relations, such as a gift certificate, that may assuage the individual (AHIMA 2010).

Modem: The modem is a port to allow the wiring of the PC to a phone line so that the computer can connect to the Internet and for facsimile purposes.

Monitor: The device on which images generated by the computer's video adapter are displayed (Microsoft Corporation 2002).

Motherboard: It is basically a system board where the circuitry chips or semiconductor chips are located.

Mouse: The mouse is a peripheral input device that is used by pointing the hand to correspond with movement on the computer screen. The concept was first developed as a pointing device and due to the device's size and tail-like cable, it was named for the mouse (White 2008, 203).

Multitasking: The computer's operating system instructions allow it to handle several tasks at once. This is called multitasking, which involves the computer CPU, or brain, working to timeshare the tasks so that several functions can be done at once, using a share of the computer's time to execute.

MyPHR.com: AHIMA views the PHR as a significant and useful tool of technology. In 2003, AHIMA created the MyPHR Web site (www.myphr.com) to promote and educate the public about the PHR and to provide guidance on how to create one (AHIMA e-HIM Personal Health Record Work Group, 2005).

National Committee on Vital and Health Statistics (NCVHS): A public policy advisory board that recommends policy to the National Center for Health Statistics and other health-related federal programs (AHIMA 2010).

National Council for Prescription Drug Programs (NCPDP): A not-for-profit ANSI-accredited standards development organization founded in 1977 that develops standards for exchanging prescription and payment information (AHIMA 2010).

National drug codes (NDC): Codes that serve as product identifiers for human drugs, currently limited to prescription drugs and a few selected over-the-counter products (AHIMA 2010).

National eHealth Collaborative (NeHC): NeHC is working with other stakeholders to address "issues and effecting the change needed to enable the secure and reliable exchange of electronic health information nationwide" (NeHC, 2009).

National Health Information Infrastructure (NHII): An infrastructure proposed by the National Committee on Vital and Health Statistics in 2002 that would be a set of technologies, standards, applications, systems, values, and laws that support all facets of provider healthcare, individual health, and public health (AHIMA 2010).

National health information network (NHIN): Interoperable information infrastructure that links various healthcare information systems together, allowing patients, physicians, healthcare institutions, and other entities nationwide to share clinical information privately and securely; network of networks (AHIMA 2010).

Natural language processing (NLP): Conversion of human language (structured or unstructured) into data that can be translated and then manipulated by computer systems; branch of artificial intelligence (AHIMA 2010).

Natural language processing technology: Conversion of human language (structured or unstructured) into data that can be translated and then manipulated by computer systems; branch of artificial intelligence (AHIMA 2010).

Natural language queries: Natural language queries allow the user to use common English words to tell the database which data are needed (Austin and Boxerman 2003). For example, the user may enter a query by typing "list all of the patients whose principal procedure is 47.01." This command would generate a list of patients who had the principal procedure of laparoscopic appendectomy.

Network database model: The type of database that uses pointers to link data.

Network security: Network security is using technology to protect the data transmitted across the network and includes fire walls, encryption, and data integrity.

Normalization: 1) A formal process applied to relational database design to determine which variables should be grouped together in a table in order to reduce data redundancy across and within the table 2) Conversion of various representational forms to standard expressions so that those that have the same meaning will be recognized by computer software as synonymous in a data search (AHIMA 2010).

Notebook computer: A type of portable computer (Hebda and Czar 2009).

Nursing information system (NIS): Nursing information systems assist in the planning and monitoring of overall patient care. A nursing information system (NIS) will document the nursing care provided to a patient.

Object-oriented database: A type of database that uses commands that act as small, self-contained instructional units (objects) that may be combined in various ways (AHIMA 2010).

Object-oriented model: The type of database that allows for the collection of audio, video, and other objects.

Office of the National Coordinator for Health Information Technology (ONC): A department of the U.S. Department of Health and Human Services established by executive order to advance the development, adoption, and implementation of healthcare information technology standards (AHIMA 2010).

Office of the National Coordinator for Health Information Technology (ONCHIT): A department of the U.S. Department of Health and Human Services established by executive order to advance the development, adoption, and implementation of healthcare information technology standards (AHIMA 2010).

One-factor authentication: Passwords are commonly used in conjunction with a user name or identifier. This is an example of a one-factor authentication as it only utilizes something you know (Burrington-Brown 2003a AHIMA 2005).

Online analytical processing (OLAP): A data access architecture that allows the user to retrieve specific information from a large volume of data (AHIMA 2010).

Open code: The term open code refers to software that is available to the general public and can be modified by anyone.

Operating system: The principal piece of software in any computer system, which consists of a master set of programs that manage the basic operations of the computer.

Optical character recognition (OCR): A method of encoding text from analog paper into bit-mapped images and translating the images into a form that is computer readable (AHIMA 2010).

Order entry/results reporting: A type of information that allows for entry of orders, which are then routed to the appropriate department for action. Once the results are available, they are routed back to the care provider for review.

ORYX by Joint Commission: The Joint Commission's initiative that supports the integration of outcomes data and other performance measurement data into the accreditation process; often referred to as ORYX (AHIMA 2010).

Outcomes and Assessment Information Set (OASIS): A standard core assessment data tool developed to measure the outcomes of adult patients receiving home health services under the Medicare and Medicaid programs (AHIMA 2010).

Page up and Page down keys: Page Up and Page Down keys enable movement through a document one page at a time.

Parallel port: Parallel ports are "unidirectional ports set up to send parallel data" (Joos et al. 2006, 26). Within parallel ports, data may travel in groups of eight bits or a byte of information (Joos et al. 2006, 26).

Passwords: A series of characters that must be entered to authenticate user identity and gain access to a computer or specified portions of a database (AHIMA 2010).

Patient monitoring system: Patient monitoring systems automatically collect and store patient data from various systems used in healthcare.

Patient provider portal: The patient provider portal is a secure method of communication between the healthcare provider and the patient, just the providers, or the provider and the payer. The patient provider portal may include secure e-mail or remote access to test results, and provide patient monitoring.

Patient registration: Patient registration systems are frequently known as ADT. This system collects data on the patient from preadmission to discharge.

Patient-specific data: 1. Data in the health record that relates to a particular patient identified by name; 2. Personal information that can be linked to a specific patient, such as age, gender, date of birth, and address-specific data (AHIMA 2010).

Payment milestone: A payment milestone is an action that once occurring triggers payment to the vendor. This payment is a specified percent of the total cost of the system.

PCI-Express: This interface allows data to move more quickly. The PCI-E is a bus architecture that can route data at greater than 8 gigabytes per second in each direction within the bandwidth (White 2008, 29).

PDA: A hand-held microcomputer, without a hard drive, that is capable of running applications such as e-mail and providing access to data and information, such as notes, phone lists, schedules, and laboratory results, primarily through a pen device (AHIMA 2010).

Peer review: 1. Review by like professionals, or peers, established according to an organization's medical staff bylaws, organizational policy and procedure, or the requirements of state law; the peer review system allows medical professionals to candidly critique and criticize the work of their colleagues without fear of reprisal; 2. The process by which experts in the field evaluate the quality of a manuscript for publication in a scientific or professional journal (AHIMA 2010).

Peer-to-peer network: If a network does not use a central server or hub, this is referred to as a peer-to-peer network and all the computers on this network can perform the duties at the same time (White 2008, 313).

Person or entity authentication: The corroboration that an entity is who it claims to be (AHIMA 2010).

Personal computer: Within the personal computer, there are three main parts: the CPU, the memory, and the storage devices of the system.

Personal health record (PHR):   An electronic or paper health record maintained and updated by an individual for himself or herself (AHIMA 2010).

Pharmacy information system (PIS):   A pharmacy information system (PIS) assists the care providers in ordering, allocating, and administering medication. With focus on patient safety issues, especially medication errors, the pharmacy information system is a key tool in providing optimal patient care.

Phishing: Phishing is an e-mail that appears from a legitimate business that asks for account number or other personal information. The e-mail is actually from a phisher who uses the account number or other information maliciously.

Physical safeguards: Measures such as locking doors to safeguard data and computer programs from undesired occurrences and exposures; a set of four standards defined by the HIPAA Security Rule including facility access controls, workstation use, workstation security, and device and media controls (AHIMA 2010).

Physician advisor (PA):   The physician advisor volunteers his or her time as part of a hospital committee to review health records for various reasons. The PA can be used for medical record reviews, utilization reviews, quality reviews, surgical case and tissue reviews, other pathological reviews, and a host of blood and laboratory reviews for various medical staff and hospital committees.

Picture archival communication system (PACS):   An integrated computer system that obtains, stores, retrieves, and displays digital images (in healthcare, radiological images) (AHIMA 2010).

Pixel: An abbreviation for the term **picture element**, which is defined by many tiny bits of data or points (AHIMA 2010).

Plasma screen: A type of screen used in computers.

Plug and Play (PnP):   An adapter card hardware that sets connections through software rather than hardware, making hardware easier to install (AHIMA 2010).

Population health: Population health is the capture and reporting of healthcare data that is are used for public health purposes. It allows the healthcare provider to report infectious diseases, immunizations, cancer, and other reportable conditions to public health officials.

Practice management system: Software designed to help medical practices run more smoothly and efficiently (AHIMA 2010).

Presentation layer: The presentation layer controls screen layout, data entry, and data retrieval. The flexibility of the presentation layer is what allows the various healthcare providers to manipulate it (Amatayakul, 2007).

Primary data: Primary data come directly from the source. The medical record is a primary data source because the information comes directly from the patient and the healthcare providers.

Primary key: An explanatory notation that uniquely identifies each row in a database table (AHIMA 2010).

Print Screen key: The Print Screen key is either used alone or with the Alt key so that the contents of the monitor's screen can be printed onto the clipboard. Once the information is on the clipboard, it then can be copied and pasted into an application program to be printed or saved.

Printer: Printers are peripheral devices that convert the text and images on the screen into text and images on paper sheets. There are two basic types of printers: impact and nonimpact printers.

Privacy: The quality or state of being hidden from, or undisturbed by, the observation or activities of other persons, or freedom from unauthorized intrusion; in healthcare-related contexts, the right of a patient to control disclosure of personal information (AHIMA 2010).

Privacy rule: The federal regulations created to implement the privacy requirements of the simplification subtitle of the Health Insurance Portability and Accountability Act of 1996 (AHIMA 2010).

Probabilistic algorithm: Probabilistic algorithms are able to identify transpositions and name changes and can use phonetic search capabilities (AHIMA MPI Task Force, 2004).

Programming languages: A set of words and symbols that allows programmers to tell the computer what operations to follow (AHIMA 2010).

Project: A project is a plan and course of action that will address a specific objective, made up of a series of activities and tasks with a defined start and stop date.

Project definition: First step in the project management life cycle that sets expectations for the what, when, and how of a project the organization wants to undertake (AHIMA 2010).

Project Evaluation and Review Technique (PERT) chart: A project management tool that diagrams a project's timelines and tasks as well as their interdependencies (AHIMA 2010).

Project management: A formal set of principles and procedures that help control the activities associated with implementing a usually large undertaking to achieve a specific goal, such as an information system project (AHIMA 2010).

Project management software: A type of application software that provides the tools to track a project (AHIMA 2010).

Project manager: The project manager is responsible for coordinating the individual project, monitoring the budget, managing the resources, conducting negotiations, and keeping the project on schedule.

Project team: A collection of individuals assigned to work on a project (AHIMA 2010).

Proprietary software: Proprietary software refers to software where the company that developed it maintains all rights to the software and will provide it to the user for a fee. Proprietary software cannot be modified without the expressed written agreement by the owner.

Protected health information (PHI):   Individually identifiable health information, transmitted electronically or maintained in any other form, that is created or received by a healthcare provider or any other entity subject to HIPAA requirements (AHIMA 2010).

Prototype: A type of rapid information system developed that uses an iterative process between the users and the developers.

Public domain software: Another type of free software that has no restrictions is public domain software. Although there is no copyright for the software (and unlike FOSS), public domain software does not come with the source code.

Quadgram: A term used in voice recognition to indicate word sequences with four words.

Qualitative analysis: A review of the health record to ensure that standards are met and to determine the adequacy of entries documenting the quality of care (AHIMA 2010).

Quantitative analysis: A review of the health record to determine its completeness and accuracy (AHIMA 2010).

Query: A query is a "search for data that meets specified criteria to allow you to retrieve certain subsets of the data" (White 2008, 121).

Query by example: Query by example (QBE) is a query method commonly used by microcomputers (Austin and Boxerman 2003). The user only has to point and click to choose tables and fields contained in the database. The system then allows the user to choose whether the entries that meet those criteria should be included or excluded from the query.

Radiofrequency identification device (RFID):   An automatic recognition technology that uses a device attached to an object to transmit data to a receiver and does not require direct contact (AHIMA 2010).

Radiology information system (RIS):   A radiology information system (RIS) is used to collect, store, and provide information on radiological tests such as ultrasound, magnetic resonance imaging, and positron emission tomography. The RIS also supports other radiological procedures performed in radiology such as ultrasound-guided biopsies and upper gastrointestinal series.

Random access memory (RAM):   Semiconductor-based memory that can be read and written by the central processing unit or other hardware devices (Microsoft Corporation 2002).

Read-only memory (ROM):   Read-Only Memory (ROM) is memory that has been programmed onto a chip at the factory and cannot be changed. When a user purchases ROM memory, it is purchased at a certain predetermined amount. No instructions or data can be changed in the memory in ROM. The computer start-up instructions are in the ROM memory. A computer cannot write new information to ROM memory.

Redundancy: The concept of building a backup computer system that is an exact version of the primary system and that can replace it in the event of a primary system failure (AHIMA 2010).

Reengineering: Fundamental rethinking and radical redesign of business processes to achieve significant performance improvements (AHIMA 2010).

Regional health information organizations (RHIOs):   An organization that manages the local deployment of systems promoting and facilitating the exchange of healthcare data within a national health information network (AHIMA 2010).

Registered health information administrator (RHIA):   A type of certification granted after completion of an AHIMA-accredited four-year program in health information management and a credentialing examination (AHIMA 2010).

Registered health information technician (RHIT):   A type of certification granted after completion of an AHIMA-accredited two-year program in health information management and a credentialing examination (AHIMA 2010).

Registration data of the admission, discharge, transfer (R-ADT):   A type of administrative information system that stores demographic information and performs functionality related to registration, admission, discharge, and transfer of patients within the organization.

Relational database model: A type of database that stores data in predefined tables made up of rows and columns (AHIMA 2010).

Relational model: A data model in which the data is organized in relations (tables). This is the model implemented in most modern database management systems (Microsoft Corporation 2002).

Release of Information system: The release of information (ROI) system is designed to manage all aspects of requests for protected health information received and processed by the HIM department.

Report design: Report design is the process of creating and formatting a report. This design includes the content of the report, the order of the data on the report, and any desired formatting specifications.

Request for information (RFI):   A written communication often sent to a comprehensive list of vendors during the design phase of the systems development life cycle to ask for general product information (AHIMA 2010).

Request for proposal (RFP):   A type of business correspondence asking for very specific product and contract information that is often sent to a narrow list of vendors that have been preselected after a review of requests for information during the design phase of the systems development life cycle (AHIMA 2010).

Resolution: The degree of sharpness of a computer-generated image as measured by the number of dots per linear inch on a printout or the number of pixels across and down a display screen (AHIMA 2010).

Revenue cycle: 1. The process of how patient financial and health information moves into, through, and out of the healthcare facility, culminating with the facility receiving reimbursement for services provided; 2. The regularly repeating set of events that produces revenue (AHIMA 2010).

Rich text format: Rich text format (RTF) is a "format for text and graphics interchange that is used with different output devices, operating environments, and operating systems" (Microsoft Company 2008).

Risk analysis: The process of identifying possible security threat to the organization's data and identifying which risks should be proactively addressed and which risks are lower in priority; also called risk assessment (AHIMA 2010).

Risk assessment: The process of identifying possible security threat to the organization's data and identifying which risks should be proactively addressed and which risks are lower in priority; also called risk analysis (AHIMA 2010).

Router: A device programmed to filter out or to allow certain types of data to pass through (AHIMA 2010).

Routine reports: Routine reports are those that are needed repeatedly.

Rules-based algorithm: A type of algorithm that can be used to determine the probability that a patient has duplicate medical record numbers in the master patient index.

Rules-based encoder: Rules-based encoders require the user to type in the name or portion of the name of the diagnosis/ or procedure. This entry into the encoder generates a list of suggestions from which the coder selects.

RxNorm: A clinical drug nomenclature developed by the Food and Drug Administration, the Department of Veterans Affairs, and HL7 to provide standard names for clinical drugs and administered dose forms (AHIMA 2010).

Satellite: (Chapter 2) Satellite is used in the sense of how computer data is sent through frequency cables to a user, except here the data is sent from the ground to a fixed altitude location so that no cables are used. Data is sent through electromagnetic waves bounced from the ground to the satellite and back as part of the data transmission process. As more satellites are being launched and technology develops, this area further develops.

(Chapter 8) Satellite is used in the sense of a 'satellite lab' or 'satellite clinic' such as radiology satellite meaning a smaller version of the lab or clinic or radiology department is located within the facility or near the campus for patients. Satellite clinics or other ancillary services are provided as a service for the patient for closer proximity for less time to travel, for less waiting time, and so on.

Scanner: The scanner enables the input of data that is not normally coded for computer use. This machine digitizes data so that it can be read, analyzed, and stored, if necessary, by a computer. Scanners are versatile and can be used to input text, images, and numerical and graphical data.

Scanning workstation: The scanning workstation is the personal computer (PC) that controls the scanner. Once a document is scanned, the workstation compresses the bitmap (.bmp) file created by the scanner.

Scheduling software: Scheduling software is an application for administrative processes that includes "electronic scheduling systems for hospital admissions, inpatient and outpatient procedures, and identifying eligible or potential eligible patients for clinical trials" (Thakkar and Davis 2006, 10).

Scheduling system: Scheduling systems are used to control the use of resources through the organization (Hebda, Czar, and Mascara, et al. 2002). These resources can include staff, equipment, rooms, and more. Scheduling systems may be centralized or independent.

Scope creep: A process in which the scope of a project grows while the project is in process, virtually guaranteeing that it will be over budget and behind schedule (AHIMA 2010).

Screen design: Screen design is developing screens of an information system to meet the needs of the user and to promote job efficiency.

Search engine: A software program used to search for data in databases; for example, a structured query language (AHIMA 2010).

Secondary data: Data taken from a primary source, (such as the medical record) and abstracted into another database or registry are called a secondary data source. Examples of secondary data sources are cancer registry, master patient index, and disease index.

Security: 1. The means to control access and protect information from accidental or intentional disclosure to unauthorized persons and from unauthorized alteration, destruction, or loss; 2. The physical protection of facilities and equipment from theft, damage, or unauthorized access; collectively, the policies, procedures, and safeguards designed to protect the confidentiality of information, maintain the integrity and availability of information systems, and control access to the content of these systems (AHIMA 2010).

Security awareness training: This training provides employees of the covered entities with information with and a basic knowledge of the security policies and procedures of the organization (Newby 2009).

Security event: Security events are poor security practices that have not led to harm (Amatayakul 2005b).

Security incident: Security incidents {are poor security practices that} have resulted in harm or a significant risk of harm (Amatayakul 2005b).

Security management plan: A security management plan must include the policies required to prevent, identify, control, and resolve security incidents (45 CFR 160, 162, and 164 2003DHHS, 2003, p 8346).

Security official: The security rule mandates an individual to be in charge of the security program for the covered entity. HIPAA calls this individual a security official; however, this position is frequently called chief security officer (CSO) by the covered entities.

Security rule: The federal regulations created to implement the security requirements of the Health Insurance Portability and Accountability Act of 1996 (AHIMA 2010).

Semantics: The meaning of a word or term; sometimes refers to comparable meaning, usually achieved through a standard vocabulary (AHIMA 2010).

Serial port: The serial port arranges data to travel in serial form or one bit at a time (Joos et al. 2006, 26).

Setting configuration: Setting configuration is the entry of the desired behaviors of the system into tables or setting fields.

Site preparation: Site preparation is making any needed changes to the physical location where the computer, workstations, printers, or other hardware will be installed (Abdelhak et al. 2007).

Site visits: An in-person review conducted by an accreditation survey team; the visit involves document reviews, staff interview, an examination of the organization's physical plant, and other activities (AHIMA 2010).

Smart cards: Smart cards are plastic cards, similar in appearance to a credit card, with a computer chip embedded in it. Smart cards have been widely adopted for use in banking, retail, government, and other applications.

Software license: The software license grants the organization the right to utilize a vendor's software and defines how the software may be used (Abdelhak et al. 2007).

Software piracy: Software piracy occurs when unauthorized copying or use of copyrighted software happens outside the terms of the agreement (Joos et al. 2006, 381).

Sound card: The sound card enables the computer to reproduce sound from electrical currents for speakers, headphones, the microphone, and input from peripheral devices.

Source code: Source code is the programming code that was used to develop the system.

Source system: Source systems are information systems that populate the EHR. These source systems include the electronic medication administration record, laboratory information system, radiology information system, hospital information system, and nursing information systems.

Spam filter: Software that keeps unwanted spam e-mails out of the e-mail inbox and places them in a spam folder for the user to confirm that it is spam and then delete.

Speaker dependent: A speech recognition system that is "speaker dependent" means that it has been "trained" to a particular user and already has an established vocabulary for that user.

Speech recognition technology (SRT):   Technology that translates speech to text (AHIMA 2010).

Spoliation: Unintentional destruction or alteration of evidence is called spoliation (Tomes 2005).

Spyware: Spyware may be used to track keystrokes and passwords, monitor Web sites visited, or other actions, and report these actions back to the creator of the spyware. The spyware may slow down the computer system and contribute to identify identity theft or other breaches of privacy.

Standard Generalized Markup Language (SGML):   An International Standards Organization standard that establishes rules for identifying elements within a text document (AHIMA 2010).

Standards development organization (SDO):   A private or government agency involved in the development of healthcare informatics standards at a national or international level (AHIMA 2010).

Star network: A star network is the most common of the network setups for a LAN network. All of the cables that connect to computers at any point connect to the hub or center, which is called the star. A star network is analogous to a bicycle wheel that has many spokes on it where all are outreaching yet all connect to a center hub.

Structured data: Binary, computer-readable data (AHIMA 2010).

Structured query language (SQL): A fourth-generation computer language that includes both DDL and DML components and is used to create and manipulate relational databases (AHIMA 2010).

Stylus: A pointing device, similar to a pen, used to make selections, usually by tapping, and to enter information on the touch-sensitive surface (Microsoft Corporation 2002).

Subjective data: Data that is not backed up by facts and figures.

Symbology: The term used to describe the format of a bar code.

Synchronous: Meaning "involved on the computer at the same time" (Joos et al. 2006, 326).

Syntax: A term that refers to the comparable structure or format of data, usually as they are being transmitted from one system to another (AHIMA 2010).

System analysis: System analysis is a "process of studying organizational operations and determining information systems requirements for a given applications " (Glandon et al. 2008, p 75).

System development life cycle (SDLC): Abdelhak et al. (2007, 306) define the system development life cycle (SDLC) as the "process used to identify, investigate, design, select, and implement information systems."

System evaluation: "The purpose of system evaluation is to determine whether the system functions in the way intended" (Abdelhak et al. p 337).

System files: System files are small disk files that contain software codes that are instructions for the computer and are the first files that a computer reads when "booting up."

System implementation: The third phase of the systems development life cycle (AHIMA 2010).

System selection: System selection and system implementation is the process of deciding on an information system (IS), preparing it, and training facility staff for use of the system in the healthcare facility.

Systematized Nomenclature of Medicine (SNOMED): A comprehensive clinical vocabulary developed by the College of American Pathologists, which is the most promising set of clinical terms available for a controlled vocabulary for healthcare (AHIMA 2010).

T1 line: A type of transmission that carries point-to-point digital communication circuits with 25 channels, each of which carries 64,000 bits per second, is the T1 line (White 2008, 313).

Tab keys: A key, often with both a left-pointing and a right-pointing arrow, that traditionally (as in word processing) is used to insert tab characters into a document (Microsoft Corporation 2002).

Tag: In markup languages, such as SGML and HTML, a code that identifies an element in a document, such as a heading or a paragraph, for the purposes of formatting, indexing, and linking information in the document (Microsoft Corporation 2002).

Target sheet: Target sheets are pages that are blank except for a bar code that will tell the scanner and ultimately the computer the content of the pages that follow.

Technical safeguard: Technical safeguards are defined by the security rule as "the technology and the policy and procedures for its use that protect electronic protected health information and control access to it." (45 CFR 160, 162, and 164 2003, DHHS, 2003, p 8370) Technical safeguards use technology as well as policies and procedures to protect the ePHI from unauthorized access and destruction/ or alteration.

Telehealth: Telehealth is the use of telecommunications and networks to share information between a patient and a healthcare provider located in at different locations/sites. These locations can be across town or across the world.

Telephone callback procedures: Procedures used primarily when employees have access to an organization's health information systems from a remote location that verify whether the caller's number is authorized and prevent access when it is not (AHIMA 2010).

Telesurgery: The use of robotics to perform surgery is called telesurgery. This allows surgery to be performed on a patient in a different location.

Template: A pattern used in computer-based patient records to capture data in a structured manner (AHIMA 2010).

Template-based entry: Templates-based entry is a cross between free text and structured data entry. The user is able to pick and choose data that are entered frequently, thus requiring the entry of data that change from patient to patient (Amatayakul, 2007).

Terabyte (Tb): 1,000 gigabytes.

Termination process: A HIPAA-mandated process that terminates an employee's access immediately upon separation from the facility.

Terminology asset manager: This position develops data sets, nomenclatures, and classification standards, and in order to do so the HIM professional must understand the data needs of all stakeholders.

Test environment: A section of the information system where software upgrades are tested to ensure that they work appropriately before moving the changes into production (Hebda and Czar 2009).

Testing: The act of performing an examination or evaluation (AHIMA 2010).

Thermal printer: Thermal printers use heat to transfer the ink onto the sheet of paper or other medium. Much of the thermal printing is seen in barcoding, done in the industry on large commercial printers.

Third-party license: Third-party licenses can be involved with software licensure, which means that an additional licensure is required between the user and the vendor.

Token: A physical device, such as a key card, inserted into a door to admit an authorized person or into a computer to authenticate a computer user (AHIMA 2010).

Token ring network: The token ring network is similar to a ring or circle of cable of computers in the network. There is no beginning or end within this loop. Data flows around this circle until it reaches the exact computer address that it is meant to reach.

Touch screen: Similar to the light pen in that it works by touch of the fingertip onto the monitor screen. As the screen projects images or data, the user simply touches the image or data and the computer recognizes the touch as input for the preprogrammed data of each image to be performed, calculated, or completed.

Train the trainer: A method of training certain individuals who, in turn, will be responsible for training others on a task or skill (AHIMA 2010).

Transactions and Code Sets rule: The Transaction and Code Sets rule was designed to standardize transactions performed by healthcare organizations. These standards apply to electronic transactions only; however, paper submissions are similar.

Transcription system: The transcription system is used by the transcriptionist to type the various documents dictated by the physicians. The transcription system should be interfaced with the hospital information system so that the patient name, medical record, and date of service are already populated within the system.

Transmission Control Protocol/Internet Protocol (TCP/IP): The multifaceted protocol suite, or open standard not owned by or proprietary to any company, on which the Internet runs (AHIMA 2010).

Transmission security: Transmission security is mechanisms designed to protect ePHI while the data are being transmitted between two points.

Trauma registry software: Trauma registry software tracks patients with traumatic injuries from the initial trauma treatment to death.

Tree network: The tree network is sometimes called a hierarchical network. The main computer is the root or the first level; the next level of computers that are connected is the second level. In the second level of the hierarchy, computers are connected from the second computer in the series. There can be other levels within this network but no other computers can be connected above the central computer or node in the hierarchy. A tree network must have three levels or else it would be a star network.

Trigger: A documented response that alerts a skilled nursing facility resident assessment instrument assessor to the fact that further research is needed to clarify an assessment (AHIMA 2010).

Trigram: A term used in voice recognition to indicate word sequences with three words.

Turnaround time (TAT): Turnaround time (TAT) is defined as "the elapsed time from completion of dictation to the delivery of the transcribed document either in printed medium or electronically to a repository" (AHIMA and MTIA Joint Task Force on Standards Development 2008, p. 18).

Two-factor authentication: Tokens are used in conjunction with a password to provide two-factor authentication because a token and a password are two different types of authentications—something you know and something you have (Burrington-Brown, AHIMA 2003a).

Unified Medical Language System: A program initiated by the National Library of Medicine to build an intelligent, automated system that can understand biomedical concepts, words, and expressions and their interrelationships; includes concepts and terms from many different source vocabularies (AHIMA 2010).

Uniform Ambulatory Care Data Set (UACDS): A dataset developed by the National Committee on Vital and Health Statistics consisting of a minimum set of patient/client-specific data elements to be collected in ambulatory care settings (AHIMA 2010).

Uniform Hospital Discharge Data Set (UHDDS): A core set of data elements adopted by the U.S. Department of Health, Education, and Welfare in 1974 that are collected by hospitals on all discharges and all discharge abstract systems (AHIMA 2010).

Uniform Resource Locator (URL): A URL is a Web site address that will take the Web browser directly to the document located on a Web page.

Universal serial bus (USB) port: USB ports are used for connecting devices such as flash drives, digital cameras, and iPods. The USB ports are built on the outside of computers, usually on the front, where access is easy for the user so that peripheral devices can easily be connected without interrupting any other resources in the computer.

Unstructured data: Nonbinary, human-readable data (AHIMA 2010).

Use case: A technique that develops scenarios based on how users will use information to assist in developing information systems that support the information requirements (AHIMA 2010).

User preparation: User preparation is providing the users with enough information about the system being implemented so that they are prepared both psychologically and through training to use the system.

User task force: The user task force is a group of users, who will ultimately be using the system, that tests the system and performs other project-related tasks for which the committee receives feedback.

Username: A unique identifier assigned to each user.

Video card: A component of a computer that controls the display on the screen.

Virus: A computer program, typically hidden, that attaches itself to other programs and has the ability to replicate and cause various forms of harm to the data (AHIMA 2010).

Vocabulary standards: A list or collection of clinical words or phrases with their meanings; also, the set of words used by an individual or group within a particular subject field (AHIMA 2010).

VoiceXML (VXML):   The Voice Extensible Markup Language or VoiceXML is the standard "with which voice applications are developed" (ATRC 2009, 5).

Web page: A Web page is the text written on a Web site and displayed on the Internet or World Wide Web.

Weighted system: With the weighted system each function would be listed along with a score showing how important the functionality is. The project team would give each function a score and the score would be multiplied by the weight. The weighted scores would then be totaled.

What you see is what you get (WYSIWYG):   The screen mimics the output of the printer, so the user can see what the final output of the document will be.

Wide area network (WAN):   Networks that are not geographically located near each other are called wide area networks (WANs). These can reach across offices or buildings (White 2008, 313).

Wi-Fi: A wireless technology that allows access to the Internet.

Wireless card: A wireless network interface card or simply wireless card is a device for a plug-in for the PC, laptop, or PDA to communicate to the network. These come in various sizes and shapes depending on the type of computer for which the card will be used.

Wireless Markup Language (WML):   Similar to Hypertext Markup Language (HTML), the language used on the Internet, but with WML there is no need for a keyboard or a mouse for input because the WAP cards are used as the input data.

Work and data flow analyst: The work and data flow analyst must be able to study the flow of data into the system and its associated processes and look for ways to improve it. The work and data flow analyst must be able to use data flow diagrams and other tools to document the various flows of data within the facility.

Workflow technology: Technology that allows computers to add and extract value from document content as the documents move throughout an organization (AHIMA 2010).

Workforce clearance procedure: The workforce clearance procedure ensures that each member of the workforce's level of access is appropriate (Newby 2009).

Workgroup for Electronic Data Interchange (WEDI):   A subgroup of Accreditation Standards Committee X12 that has been involved in developing electronic data interchange standards for billing transactions (AHIMA 2010).

World Wide Web (WWW):   A portion of the Internet that connects large databases and servers to support electronic mail and other communications (AHIMA 2010).

Worm: A special type of computer virus, usually transferred from computer to computer via e-mail, that can replicate itself and use memory but cannot attach itself to other programs (AHIMA 2010).

WORM technology: WORM is an acronym for write once, read many. The use of this technology prevents the user from altering what is stored, but the data can be viewed as many times as necessary.

Write once read many (WORM):   Optical disk technology uses a format that is known as write once read many (WORM) technology (Abdelhak et al. 2007, 257). Optical disks are etched by a laser onto a disk platter. Data cannot be altered or misfiled on health records once it has been permanently etched onto a laser disk with WORM technology.

Zip: A computer utility that combines two or more files into one and reduces the size of the file.

References

3M. 2009. What we do: Health information management. http://solutions.3m.com/wps/portal/3M/en_US/3M_Health_Information_Systems/HIS/What_We_Do/Health_Info_Management/.

45 CFR 160, 162, and 164. Healthcare Reform: Security Standards; Final Rule. 2003 (Feb. 20) http://www.cms.hhs.gov/SecurityStandard/Downloads/securityfinalrule.pdf.

Abdelhak, M., S. Grostick, M.A. Hanken, and E. Jacobs. 2007. *Health Information: Management of a Strategic Resource.* St. Louis, MO: Saunders Elsevier.

Adaptive Technology Resource Centre. 2009. Technical glossary: Voice Recognition. http://atrc.utoronto.ca/index.php?option=com_content&task=view&id=50&Itemid=9.

AHIMA e-HIM Personal Health Record Work Group. 2005. The role of the personal health record in the EHR. *Journal of AHIMA* 76(7):64A-D.

AHIMA MPI Task Force. 2004. Practice brief: Building an enterprise master person index. *Journal of AHIMA* 75(1):56A-D.

American Health Information Management Association. 2006. Wordpower: A glossary of software licensing terms. *Journal of AHIMA* 77(4):42, 44.

American Health Information Management Association. 2010. *Pocket Glossary of Health Information Management and Technology.* 2nd ed. Chicago: AHIMA.

American Health Information Management Association and Medical Transcription Industry Association Joint Task Force on Standards Development. 2008. (Summer). Transcription turnaround time for common document types. *Perspectives in Health Information Management.*

American Health Information Management Association and Medical Transcription Industry Association Joint Task Force on Standards Development. 2008. (Summer). Transcription turnaround time for common document types. *Perspectives in Health Information Management.*

Amatayakul, M. 2004b. The trouble with audit controls. *Journal of AHIMA* 75(9):78–79.

Amatayakul, M. 2005b Reporting security incidents. *Journal of AHIMA* 76((3):60.

Amatayakul, M.S. 2007. *Electronic Health Records: A Practical Guide for Professionals and Organizations.* Chicago: AHIMA.

Amatayakul, M.S. 2009. *Electronic Health Records: A Practical Guide for Professionals and Organizations.* Chicago: AHIMA.

Austin, C.J. and S.B. Boxerman. 2003. *Information Systems for Healthcare Management.* Chicago: Health Administration Press.

Bliss, M.F. 2005. *Speech Recognition for the Health Professions.* Upper Saddle River, NJ: Pearson Prentice Hall.

Burrington-Brown, J. 2003a. On the line—Professional Practice solutions: What is multi-factor authentication? *Journal of AHIMA* 74(5):64.

Derhak, M. 2003. Uncovering the enemy within: Utilizing incident response, forensics. *In Confidence* 11(9):1–2.

Englebardt, S.P. and R. Nelson. 2002. *Healthcare Informatics: An Interdisciplinary Approach.* St. Louis, MO: Moseby.

Fenton, S., K. Giannangelo, C. Kale, and R. Scichilone. 2007. Data standards, data quality, and interoperability. *Journal of AHIMA* 78(2):extended online edition.

Giannangelo, K. 2006. *Healthcare Code Sets, Clinical Terminologies, and Classification Systems*. Chicago: AHIMA.

Glandon, G.L., D.H. Smaltz, and D.J. Slovensky. 2008. *Austin and Boxerman's Information Systems for Healthcare Management*. Chicago: Health Administration Press/ AUPHA.

Hebda, T. and P. Czar. 2009. *Handbook of Informatics for Nurses & Healthcare Professionals*. Upper Saddle River, NJ: Pearson Prentice Hall.

Johns, M.L. 2006. *Health Information Management Technology: An Applied Approach*. Chicago: AHIMA.

Joint NEMS/COCIR/JIRA Security and Privacy Committee. 2003. Defending medical information systems against malicious software. http://medicalimaging.org/documents/medical-defending.pdf.

Joos, I., N.I. Whitman, M.J. Smith, and R. Nelson. 2006. *Introduction to Computers for Healthcare Professionals*, 4th ed. Sudbury, MA: Jones & Bartlett, Publishers.

McWay, D.C. 2008. *Today's Health Information Management: An Integrated Approach*. Clifton Park, NY: Thomson Delmar Learning.

Microsoft Company. 2008. Word 2007: Rich Text Format (RTF) Specification, version 1.9.1. http://www.microsoft.com/downloads/details.aspx?familyid=dd422b8d-ff06-4207-b476-6b5396a18a2b&displaylang=en #RelatedLinks.

Microsoft Corporation. 2002. *Microsoft Computer Dictionary*, 2nd ed. Redmond, WA: Microsoft Press.

National eHealth Collaborative. 2009. http://www.nationalehealth.org.

Newby, C. 2009. *HIPAA for Allied Health Careers*. Boston: McGraw-Hill Higher Education.

Rada, R. 2003. *Health Information Security: HIPAA*. Chicago: HIPAA-IT LLC and Healthcare Information and Management Systems Society.

Ruano, M. 2003. Understanding telecommunications, network security, and HIPAA. *In Confidence* 11(5):5.

Thakkar, M. and D.C. Davis. 2006. Risks, barriers, and benefits of EHR systems: A comparative study based on size of hospital. *Perspectives in Health Information Management*. 13(5):10.

Tomes, J.P. 2005. Spoilation of medical evidence. *Journal of AHIMA* 76(9):68–72.

Voice Perfect Systems. 2008. How NaturallySpeaking works. http://www.voiceperfect.com/naturallyspeaking/howitworks.

Wager, K.A., F.W. Lee, and J.P. Glaser. 2005. *Managing Health Care Information Systems*. San Francisco: Jossey-Bass.

White, R. *How Computers Work*, 9th ed. 2008. Indianapolis, IN: QUE, Publishing.

White, R. 2008. *How Computers Work*, 9th ed. Indianapolis, IN: QUE Publishing.

Index